Recognition of
Child Abuse
for the Mandated Reporter

G. W. Medical Publishing, Inc.

Mosby–Year Book, Inc.

St. Louis Baltimore Berlin Boston Carlsbad Chicago London Madrid
Naples New York Philadelphia Sydney Tokyo Toronto

Recognition of
Child Abuse
for the Mandated Reporter

JAMES A. MONTELEONE, M.D.
Professor of Pediatrics and Gynecology
St. Louis University School of Medicine
Director of the Division of Child Protection
Cardinal Glennon Children's Hospital
St. Louis, Missouri

SECOND EDITION

G.W. Medical Publishing, Inc.
St. Louis, Missouri 1996

Publisher: Marianne and Glenn Whaley

Design Director: Glenn Whaley

Developmental Editor: Elaine Steinborn

Production Manager: Charles J. Seibel III

–Book Design/Page Layout: Dee Ann Lange
–Cover Design: D. Scott Tjaden
–Production: Christine Bauer

Indexer: Linda Caravelli

SECOND EDITION

Copyright © 1996 by G. W. Medical Publishing, Inc.
Second Edition Printed in 1996

Printed in the United States of America

G. W. Medical Publishing, Inc.
2601 Metro Blvd., St. Louis, Missouri 63043

Library of Congress Cataloging in Publication Data
Monteleone, James A.
  Recognition of child abuse for the mandated reporter/ James A. Monteleone. -- 2nd ed.
        p.   cm.
  Includes bibliographical reference and index.
  ISBN 1-878060-24-4 (pbk. : alk. paper)
  1. Battered child syndrome. 2. Chils abuse.   I. Title.
RA1122.5.R44 1996
618.92'858223--dc20

                                          96-32412
                                            CIP

ISBN 1-878060-24-4

CONTRIBUTORS

Pasquale J. Accardo, M.D.
Professor of Pediatrics
St. Louis University School of Medicine
Medical Director, Knights of Columbus Developmental Center
Cardinal Glennon Children's Hospital
St. Louis, Missouri

Armand E. Brodeur, M.D., M.Rd., L.L.D., F.A.C.R., F.A.A.P.
Professor Emeritus of Radiology and Pediatrics
St. Louis University School of Medicine
Emeritus Director of Pediatric Radiology
Cardinal Glennon Children's Hospital
Director of Radiology
Shriners Hospital for Crippled Children
St. Louis Unit
St. Louis, Missouri

Cassandra K. Dolgin, B.A., J.D.
Member of the Missouri Bar
St. Louis, Missouri

Jesse A. Goldner, M.A., J.D.
Professor of Law
Director of the Center for Health Law Studies
St. Louis University School of Law
Professor of Pediatrics
Professor of Law in Psychiatry
St. Louis University School of Medicine
St. Louis, Missouri

Gus H. Kolilis, B.S., Education
International Police Chief's Association
Missouri Police Chief's Association
St. Louis Police Officers Association (Charter and Life Member since 1968)
St. Louis Fraternal Order of Police (Life Member)
International Police Association, Region 8
University of Missouri-Columbia Alumni Association (Life Member)
American Professional Society on the Abuse of Children

Sandra H. Manske, R.N., M.A., J.D.
Member of the Missouri Bar
St. Louis, Missouri

Vicki McNeese, M.S.
Staff Psychologist
Cardinal Glennon Children's Hospital
Adjunct Instructor of Psychology
St. Louis University
St. Louis, Missouri

James A. Monteleone, M.D.
Professor of Pediatrics and Gynecology
St. Louis University School of Medicine
Director of the Division of Child Protection
Cardinal Glennon Children's Hospital
St. Louis, Missouri

Lynn Douglas Mouden, DDS, MPH, PICD, FACD
Associate Chief, Bureau of Dental Health,
Missouri Department of Health
Jefferson City, Missouri

Wayne I. Munkel, M.S.W., L.C.S.W.
Medical Social Consultant
Department of Social Service
Cardinal Glennon Children's Hospital
St. Louis, Missouri

Peggy S. Pearl, Ed.D.
Professor, Department of Consumer and Family Studies
Southwest Missouri State University
Springfield, Missouri

Colette M. Rickert, LPCC, A.T.R.-BC
American Art Therapy Association
American Counseling Association

Anthony J. Scalzo, M.D.
Associate Professor of Pediatrics
Division of Emergency Medicine
St. Louis University School of Medicine
Clinical Toxicologist
Director of Regional Poison Control Center
Cardinal Glennon Children's Hospital
St. Louis, Missouri

Barbara Y. Whitman, Ph.D.
Associate Professor of Pediatrics
St. Louis University School of Medicine
Director, Family Services and Family Studies
Knights of Columbus Developmental Center
Cardinal Glennon Children's Hospital
St. Louis, Missouri

James J. Williams, M.D.
Staff Pediatrician
The Permanente Medical Group
Redwood City, California
Attending Pediatrician
San Francisco General Hospital
San Francisco, California

FOREWORD TO THE FIRST EDITION

We live in a society beset by escalating violence. According to recent FBI statistics, the annual incidence of reported violent crimes has risen from 161 per 100,000 persons in 1960 to 758 per 100,000 in 1992. These crimes, which include child abuse, are estimated by the National Committee for Prevention of Child Abuse to have risen by 40% between 1985 and 1991. However, the true number of victims is far greater than reported, and the deleterious effects on those children who survive these acts of abuse and neglect persist for a lifetime.

Dr. Monteleone and his collaborators provide a compelling litany of information to assist in realistically confronting the problem. They underscore risk factors that contribute to abuse, and national statistics show that many of these are dramatically increasing. For example, there has been a doubling of single parent households over the past 23 years, from 4 million to 8 million. Over the same period, the proportion of births out of wedlock has increased from about 11% to nearly 30%.

The authors further illustrate a frequent dilemma—protecting the child while assuring that caregivers are not unjustly accused. All too often this task can seem impossible, the effort and personal emotional risks too great, and the frustrations inevitable.

The importance of strong commitments to accuracy and action goes beyond merely providing a child the right to survive and thrive to adulthood. The long-term consequences of our failure to do so have been made abundantly clear: the abused later become the abusers, and, if unchecked, the whole process will be repeated and amplified in future generations. All who are committed to child health, social improvement, and legal protection must educate themselves carefully about these difficult issues. We must accept the responsibility as advocates for all children at risk. Without our help, they can neither run nor hide from the perpetrators of their misery.

C. George Ray, M.D.
Professor and Chairman
Department of Pediatrics
St. Louis University School
of Medicine
St. Louis, Missouri

PREFACE TO THE FIRST EDITION

This reference was created to help mandated reporters recognize child maltreatment, identify those children who are at high risk for abuse and neglect, and realize strategies for preventing and intervening in abuse situations. The information presented here will be beneficial to teachers, school nurses, day-care workers, social service workers, attorneys, law enforcement personnel, and other professionals involved with children and morally, if not legally, obligated to report suspected abuse. This single volume contains information concerning physical and psychological abuse, neglect, sexual abuse, and legal aspects.

In the mid-1980s I was involved, along with the St. Louis Child Abuse Network, in a project to review deaths and catastrophic injuries to children due to abuse. One objective of the study was to create a profile of the child at risk and his or her caregivers. The results of that study were released to the media and presented at several conferences, but not published. This study was unique in that it collected data on both severely abused children and their families and on control groups of mildly abused and nonabused children and their families. Along with other studies at that time, it showed the value of reviewing not only the circumstances of the deaths of abused children but also the circumstances of suspicious deaths. In 1992 the State of Missouri enacted legislation providing for the establishment of death review teams throughout the state. The information presented will enable those dealing with children and families to recognize high-risk situations and hopefully provide help before abuse occurs. In addition, when an injury is suspicious, the data from this review process will allow responsible individuals to decide if an injury is abuse and should be reported.

In the past, few, if any, books focused on the needs of the mandated reporter outside of the health care system. Those books available concentrated on the social aspects of child abuse—the "why" and "who" of abuse. Teachers and other mandated reporters have communicated their need to be able to recognize abuse and know what to do after they decide they have reason to suspect abuse—the "what" and "how" of abuse. This book attempts to address these issues, providing guidance and important information about how the legal and social systems process a child abuse case, and preparing the mandated reporter for the procedures involved in protecting children from abuse.

Sexually abused children often first disclose their abuse to a teacher or other counselor. The most important aspect of evaluating the sexually abused child is the disclosure, and all other elements, including the physical examination, depend on what the child says. Handling that disclosure sets the direction for the rest of the investigation and helps determine the credibility of the child's statement. This area is well covered in this reference, representing the most comprehensive presentation of this topic currently available.

The contributors to this volume are experts in their fields. I felt strongly that no one person could effectively address all aspects of child abuse, and I have recruited individuals who have extensive experience in child protection and are well-recognized by their peers and the legal system.

I believe that this text is an essential resource for all adults responsible for the care of children. It will help them to identify problems in the lives of children and empower them to report suspected cases in appropriate and meaningful ways. Throughout my career I have been touched by the plight of innocent victims of abuse. It is my hope that the future will see children valued and protected from abuse by adults. I offer this book as a contribution to the important work of caring for the least members of society—our children.

James A. Monteleone

TABLE OF CONTENTS

CHAPTER 14: WORKING WITH CHILD ABUSE VICTIMS IN THE CLASSROOM

CHAPTER 15: PREVENTION

Recognition of
Child Abuse
for the Mandated Reporter

Chapter 1

IDENTIFYING PHYSICAL ABUSE

JAMES A. MONTELEONE, M.D.
ARMAND E. BRODEUR, M.D.

Child abuse involves every segment of society and crosses all social, ethnic, religious, and professional lines. The definition of child abuse can range from a narrow focus, limited to intentional inflicted injury, to a broad scope, covering any act that adversely affects the developmental potential of a child. Included in the definition are neglect (acts of omission) and physical, psychological, or sexual injury (acts of commission) by a parent or caretaker. Intent is not considered in reporting abuse; protection of the child is paramount.

According to the United States Department of Health and Human Services report (1980), the national incidence of countable child maltreatment was 9.8 children per 1,000 population. This totaled about 625,100 children. In 1988 this agency reported that 16.3 children per 1,000 population, or 1,025,900 children, were maltreated. Whether these data reflect an increase in the occurrence of child maltreatment or an increase in the ability of professionals to recognize and report cases has not yet been determined.

We live in a violent society. Children are often the targets of that violence. The violence is most apt to occur in the home and be carried out by a family member. Some studies suggest that people who were abused as children are more apt as adults to become abusers than are those who were not abused as children. Social factors—poverty, unemployment, and isolation—are major factors that increase the risk of child abuse.

Effective strategies to deal with and prevent abuse must involve a concerted effort by many disciplines. No one individual can have all of the answers and consistently make correct decisions without the input from the various members of a team of child care workers and professionals.

Previously, books dealing with child abuse have concentrated on the social factors—the *who* and the *why* of child abuse. This book, while not ignoring the who and the why, emphasizes the *what* and the *how*: *what* is abuse, *what* to do when you suspect abuse, and *how* to do it.

◆NORMAL CHILD DEVELOPMENT AND BEHAVIOR

In evaluating injuries, the age of the child is crucial. Infants who are basically immobile and who are receiving good care rarely suffer injury. When they are learning to walk or crawl, single bruises are generally found as a result of their many falls. Multiple bruises, involving more than one body area, require several impacts and the history should reflect this.

With some exceptions, a child cannot roll over until at least 4 months of age, often not until about 6 months of age. A child will not crawl until about 10 months or walk until about a year old. He will not run well until age 2 years, and cannot ride a tricycle until about 3 years. It is also about this time that the child climbs the stairs, alternating feet.

Accidental injuries require specific motor skills on the part of a child. A fall from a bed is not possible before the child can roll over; a fall down the stairs is not plausible until the child can crawl. The ability to turn a circular-motion hot water knob is not achieved until approximately 2 years of age. Therefore a 2-month-old infant cannot roll over, let alone crawl, to a radiator to sustain a burn or get into a poisonous substance, and a 2-year-old child who has severe buttock burns could not have ridden a tricycle into a space heater.

Occasionally an injury is blamed on a brother or sister. This explanation is believable because children often are abusive to their siblings. However, it must be determined if the injury could have occurred as described and if the brother or sister is developmentally mature enough to have caused the injury. It may be necessary to test the child or sibling to see if the action attributed to him or her is possible.

Explanations of injuries must be evaluated using common sense and a sound knowledge of the results of routine accidents in the home. For example, a 17-month-old cannot burn his buttocks by climbing onto a space heater and sitting on the top without burning his hands and legs in the climb—assuming he can climb. Similarly, a 5-month-old cannot spontaneously suffer a severe rectal tear and dilated anus, nor can he suffer multiple skull fractures and internal abdominal injuries in a fall from the couch. Finally, a fractured femur does not generally occur when a 5-month-old infant tangles his leg in a blanket while rolling over.

◆ Conditions That Have Been Confused With Abuse

A number of conditions over the years have been mistaken for child abuse and have been reported to state protective agencies. It is important that you know these conditions and make an effort to identify them. Although it is tragic to miss recognizing a child who has been abused, it is equally tragic to falsely accuse a caregiver of abuse, especially when the child is ill. Such allegations only add to the caregiver's concerns for the child.

A number of systems can be involved: the skin, which bruises easily or could have burns; the skeletal system, where fractures and other bony changes are possible; the eye; and the central nervous system. A list of conditions that have been encountered is given in **Table 1-1**.

Table 1-1. Conditions Which Have Been Mistaken for Abuse

Condition	Appearance
Mongolian spots	Apparent bruising to back and buttocks
Postmortem lividity	Bluish discoloration to dependent areas (buttocks, back, ankles) after death
Folk Medicine	
Vietnamese	
Coining, Cao Gio	Bruises along bony prominences of rib cage, back, and chest
Chinese	
Spoon rubbing	Can include blood in the urine
Moxibustion	Small circular incense burns at therapeutic points
Russian	
Cupping	Circular area of ruptured blood vessels on the back
Latin American	
Cupping (ventosos)	Circular first-degree burns on the back, abdomen, or chest
Arabs and Jews	
Maquas	Small deep burns at the site of disease
Mexican	
Caida de Mollera (fallen fontanelle)	Shaken infant syndrome, closed head injury
Phytophotodermatitis psoralens in plants (limes, parsnips, figs, etc.)	Streaks on the skin of the face, hands, chest, and lower legs; these may blister Hand prints may form where the adult touches the child
Easy Bruisability	
Hemophilia	Areas of ruptured blood vessels in various parts of the body at various stages of healing
Vitamin K deficiency	Hemorrhages under the skin or internally
Leukemia	Areas of ruptured blood vessels, bruises, death of the child
Henoch-Schonlein purpura	Purplish discoloration on various areas of the body, such as the face, eyes, arms, or legs
Disseminated intravascular coagulation, meningitis	Multiple bruises, death of the child
Erythema multiforme	Bruises and purplish discoloration on various areas of the body

Table 1-1. Conditions Which Have Been Mistaken for Abuse *(continued)*

Condition	Appearance
Ehlers-Danlos syndrome	Bruises, scars, open wounds on the head, knees, elbows, or chin
Burns and Burn-like Lesions	
Epidermolysis bullosa	Blisters to pressure areas
Impetigo	Blisters resembling cigarette burns
Car seat burn	Blisters, first- and second-degree burns on the back, neck, and/or extremities
Frostbite	Linear burns at moisture points, such as the cheeks, chin, lips, and glove and sock line
Wringer injury	Burns under the arms
Congenital indifference to pain	Numerous old and recent cuts, scars, bruises, or burns
Brain tumor or brain aneurysm	Shaken infant syndrome
Osteogenesis imperfecta	Multiple unexplained fractures
Hypogammaglobulinemia or cystic fibrosis	Failure to thrive
Hair tourniquet	Swelling and redness of the toe or penis
Genetic Disorders	
Mitochondrial disorder, congenital adrenal hyperplasia in a male, diabetes insipidus	Multiple SIDS babies, severe dehydration, failure to thrive
Methylmalonic acidemia	Poisoning
Congenital syphilis	Periosteal reaction, fractures
Copper deficiency	Multiple bony abnormalities
Vitamin C or D deficiency	Fractures, changes in the bone
Caffey's disease	Swelling of the lower limbs
Toddler's fracture	Spiral fracture of the lower one-third of the tibia in toddlers
Fractures from passive exercise	Stress fracture of the long bones seen in cerebral palsy patients who are receiving physical therapy
Self-inflicted Injuries	
Cornelia De Lange syndrome, Lesch-Nyhan syndrome, head-bangers	Various cutaneous injuries, bites, burns, and bruises

Many of the conditions listed in **Table 1-1** are one-time occurrences. However, the potential for mistakes is enormous. *Mistakes can be avoided by carefully listening to the personal and family history and observing and describing the injuries seen.* Referral to a health care practitioner for a thorough physical examination is required.

FOLK MEDICINE

Some folk medicine practices may resemble abuse. If there are immigrants in the community it is necessary to be aware of their medical beliefs and practices and make efforts to educate these individuals concerning acceptable medical care. *Among the practices that have been found are the following:*

> *Cao Gio* is a form of folk medicine practiced by Southeast Asians. The healers follow traditional folk medicine when they rub a coin or a spoon heated in oil on an ill child's neck, spine, and ribs. The practice can cause a burn or abrasion (**Figure 1-1**).

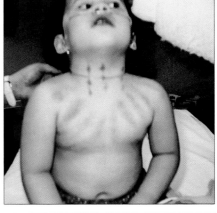

> In *Caida de Mollera* (fallen fontanelle), which is practiced by Hispanics, an attempt is made to elevate the fontanelle in children dehydrated from diarrhea and vomiting by holding the child upside down. Retinal hemorrhages may result.

> *Cupping* (ventosos) is practiced by some Latin American and Russian cultures. A vacuum is created under a cup or glass by placing a small amount of material under the vessel on the skin and burning the material. First- or second-degree burns of the area can result.

> *Moxibustion*, practiced by Southeast Asians, is a form of acupuncture in which lighted sticks of incense or other material from the herb artemisia are used to make small circular burns on the skin at therapeutic points.

> Bedoins, Arabs, and Jews use treatment called *maquas*, in which hot metal spits or coals are applied to areas near the site of disease or on a traditional "draining point." Small burns are produced at the site.

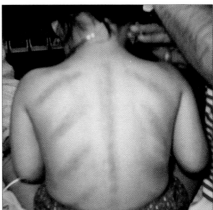

All of these forms of folk medicine are abusive practices done out of ignorance. Every effort should be made to prevent their continuance.

Some states have legislation declaring that it is acceptable to treat an ill child with prayer instead of medical care, provided the religious treatment is in accord with the tenets and practices of a recognized religion, such as Christian Science. However, certain states have removed the faith healing exemptions from their child protective statutes, and other states may follow.

Figure 1-1a,b. This is a 4-year-old South Asian girl with severe asthma. Note the typical lesions of coining along the rib cage, back and front. The neck injuries are typical, but are also coining lesions.

◆ ACCIDENTAL VERSUS INFLICTED INJURIES

Differentiating accidental injuries from inflicted injuries is important. Errors in recognizing these differences can be catastrophic and costly for the child and the family. If inflicted injury is not recognized, the child is left in the care of persons who may injure him again. If the injury was accidental, the parents are wrongfully accused and investigated, and the child and parents may be separated.

A caregiver rarely reports that he has abused his child. He will try to convince you that the injury resulted from an accident initiated by the child. To recognize abuse you must first believe that abuse is a possibility and effectively eliminate the potential of an accident having produced the injury(ies) seen.

Children explore those things that are in front of them and generally move forward; therefore, most accidental injuries involve only the front of the body. Specific locations affected are the forehead, nose, chin, palms, elbows, and shins—areas where the bone is close to the skin.

Injuries to the palms of the hands can be accidental, occurring when the child is breaking a fall or exploring a dangerous object, such as a hot iron or a piece of machinery. However, both the palms and the backs of the hands are common areas where punishment is inflicted, and you must be alert to the possibility of abuse when there are injuries in these areas.

Injuries to the buttocks, genitalia, abdomen, back, and side areas of the body, especially the sides of the face, frequently indicate abuse. Abdominal bruising is unusual even with blunt trauma. Bruising around the genitals or anal area is usually intentional.

You must determine if the injury could have occurred as the caregiver or child describes. Then you must decide if this particular child is developmentally mature enough to have caused the injury. If the parents state that the child was injured by doing something that he is not developmentally able to do or if the injury is too severe to be caused by the incident described, then the history given is incorrect and you must conclude that the injury was nonaccidental.

Why does an abusive injury or situation go unrecognized? Several reasons may be cited:

1. You may not be able to accept that a parent could abuse a child.
2. You may not want to get involved or interfere in what you believe is, rightfully, a family situation.
3. Without proper training in observation, you may overlook the signs of abuse.
4. In general, people tend to believe what they are told and base decisions on that belief.

◆ INTERPRETING ABUSE INJURIES

SKIN INJURIES
Skin injuries are the most common and easily recognized signs of maltreatment in children. Human bites strongly indicate abuse. Skin injuries can vary from superficial injuries, such as first-degree burns and abrasions, to deeper injuries, ranging from cuts to second- and third-degree burns. Patterns and locations of these injuries are clues to suspecting child abuse.

HUMAN BITES
Human bites are intentional and are common injuries in abuse. Recognizing human bite marks is particularly important in child abuse cases because forensic dentists can study them and help determine who actually abused the child.

Human bite marks can be easily overlooked if you are unaware of their characteristics. The location of bite marks on infants tends to differ from the location on older children. Bite marks around the genitals or buttocks are usually seen in infants and are inflicted as punishment. Older children have bites associated with assault or sexual abuse; there are generally more than one, they occur at random, their appearance is well-defined, and they may be associated with a sucking mark. The sucking mark may be the only indicator noted if sexual abuse has occurred.

There are three components of a human bite to look for: the bite mark, the suck mark, and the thrust mark (**Figure 1-2**). Bite marks are ovoid areas with tooth imprints, and shape and size are significant. The suck mark is caused when the person biting pulls the skin into his mouth, creating a negative pressure. The

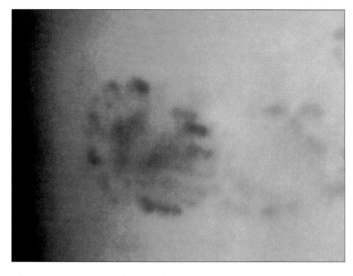

Figure 1-2. Bite injury showing three components.

thrust mark is caused when the tongue pushes against the skin, which is trapped behind the teeth. The inner portion of the bite mark may show no abnormality or may contain the suck or thrust mark. These two marks are similar in appearance in that each resembles a bruise in the center of the mark.

The front teeth give the human bite mark its configuration, which is the shape of the dental arch. Generally, no one tooth stands out (unlike animal bites), and the marks are irregular in size, shape, and position. The incisor teeth leave narrow rectangles, the canines leave triangular shapes, and the premolars make circular marks. The canines are more likely to be recognizable in bites from adults than in bites from children. Early recognition of a human bite mark supplies valuable information. A child's bite can be distinguished from an adult's bite by measuring arch and tooth widths. If puncture marks from the canines are visible in the bite, it is possible to distinguish bites of permanent teeth (older than age 8 years) from primary teeth bites because the distance of separation is greater than 30 mm.

BRUISES

The skin can be a window to deeper injuries. Hemorrhage into deeper tissues, such as muscle, will work its way to the surface. The accumulation of blood under the skin will be evident for a number of days, changing color as it ages. A fresh injury is red to blue; in 1 to 3 days it becomes deep black or purple; in 3 to 6 days the color changes to green and gradually brown; in 6 to 15 days it passes from green to tan to yellow to faded; and finally it disappears. The younger the child, the quicker the color resolves.

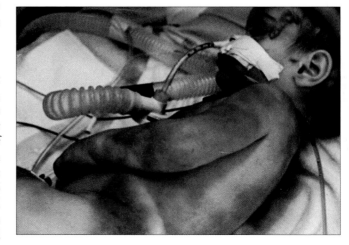

Figure 1-3. Child with multiple bruises involving multiple surfaces, on inaccessible places, and in various stages of healing.

Multiple bruises or bruises in inaccessible places are indications that the child has been abused (**Figure 1-3**). In addition, babies who are not mobile do not usually have bruising. The toddler who is learning to walk typically has bruises on the front parts of his body, as stated earlier. Severe bruising is unlikely. In the older child (age 2 to 5 years), some parts of the body, such as the knees, shins, foreheads, and elbows, are bruised often because these portions of the body are contact points.

Bruises and broken blood vessels detected under the skin result from abuse when they occur in areas of the body that are unlikely to be injured accidentally. Multiple bruises and bruises of the buttocks or the genital area are usually not accidental. Bruises in different stages of healing are the result of repeated trauma and indicate abuse when the parents give a history describing a single accident. **A significant discrepancy between the physical findings and the history is the cardinal sign of abuse.**

Bruises that take the shape of a recognizable object are generally not accidental. Loop marks are caused by a flexible object, such as a belt, electric cord, or clothesline, folded on itself and used to beat the child (**Figure 1-4**). Multiple curved loop marks on the child clearly indicate abuse. These bruises are usually reddened with broken blood vessels under the skin, but there can be actual cuts or scrapes. A hand imprint on a child's face after a slap and finger and thumb marks on an arm or leg where the child was grabbed or squeezed are inflicted injuries. Belt buckles and similar objects used to inflict punishment leave recognizable imprints on the child's skin. Rope burns, bruises, or scars around the arms, ankles, neck, or waist are evidence that the child was tied (**Figure 1-5**). Many of these injuries leave long lasting scars. There have been incidences where the penis is tied to prevent bed-wetting or pinched as punishment for soiling (**Figure 1-6**).

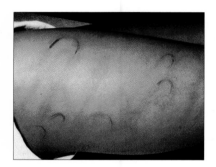

***Figure 1-4**. Loop marks caused by whipping with extension cord.*

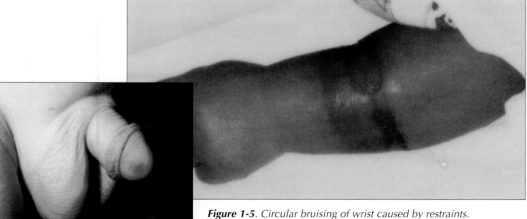

***Figure 1-5**. Circular bruising of wrist caused by restraints.*

***Figure 1-6**. Broken blood vessels on the penis caused by pinching. Child was disciplined for soiling himself.*

Parents can claim that a child suspected of abuse bruises easily. Bleeding disorders, such as hemophilia, are usually diagnosed at an early age but occasionally a mild form is not apparent until the child is older. The usual age for a bleeding disorder to become evident is when the child begins to walk and cruise, or with the eruption of the first tooth. This, coincidentally, is also the age when child abuse occurs frequently. It is important to note that hemophilia is a stress-producing disease and that hemophiliac children are at increased risk for being abused. Their tendency for easy bruising can mask an intentional injury.

HAIR LOSS

Hair loss can be a manifestation of child maltreatment. It can occur when parents pull their child's hair, frequently using the hair as a handle to grab the child and jerk or drag him. The result of the pulling on the scalp can cause the blood vessels under the skin to break. An accumulation of blood can help differentiate between abusive and nonabusive loss of hair.

Traumatic hair loss is defined as the forceful pulling of hair or the breaking of hair shafts by friction, traction, or other physical trauma. The usual causes are extreme cosmetic practices or the child's habit of consciously or subconsciously plucking, pulling, breaking, or cutting the hair. This usually occurs with the hair on the head, but the eyebrows and eyelashes may also be affected. The child may pluck, twirl, or rub areas where the hair is growing, resulting in the loss or breakage of hair shafts. Most affected individuals are under varying degrees of emotional stress. Some have severe psychological problems.

Extreme cosmetic practices that can cause this condition are tight braiding or pony-tails; the use of tight rollers, barrettes, head bands, or rubber bands; hair straightening practices such as teasing or pulling; frequent brushing with nylon bristles; and the use of hot combs and gel. Other common causes of traumatic hair loss include pressure, as is seen in infants who lie on their backs or are in the habit of "head-banging"; prolonged bed rest in one position, as in chronically ill persons or neglected children; thermal or electric burns; repeated vigorous massage; a severe blow to the scalp; and abusive hair-pulling.

A common disorder involves the sudden appearance of sharply defined round or oval patches of hair loss. Recent evidence suggests that a disease may cause this disorder. Another possible cause of bald patches is fungal infections, for example, ringworm. One or more round or oval well-circumscribed and clearly defined patches are usual. Occasionally the first patches seen do not conform to this typical appearance. This usually distinguishes it from other forms of hair loss.

FALLS

In most cases, a minor injury occurs when a child has a routine fall in the home, such as out of bed, from a sofa, off a chair, or down the stairs. There is usually no object, such as a tricycle or stroller, involved. Sometimes a single skull fracture occurs. If a child is reported to have had a routine fall but has what appear to be severe injuries, the inconsistency of the history with the injury indicates child abuse.

A fall down the stairs, especially when the stairs are not padded, will cause a series of bruises the size and shape of the stair edge. The bruises are usually on several body surfaces. **Children who fall down the stairs rarely have life-threatening injuries and do not require admission to an intensive care unit.**

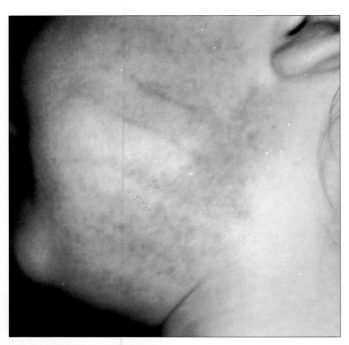

Figure 1-7. *Face injury caused by blow to the side of the face. Linear marks are caused by fingers.*

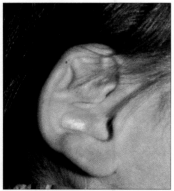

Figure 1-8. *Injuries to ear, **a**, old, and **b**, recent, caused by a blow to the side of the face. When the injury heals without medical intervention it leaves a distortion of the ear cartilage often called "cauliflower" ear.*

Injuries caused by a fall from a car generally include scrapes. The wounds are usually dirty and contain sand, dirt, gravel, and other matter from the road surface and shoulder. The injuries can involve more than one body surface area because, depending on the speed of the vehicle, the child will roll when he strikes the ground. His clothes should show evidence of the experience.

Vehicular accidents are usually reported to the police. In suspicious cases, if the police are unaware of the existence of such an accident, further investigation is warranted.

EXTERNAL HEAD, FACIAL, AND ORAL INJURIES

The head is a common area of injury; approximately 50% of physical abuse patients have head or facial injuries. Injuries to the mouth are rarely reported, most likely because the mouth is often not examined.

As stated earlier, accidental injuries to the face are usually to the front part of the body and involve the forehead, nose, chin, and incisor teeth. However, not all of these injuries are accidental, and a careful history is needed to evaluate whether the injury is plausible and consistent with the physical injuries that are seen.

Injuries to the sides of the face, including the ears, cheeks, and temple area, are highly suspicious for abuse (**Figure 1-7**). Bleeding around the ear and ear lobe or inside the ear canal are also important indicators of abuse.

Cuts, bleeding, and redness or swelling of the external ear canal may be evidence of a severe blow to the ear. Such a blow may cause rupture of the tympanic membrane, with resultant hearing loss or ear infection. Injuries to external ear structures are often abusive (**Figure 1-8**).

Tears of the lips can occur through two mechanisms:

1. There may be a direct blow to the mouth. In this case you might see a linear or ragged tear. There may also be contusions, broken teeth, and facial fractures.

2. At feeding time, the caregiver may force or jam a spoon or bottle into the baby's mouth, tearing the lip(s). Other trauma rarely accompanies this injury.

The tissues of the lip can be torn accidentally if the child falls and strikes a sharp edge, for example, a coffee table, as is common among toddlers. When a tear of these tissues is found in an infant who is not crawling or walking, the case should be evaluated for other evidence of abuse.

Lip injuries are the most frequently seen oral injuries and appear as bruises, tears, cuts, scrapes, or burns. These injuries are caused when the lip is caught between a blow and the teeth. Lip burns are caused by hot liquid or hot objects such as utensils or cigarettes.

Traumatic injuries to the teeth of children are common and often accidental. A tooth may be loosened but remain in the socket. If one tooth appears to be loose, all of the teeth must be examined. The child should be referred to a dentist as soon as possible when several teeth are very loose.

A tooth may also be forced back into the alveolar bone. It will appear shorter than the rest of the teeth, or, if the blow that caused this injury was extremely hard, the tooth may be driven completely into the bone and not be visible. The child will complain of pain in the area.

The tooth may also be removed from the socket when the child is hit from the front; this occurs more commonly with permanent teeth. Try to locate the missing tooth to make sure that it has not been swallowed or aspirated. The tooth should be saved in case dental restoration is possible.

Fracture of the front teeth in children is common and usually not intentional. Fracture may be caused by a sharp blow to the teeth with a hard object and can occur during a fall or when the child is struck. If there are missing pieces, check the child's mouth and immediate surroundings. Children with fractured teeth need prompt attention.

The tongue can be injured with a blow to the jaw, trapping it between the teeth. Most injuries are on the side and appear as cuts or crushed tissue, frequently with jagged edges.

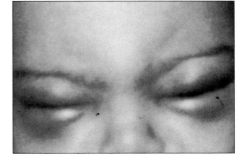

If a black eye is present, the history must detail an appropriate injury to that side. It is difficult to break the tissues around the eye without damaging the nose as well, unless the black eye results from a direct blow, as from a fist. It is unlikely that a child will suffer two black eyes as the result of a fall unless the nose is broken also. If the child falls on the center of the face, injury to the nose will occur. This position of contact protects one or both eyes, and they should not be blackened (**Figure 1-9**). When there has been a blow to the forehead, possibly from a swing or the corner of a table, the area under the eye may also appear dark.

Figure 1-9. Bilateral black eyes, when there is no broken nose, must be caused by at least two blows and cannot be explained by a single incident.

Bleeding in the upper eyelid often results when blood seeps down into tissues surrounding the eye after an injury to the forehead. Bleeding around the entire eye as the result of a forehead injury is unlikely.

SHAKEN INFANT SYNDROME

Shaken infant syndrome is responsible for at least 50% of the deaths of children caused by nonaccidental trauma and also causes the most severe results of abuse. Shaking produces a whiplash injury to the brain. This form of abuse is comparable to those injuries seen in car accidents that result from acceleration-deceleration phenomena. The shaking produces a stretching and breaking of blood vessels internally and the possibility of bruising of the brain or actual tearing of the brain tissue as the brain moves within the skull.

Impact against a soft surface will not change the amount of the force against the brain but can minimize the damage to the outer soft tissues. A boxer may be knocked unconscious, with injury to the brain, after impact from a gloved and cushioned hand yet suffer no facial bruising. In like manner, a child thrown against a soft crib mattress, bed, or carpeted floor can sustain severe brain injuries with no evidence of external damage.

Children under 2 years of age are prone to brain injury during severe shaking because at this age the head is quite large when compared to the body, the neck muscles are relatively weak, the child has poor head and neck control, there is more water in the infant brain, and the area is not as well protected physically.

What makes the shaken infant syndrome more difficult to recognize and diagnose than other forms of infant trauma is that there is usually no obvious evidence of trauma. In addition, the history given by the caregiver is usually deliberately misleading.

You must question the caregiver regarding how the injury occurred. Remember that, as in other forms of child abuse, the history is apt to be misleading, false, or not available. If a minor fall is given to explain an injury that has resulted in an unconscious child, child abuse should be suspected. As discussed earlier in this chapter, infants under 1 year of age rarely sustain devastating accidental head injury, and accidental severe head injury, as seen in an automobile accident, is usually witnessed. Abdominal or chest trauma may also be present.

Catastrophic injuries to children are costly in terms of survivor outcome. One third of these children die; one third, although they survive, are mentally and/or physically disabled and often require a lifetime of care; and one third will have a good recovery. As we look at the three outcomes, the third, good recovery, is likely to be the most costly. The survivors often have severe emotional problems and may even become abusive themselves or end up in prison. Prevention through the early recognition of potential abusers is essential. Even apparent survivors should receive extensive counseling.

DROWNING

Drowning resulting from child abuse is difficult to distinguish from accidental submersion or from sudden and unexpected natural causes. Accidental drownings usually involve toddlers or older children in public areas—swimming pools, drainage ditches, lakes, and rivers—especially in rural areas. In cities, bathtubs are the major site of accidental childhood drownings. Homicidal drownings usually occur in the home; the victims are young, either infants or toddlers.

Several features serve to differentiate accidental from nonaccidental drowning:

1. Accidental drowning occurs during the usual bath time when more than one child is present in the tub, and generally any older children have left the youngest. The household routine is usually upset, resulting in a lapse of supervision.

2. Nonaccidental drownings or near-drownings occur in the bathtub at an unusual time of day with the drowned child alone in the bath.

3. The parents fit the profile of abusing caretakers, and a precipitating crisis, often a domestic problem, is present in nonaccidental drownings.

4. The abused children are older, usually between 15 and 30 months of age, compared with the usual age of 9 to 15 months for accidental drowning.

5. The depth of the bath water ranges from 2 to 14 inches, and those children immersed 5 minutes or more die.

6. There is often a history of previous abusive behavior by the parent or guardian or a history of alcohol and drug abuse in nonaccidental drownings.

7. There is a delay between the event and calling for help or finding the child in nonaccidental drownings.

Irrigation ditch drownings are more prevalent among the toddler group, whereas lakes, rivers, and swimming pools are the prime locations among older children. Bathtub drownings of older children often involve children with cerebral palsy or epilepsy. In bathtub drownings of younger children the child is generally left alone in the tub by the parent or older sibling for a short period of time. In bucket deaths, the child may be a toddler who is tall enough to tip himself into the pail, but not large enough to knock it over. The water in the bucket is heavy enough to weigh it down and deep enough to cover the child's nose and mouth.

Fetal Abuse

Fetal abuse involves a range of behaviors in pregnant women, or their partners, characterized by the nonaccidental performance of acts that can be detrimental to the fetus. These acts include hitting the abdominal wall and, through it, the fetus, insertion of injurious substances or instruments via the vagina, or a failure to protect the fetus from an indirect assault, as with alcohol, nicotine, or drugs.

The cost of fetal abuse to society is considerable. It has been estimated that the risks to the fetus from maternal alcohol and nicotine abuse outweigh the risks of many other medical conditions. No one knows what significance physical assault of the fetus has on abortion, prematurity, stillbirth, deformity, or mental retardation.

Parents' attitudes toward "being pregnant" often bear little relationship to those toward the fetus itself. Whether the child is "wanted" or "unwanted" does not appear to determine whether or not he or she will be abused. Even a "wanted" fetus may become the victim of abuse.

A strong association exists between alcohol and cigarette use during pregnancy. Both can have adverse effects on the child after birth.

The impulse to harm the fetus is not uncommon in pregnant women. Although spouse abuse of pregnant women has been reported, it may be that the fetus is sometimes the target in spouse abuse of pregnant women.

The risk of assaultive behavior is greatest in late pregnancy because of the stresses of the third trimester and because the parents both become tired of the pregnancy state in the final 2 to 3 months. Fetal abuse may be triggered by the mother's feeling of rejection by her spouse, family, or doctor because they pay attention to the fetus and not her. She may respond to this perceived rejection by physically attacking her "rival" or may neglect giving herself and the fetus proper care, dealing with the situation passively but with equally serious consequences. This is similar to the situation with older children who are neglected by their mothers.

FETAL ABUSE AND NEONATICIDE

Neonaticide is defined as murder of the baby during the first 24 hours of life. Neonaticide is usually committed because the child is not wanted. In fetal abuse, it is likely that passive acceptance, or denial, of an unwanted pregnancy is common and consequently elective abortion is not sought. Mothers who commit neonaticide suppress the reality of their pregnancy and make no preparations. They murder the infant when the reality of birth breaks through their defenses.

SUFFOCATION

The number of young children suffocated by their parents is unknown, but smothering is being reported in increasing numbers. The families involved generally have a high incidence of sudden death of other siblings; investigation determines that some of the siblings were also suffocated.

Since many of the dead children and their siblings had an initial diagnosis of sudden infant death syndrome (SIDS), the features of suffocation must be compared with those of SIDS. The classic features of SIDS are young age, previous good health of the child, lack of previous breathing problems or other illness, and rare positive family history. In suffocation cases, it is common to find a child more than 6 months old with previous breathing problem episodes, previous unexplained disorders, and a dead sibling.

There are families who have increased risk for multiple SIDS, so this possibility must be explored. Recurrent SIDS is probably more an environmental problem than a genetic one.

NEGLECT

While not an injury, neglect is a feature in many abuse cases. The symptoms of neglect reflect a lack of both physical and medical care. An unclean baby can be a strong factor in determining neglect, although the ability to accumulate dirt in skin creases and other unreachable places is a natural characteristic of infants and children. There are degrees of uncleanliness. Most babies get dirty during normal play and a bath removes the dirt. The degree of dirtiness that suggests neglect requires several baths to begin to remove it and is accompanied by an offensive odor. Feces and dirt in the skin folds and under the nails may be evidence of failure to provide for the child's basic needs.

Diaper rash can be a key to the attentiveness and care attitudes of the parents. The skin of some babies is extremely sensitive and some irritation and peeling of the skin occur. However, the diaper rash in these cases shows evidence of being cared for and seldom reaches the point where the skin is peeling, cracked, and bleeding. A baby with a constantly dirty genital area who is left in wet diapers long enough for ammonia burns to occur is not being cared for adequately.

Multiple cat or dog bites and scratches indicate that the child may be left unattended for long periods, another factor in neglect. If a parent fails to bring a child to a physician when the child has an infection of the skin and there is evidence that the illness has been present for some time, or if the child's condition is not improving with the treatment prescribed, assuming the diagnosis and treatment are correct, the parents are probably not following the doctor's instructions, which constitutes medical neglect.

♦REPORTING SUSPECTED ABUSE

Mandated reporters include physicians, dentists, podiatrists, nurses, psychologists, speech pathologists, coroners, medical examiners, child day-care center employees, children's services workers, social workers, and schoolteachers. Any of these mandated reporters may be asked to testify.

QUESTIONING THE HISTORY

You must remember that an explanation for an injury should not change when it is questioned or challenged. If the history differs from parent to parent, when different people ask, or when the story is challenged, it is very likely fabricated.

Some parent advocacy groups do not consider any punishment of a child under the guise of discipline as child abuse. These groups consider the intent of the parent when the child was injured. Parents usually believe they are doing what is best for the child. Unfortunately, the injured child is not aware of the good intentions of the parent. As stated earlier, when deciding to report an injury, the mandated reporter concerned about a child's well-being should not be influenced by the caregiver's intent. The courts, law enforcement, and social services will decide what is best for the child and what influence intent will have.

FALSE ALLEGATIONS

False reports of child sexual abuse are uncommon and represent only a small proportion of cases. There is concern that many of the reports of sexual abuse that are later determined to be unsubstantiated may be false. Even if false reports are uncommon, they should be a serious concern, not only because of the potential legal consequences of a false accusation, but also because of the distress caused the family and the child.

Alleged abuse of children, physical and sexual, is more common in divorce and separation situations than in stable families. An allegation of abuse is difficult to deal with when made between separated parents and must be carefully evaluated. It can be a powerful weapon one parent uses against the other or may become a ploy to use against each other, calling the authorities at each return of the child, who is trapped in a compromising situation. It can also be a true allegation of abuse and the child and family in need of help.

Sexual abuse is usually secretive, involving two witnesses: abused and abuser. For good reasons, both parties may forget, or want to forget, the experience. Without a confession of guilt, one of those witnesses is lying.

WHAT TO REPORT

Children's hospitals must have a Child Protection Team and must establish guidelines for recognizing and reporting child abuse. Knowing what and when to report requires a sound knowledge of what child abuse is, a familiarity with child development and behavior, an acquaintance with the child protection system, a knowledge of adult behavior, common sense, and a smattering of physics and biomechanics (**Tables 1-2, 1-3, and 1-4**).

Table 1-2. Caretaker Indicators

Strong Indicators
Explanation of injury not believable
Explanations are inconsistent/changing story
Paramour in the home
Previously suspected of abuse
Caretaker(s) understates the seriousness of child's condition
Caretaker(s) projects blame to third party
Caretaker(s) has delayed bringing child to hospital
Caretaker(s) cannot be located
History of substance abuse
Caretaker(s) unable to function
Child is not up-to-date on immunizations
Child has severe diaper rash, is poorly kept, dirty
Caretaker(s) is psychotic

Nonspecific Indicators
Caretaker(s) is hostile and aggressive
Caretaker(s) is compulsive, inflexible, unreasonable, and cold
Caretaker(s) is passive and dependent
Father is unemployed
History of unwanted baby
Caretaker(s) has unrealistic expectations of child
Caretaker(s) is hospital shopper
Frequent visits to the pediatrician without a medical reason
Caregiver(s) overreacts to child's misbehavior

Table 1-3. Situations That are Possibly Child Abuse and Dictate a Report to the Authorities

Death of an Infant with Unknown Cause and Poor or Questionable History

Evidence of Emotional Abuse
Hair loss
Suicide, runaway
Drug use
Child perpetrator
Child has flat affect, is passive, fails to thrive

Neglect
Medical treatment delayed (depends on seriousness of condition)
Failure to thrive with no medical condition to explain it
First drug or toxin ingestion with suspicious history

Repeated drug or toxin ingestion
Small child(ren) supervised by child under 12
Severe dehydration, underweight with no medical condition to explain it

Head Injury
Subdural hematoma without appropriate history
Fracture of the skull with suspicious or no history

Thermal Injuries
Burns that involve neglect
Burns with poor or no history

Skeletal Injuries
Fractured long bone with no appropriate history

Table 1-3. Situations That are Possibly Child Abuse and Dictate a Report to the Authorities *(continued)*

Bruises
Multiple bruises
Injuries that suggest the use of an instrument
Injuries resulting from discipline in child over
  1 year of age

Intrauterine Abuse
Fetal neglect, no prenatal checkups, suspicion
  of drug or alcohol abuse, poor nutrition
Psychotic mother who gives reason to suspect
  fetus is in danger
Battered mother

Sexual Abuse
Genital injuries
Child prostitution

Table 1-4. Situations That are Child Abuse and Dictate a Report to the Authorities

Severe Neglect
  Abandonment
  Long periods with no supervision. Children
    from infancy to 8 years old left unattended
  Long delay in obtaining medical help for a
    serious injury
  Maternal deprivation

Head Injury
  Evidence of shaken infant syndrome
    –Altered level of consciousness
    –Closed head injury
    –CNS hemorrhaging
    –Retinal hemorrhages
  Catastrophic injury explained by routine fall

Deliberate Thermal Injuries
  Multiple cigarette burns in varying stages
    of healing
  Glove-and-sock pattern liquid burn
  Iron burns (shows iron pattern) on back, back
    of hand, or buttocks or curling iron burns in
    same areas
  Diaper area burns and doughnut-shaped burns
  Burns to the back of the hand
  Bilateral burns or injuries to hands

Skeletal Injuries
  Rupture of the costovertebral junction
  Posterior rib fractures
  Metaphyseal avulsion fracture

  Two or more fractures in different stages
    of healing
  Multiple skull fractures
  Long bone fracture in a nonambulating child

Bruises
  Bilateral black eyes without broken nose
  Skin bruises and lacerations in recognizable
    shapes, such as whip, belt, stick, fist, fingers,
    buckle, rope, or teeth
  Circumferential injuries (burns, bruises,
    lacerations, or scars) of the wrists, arms,
    ankles, legs, and neck
  Multiple bruises in inaccessible places, in
    different stages of healing
  Injury resulting from discipline in a child
    less than 1 year of age

Trauma
  Blunt trauma to abdomen or chest with
    inappropriate or no history
  Intrauterine abuse
  Crack baby or one born to mother with drug-
    dependency
  Evidence of fetal injury or self-injury

Sexual Abuse
  Category IV of sexual molestation
  Credible disclosure of abuse by child

♦ SUGGESTED READINGS

Caffey, J: The whiplash-shaken-infant syndrome: Mutual shaking by the extremities with whiplash-induced intracranial intraocular bleedings, linked with residual permanent brain damage and mental retardation, *Pediatrics* 54:396-493, 1974.

Holbourn, AHS: Mechanics of head injuries, *Lancet* 2:438, 1943.

Hurwitz, A, and Castells, S: Misdiagnosed child abuse and metabolic disorders, *Pediatr Nurs* 13:33-36, 1987.

Magid, K, and McKelvey, CA: *High Risk: Children Without a Conscience*, Bantam Books, New York, 1987.

Oates RK: Overturning the diagnosis of child abuse, *Arch Dis Child* 59:665-667, 1984.

Williams, RA: Injuries in infants and small children resulting from witnessed and corroborated free falls, *J Trauma* 31(10):1350-1352, 1991.

Chapter 2

BURns

Anthony J. Scalzo, M.D.

"To intentionally burn a child implies a sustained anger or hostility and appears to be a controlled, premeditated, or even sadistic action." (From Fowler, J: Child maltreatment by burning, *Burns Incl Therm Inj* 5:83-86, 1979.)

Others echo these sentiments and suggest that society must intervene to address the multiple problems of the abusively burned child. Abusive burns should be handled as top priority according to the severity of injury. The severity of later injuries in burned children suggests that the abuse pattern may be well ingrained by the time the child is burned.

The stigma of the burn does not end when the child is removed from the home of the abusing parent or discharged from the hospital; it may persist for years. Many victims of house fires die, but victims of scalds often survive with permanent disfigurement, motion disabilities due to contractures, and psychological damage. Children who were victims of abusive burns can exhibit aggressive behavior ranging from biting another child to attacking a sibling with an axe. Depression can be manifest by crying without reason, refusing to socialize, or attempting suicide. Withdrawal and other behavioral problems are all aspects of post-treatment adjustment in severely burned children.

◆ How Often Does Burning Happen?
Who Is at Risk?

Children 1 to 5 years old comprise the peak age category when burns occur. Statistics from the U.S. Consumer Products Safety Commission reveal that 37,000 children under 14 years of age were treated for hot liquid or food and tap water scalds in 1988; nearly half, 16,000 of these children, who were treated in emergency departments were under 5 years of age. Of these children, 5,000 were scalded by hot tap water, most often in the bathtub. Although flame injury usually results in a burn involving a larger surface area and is therefore more severe, it is not seen as frequently as scalds.

The National Safe Kids Coalition estimates that burns are the third most common form of childhood accidental death in the United States. The National Safety Council noted that burns cause more than 1,300 childhood deaths per year in the United States and rank only behind motor vehicle and drowning accidents. Other estimates note that more than 23,000 children were hospitalized and 440,000 were treated for burns, bringing the total cost to society from childhood burn deaths and injuries to approximately $3.5 billion dollars. Each year about 100,000 children in the United States are hospitalized for the treatment of burn injuries, and several hundred thousand are treated as outpatients. The number of burns not brought to medical attention and those that go unreported as abuse are probably significant.

The victim of abusive burning is usually a young child, 3 to 4 years of age or younger. There may also be a link between abusive burning and educationally or culturally deprived maternal background, single or divorced marital status, unemployment, physical abuse of mother (wife battery), and other characteristics of the mother, such as isolation, suspiciousness, rigidity, dependence, and immaturity.

Most burns occur in the home. These burns may occur at peak times of stress in the parents' day, specifically between 6 PM and midnight. Another peak time may be in the late afternoon and morning hours.

Regardless of the parents' educational level, scald burns occur more often in poorer socioeconomic housing or multi-unit buildings, where units close to the complexes' heating plant receive hotter water than those more distant from the heat source. With poor insulation and inefficient heat sources, the hot water heater's temperature may be increased to satisfy the demands in more distant units, meaning that those units close to the source can receive dangerously hot water.

◆TYPES OF BURNS AND PHYSICAL CONCEPTS

There are six categories of burn injuries: flame, scald, contact (with hot object), electrical, chemical, and ultraviolet radiation (sun). Abusive burns are generally concentrated in the scald and contact categories, although rarer instances of flame (matches, cigarette lighters, or stove), chemical, microwave (actually placing an infant inside a microwave), or even hair dryer–inflicted burns have been reported.

Scald burns result from exposure to a hot liquid. They can burn the skin to varying thicknesses; however, if serious burns occur on the buttocks, genital area, and hands or feet, child abuse should be suspected.

Since scalds are the most common cause of death from burns in children, we must examine why scalds occur. More scald burns occur in the bathroom than in the kitchen; therefore, hot water temperature in the bathtub is important. Length of time in the hot water and repeated exposures are also important factors in many of these burns. At 49°C (120°F), the lowest setting on most gas water heater thermostats, it takes 5 to 10 minutes to cause deep burn injury to adult skin. However, at 51°C (124°F) it takes 4 minutes. At 52°C (125°F) it takes 2 minutes, and at 54°C (130°F) it takes only 30 seconds to result in a scald. Water at 60°C (140°F), an average temperature for most households, will take 5 seconds to produce a scald burn. It is interesting to note that 140°F is generally the recommended intake temperature for many home dishwashers, although some commercial dishwashing detergents will dissolve and sanitize at 130°F. At 70°C (158°F), which is found in some homes, a serious burn will occur in less than 1 second. Temperature versus time-to-scalding data are given in **Table 2-1.**

Table 2-1. Temperature Versus Time Burn Chart	
Temperature (°F)	Time to Produce Scald *(partial thickness)* Burn in Adults *(less time in children)*
120°	5-10 minutes
125°	2 minutes
130°	30 seconds
135°	10 seconds
140°	5 seconds
145°	3 seconds
150°	1.5 seconds
155°	1 second or less

Adapted from Appendix D, Scald Burn Prevention Strategy Manual, National Safe Kids Campaign, Washington, D.C., 1990.

It is helpful to remember that children's skin is thinner than adults' skin, so serious burning occurs more rapidly and at lower temperatures. Furthermore, exposure to hot water for less than the time it takes to burn and at a lower than burning temperature can still cause significant burns if the contact is repeated with little time between exposures. Water at 49°C applied to skin for 3 minutes can be tolerated, but an application of 9 minutes' duration can result in a full-thickness skin burn.

◆ Is It an Abusive Burn?

Differentiating inflicted from accidental injury must begin with definitions. These definitions have both medical and legal implications. The requirement to report abuse, which is law in all 50 states, depends on the ability to recognize abuse.

The definition of physical abuse offered here does not exclude reasonable corporal punishment by parents. Physical abuse is "an injury to a child caused by a caretaker, for any reason, including injury resulting from a caretaker's reaction to an unwanted behavior. Injury includes tissue damage beyond erythema or redness from a slap to any area other than the hand or buttocks. Physical discipline should not be used on children who are under 12 months of age. The child should be normal developmentally, emotionally, and physically. Tissue damage includes bruises, burns, tears, punctures, fractures, ruptures of organs, and disruption of functions. The use of an instrument on any part of the body is abuse. The injury may be caused by impact, penetration, heat, a caustic, a chemical or a drug." (From Johnson, CF: Inflicted injury versus accidental injury, *Pediatr Clin North Am* 37:791-814, 1990.)

This definition leaves no confusion about defining any physical abuse situation, including burns. An instrument is defined to include devices, gadgets, and implements and mediums of delivery.

Suspicious burns in a child with a prior history of abuse or other physical signs of abuse places that child at high risk for lethal abuse.

ABUSIVE BURN PATTERNS
SCALD AND IMMERSION BURNS

The scald is generally considered the most common type of abusive burning. Inflicted scald burns are most frequently caused by hot tap water; sometimes coffee, tea, or cooking grease is involved.

Immersion burns to the buttocks or genitals are often inflicted to punish the child for soiling or wetting his or her pants. This occurs in families where the caregivers are rigid in toilet training beliefs. Cigarette burns inflicted in the pubic area as well as blows to the penis with hairbrush bristles have also been used to discipline a child during toilet training.

Scalds may involve the back, buttocks, perineum, and genitalia or may spare these areas and involve "stocking"- or "glove"-like burns of the hands and feet. Children held in a bathtub of shallow water may raise up on their hands and feet to protect themselves. This may leave characteristic patterns of third-degree burns to the hands and/or feet if the water temperature exceeds 150°F.

Sometimes the child is held by the head and legs and immersed back first into hot water. Additionally, the child may be forced down against the tub or sink and sustain a burn with a distinct line across the back, part of the buttocks, and the side, but with no burn in the center of the buttocks. This so-called doughnut-shaped burn is seen only infrequently.

SPLASH BURN INJURIES

Splash burns occur when a hot liquid is thrown or poured onto a victim. The depth of burning is usually less than with the immersion type due to the cooling effect of the liquid as it spreads out or falls down the body. Splash burns often involve the back, the lateral side of the face, and the back shoulder area. The front lower side of the face, neck, and shoulder as well as the front of the chest and trunk are commonly the areas burned during an accidental spill from a kettle or saucepan. As the hot liquid drips downward, it often burns in the shape of a "V" (arrow sign). This burn pattern occurs when the hot liquid initially contacts the skin and then spreads down the body, cooling as it goes. The edges cool faster than the central tract of hot fluid. The direction of the "arrow" or combination of "arrow signs" seen with burns in more than one area can aid in determining whether the child was abused. By studying the flow pattern of the hot liquid, clues can be gained that indicate the direction the liquid came from as well as the position of the child. If the history does not coincide with these physical characteristics, child abuse should be suspected.

The classic arrow sign may not be present, however, with hot grease spills. Grease becomes hotter than water and sticks to the skin rather than running off the surface. It may cause a deep, serious burn. The arrow sign may also be absent when the child is forced under hot running water from a faucet. The continuous flow of hot water from the faucet serves as a constant source of heat energy, referred to as an "energy sink." This may cause uniform third-degree burns without a cooling pattern, as described above. If the child is developmentally old enough to turn on the hot water faucet, he may accidentally sustain such a burn on the front of his abdomen and legs. Therefore, when given that history, the patterns of the burn, the child's developmental skills, and the presence of other associated findings must be analyzed in order to clearly differentiate abusive from accidental causes of injury.

FLEXION BURNS

Another pattern of abusive burning seen in either of the two types discussed above (immersion or splash) is the flexion burn. This type of burn pattern may occur when a hot liquid is intentionally poured onto the body or the victim is immersed in a hot liquid with the hips or other body parts fully flexed. The skin within the flexed body area is spared from contact with the burning agent.

This may occur in one area or in several parallel to each other, yielding alternating areas of burn and spared skin or a "zebra" pattern. Partial contact with grills or repeated application of curling irons to the skin on an area of the body may also give an alternating "zebra" pattern. Additionally, hot water scalds to limbs partially protected by clothes such as socks may yield alternating patterns of burned and spared skin. These, however, have patterns distinct from scald immersion lines.

CONTACT BURNS

Contact burns comprise a unique group of pattern burns. The child care worker may need to assume the role of a detective in order to accurately diagnose the cause of these inflicted burns. Curling irons, steam irons, cigarettes and cigarette lighters, and space heater grills are a few of the implements used in abusive burning. Hot plates, light bulbs, and knives have also been used.

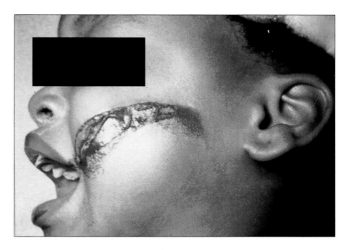

Figure 2-1a. Burn on the left lateral cheek of a child who pulled a hot clothes iron down onto her face by pulling on the cord. Note the irregular shape of the lower half of the burn, which is consistent with a hot object contacting the patient's face but then causing a glancing type of injury as it falls.

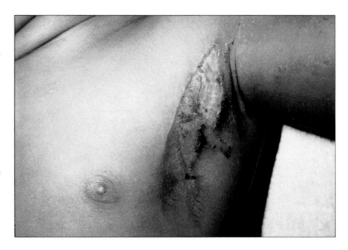

Figure 2-1b. Same child as in Figure 2-1a. The hot iron fell downward and caused a burn to the chest.

The shape of the object is branded on the child's skin. Hot objects can also cause accidental burns; however, the patterns are generally not uniform, but rather appear to be a glancing (brushing against) type of injury. The child in **Figure 2-1a,b** sustained a glancing type injury with a nonuniform burning pattern when she pulled on the cord of an iron, causing it to accidentally fall onto the skin. Here the child sustained a partial and irregular burn to the face and then, as the iron continued its fall, to the skin in front of the underarm area and to the chest area. A careful history and analysis of the burn as well as recognition of accidental patterns of burning is essential in a case such as this. This must be compared to the clearly demarcated and inflicted burn pattern seen in **Figure 2-2.** Also, you should be aware of what

Figure 2-2. *Inflicted steam iron burn on the lateral surface of the left arm of a 2-year-old child. Note the sharply demarcated edges and the pattern of steam vent holes "branded" onto the skin. The father claimed that the burn was accidental, but he admitted to spanking the child for "messing her pants."*

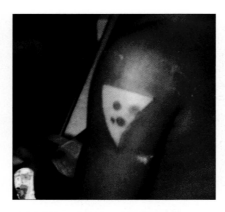

Figure 2-3. *Old clothes iron burn scar of the left buttock with depigmentation. Also note the whip and lash marks on the back of the legs.*

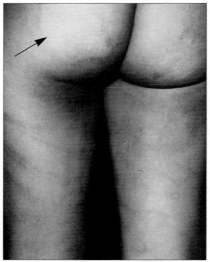

well-healed iron burns look like years later. **Figure 2-3** shows a well-healed, iron-shaped burn scar on the left buttock of a child being evaluated for additional signs of abuse, such as old loop and lash marks.

Wood burning stoves are another cause of contact burns, one that is quite prevalent in some areas; it is estimated that 13 million wood stoves are used in the United States today. The location of the burn on the body aids in the evaluation of suspected abuse versus accidental injury. The functional position of the hand at the time of the burn yields a recognizable burn pattern.

HISTORY

Your first responsibility is to obtain care for the child's injury. First aid and primary medical care are discussed in books devoted to burn treatment. While these needs are vital, the focus of this book is on what you can do to identify abuse and integrate your findings into a plan of action.

Talk with the child and parents to obtain a *history* to be reported to medical personnel. A careful history outlines the time, nature, extent, and location where the burn occurred. *Once you have completed questioning the child and/or parents about the burn, you must compare the history you have compiled with the physical evidence, taking into account the following points:*

First, evaluate the patient's developmental skills. Could he or she have done what is reported?

Second, analyze what type of burn it is and where it is located. Could it have occurred in the way reported? For example, a scald burn on the front part of the body with a pattern of cooling as it descends is consistent with a child pulling a hot liquid from a vessel onto himself. However, a burn located behind the ear or on the back and shoulder suggests a liquid thrown from behind (**Figure 2-4a,b**). Scald burns on the buttocks usually occur from being forced to sit in hot water, so a history of an accidental fall into the bathtub is suspect. Full-thickness scald burns with a distinct pattern resembling a stocking or glove or circular or oval patterns on the buttocks are not likely to be accidental (**Figures 2-5 and 2-6**).

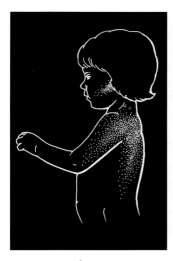 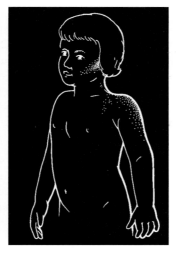

Figure 2-4a,b. *Drawing depicting the pattern of burn forming "arrow" signs on the cheek and back. This may occur when hot water is thrown from behind.*

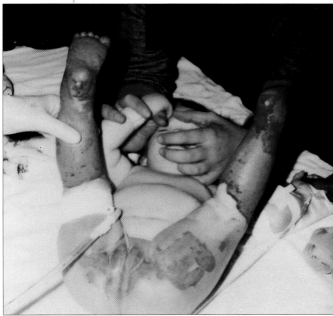

Figure 2-5. *Posterior aspect of the legs demonstrating a "stocking like" distribution of the burn. Also note the burns to the genital area.*

Figure 2-6. *"Stocking" type burn to the foot. Note the sharp demarcation of the immersion line.*

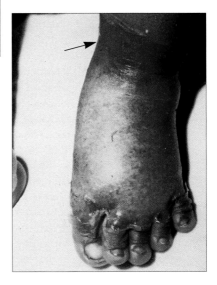

Remember, you are not responsible for classifying the type of burn you see according to specific characteristics for a formal report to the medical personnel involved. It is important for you to be observant of the burn and note whatever characteristics you see, making notes if necessary to help in answering questions for both medical and legal authorities.

Relying on a single source for the history or information regarding the injuries can limit your ability to correctly distinguish between accidental and suspicious or intentional burns. A cooperative effort between child care workers, law enforcement, social services, and medical staff is needed. All those involved should consider the plausibility of the parents' or guardian's description of how any given injury occurred.

In suspicious burns, it may be necessary for trained social workers and detectives to visit the scene of the burn or analyze photographs taken by police to ascertain if the burn could have occurred in the manner reported. This procedure should be requested by medical personnel before final conclusions regarding the cause of the burn are made. Having the caregiver review the events while walking through the area and demonstrating with a doll the child's position, describing the depth of the water, etc., helps medical personnel to determine whether the injury was accidental.

An interdisciplinary approach was used in the following case:

Case History

A 5-month-old girl was admitted to the emergency department. She could not breathe and required immediate placement of a breathing tube. The mother stated that 2 days before coming to the hospital an adult was pouring hot water near the baby and accidentally spilled it on the child. She treated the burn with cocoa butter. It seemed to be improving. The child's father stated that while he was cleaning the burn with alcohol the baby stopped breathing and had no heart rate. He said that he performed CPR for 2 hours while waiting for the mother to return home so that she could call an ambulance.

Physical and Laboratory Findings

On examination the child was noted to have a serious burn of the front part of the chest with some smaller burns on the chin and forearm. Further examination revealed that her abdomen was puffy and soft, her eyes were bloodshot, and there was a star-shaped cut near the vagina. Further medical studies found numerous fractures and other evidence of ongoing trauma.

Evaluation

The parents' history is not believable; it is obviously false. Furthermore, such a severe burn in a young infant normally causes a caregiver to seek medical attention immediately. The other physical injuries further indicated only one cause—child abuse.

In another case, emergency department staff were given the history that a 23-month-old boy, while riding his tricycle, was caught between a space heater and a wall. The child suffered third-degree burns to his buttocks and second-degree burns to the backs of his legs. The family did not seek medical attention for 2 1/2 weeks. After the parents dropped the child off to leave on vacation, he was taken to the emergency department by his grandparents when they noted the injury while bathing him. Analysis of the information gathered at the scene as well as other points of the history led to the conclusion that the burn could not have occurred in the manner reported. The child was unable to ride a tricycle. The temperature of the space heater at the level of the burn would have required 20 minutes to develop a third-degree burn; only the top of the heater had temperatures hot enough to cause a burn that severe. Using a doll, no position could explain how the combination of the buttock and leg burns could have happened. Investigation revealed that a better source for the burn was the kitchen stove. Measuring the size of the burn and noting its shape, investigators were able to determine that the circular heating plate of the stove was most likely the source of the buttocks injury. Assuming that the child was intentionally placed on the stove, his calves would align with the hot front door of the stove. In addition, other facts supported abuse as the cause: The child was being toilet trained, the area was typical for disciplinary abuse, there was a long delay before seeking medical assistance, and only a third party, the grandparents, sought help.

♦REPORTING CRITERIA

Burns themselves are often emotionally as well as physically devastating to the child. Therefore extreme care must be exercised to avoid contributing to the emotional trauma by *incorrectly* accusing a parent of abuse. To effectively develop and use criteria for diagnosing intentional burns, professionals should be familiar with the common characteristics of child abuse and neglect as well as those of inflicted burns.

Sometimes it is difficult to mentally coordinate all of the family psychosocial factors, the child's developmental milestones, any physical problems, and findings of medical personnel. *The following are guidelines for any clinician, social worker, or nurse to help differentiate accidental from abusive or neglectful burns:*

When a child comes to you with a burn and one or more of the following are found to be present, you should consider abuse:

1. Multiple bruises or scars in various stages of healing

2. Additional injuries or evidence of neglect such as malnutrition and failure to thrive (Especially suspicious are bone injuries such as old rib fractures or fractures elsewhere on the body.)

3. History of many previous hospitalizations for "accidental" trauma

4. An unexplained delay between the time of injury and the first attempt to obtain medical attention (In some cases, if the parent has medical training, such as an R.N. or M.D., the delay may be because the parents tried to care for the burn on their own.)

5. Burns appearing older than the alleged day of the accident, also indicating mixed feelings about seeking care and possibly risking exposure of the abuse

6. An account of the incident that does not match the child's age and physical abilities (An example is that of an infant who "crawled into the hot bathtub" when the infant is only a few months old and not developmentally able to do so.)

7. The responsible adults claim that there were no witnesses to the "accident" and the child was merely discovered to be burned, thus hoping to discourage any further inquiry

8. Relatives other than the parents bring the injured child to the hospital or a nonrelated adult brings the child (unless there is a good explanation for the parents' absence, such as when a child is being cared for by a baby sitter while the parents are out of town)

9. The burn is blamed on the action of a sibling or other child (Although this is often a false explanation for abusive burns, it should be noted that siblings can be abusive.)

10. The injured child is excessively withdrawn, submissive, or overly polite or does not cry during painful procedures

11. There are serious scalds of the hands or feet, often symmetrical, suggesting that the arms and/or legs were forced into a hot liquid

12. There are isolated burns of the buttocks or genital area or a doughnut-shaped burn of the buttocks, which in children can hardly ever be produced accidentally

13. The responsible adults give different stories as to the cause of the burn or change their story when questioned

Since the palm of the hand and the sole of the foot are thick and relatively resistant to thermal damage, serious burns seen here suggest prolonged immersion and therefore inflicted injury. An exception might be handicapped children, in whom the areas where feeling is reduced have thinner skin and the child may burn unexpectedly and more easily. However, handicapped children are also at increased risk of abuse. Sometimes burns or bed sores in handicapped children fall into the neglect or pseudoabusive category.

♦ ACCIDENTAL BURNS AND CONDITIONS THAT ARE NOT ABUSE

When determining whether an injury is accidental or inflicted, unusual causes of burn injuries should be considered. Unsuspecting parents may expose their children to burn injuries unintentionally.

There were an estimated 656 cases of vaporizer-related injuries in 1979. Two cases of steam vaporizer burns affected the lungs. Thermal injury to the lungs from flame or dry hot air is rare; usually the toxic gases from smoke and other gases cause inhalation injury. However, inhalation of steam can produce severe injury to the lungs as well as skin burns.

Another unexpected accidental burn may occur on deck floor tiling such as that used around outdoor pools. These tiles can become very hot after long exposure to the sun.

Inside the home, children have been injured accidentally on hot registers (grating) for floor furnaces. A burn can occur virtually instantaneously at temperatures that are normally encountered with these devices. Wall registers may also be sources of accidental burns to children. Hot floor grate registers are sources for accidental rather than inflicted injury. **Tables 2-2 and 2-3** list the estimated sources of burns.

Infant automobile restraint systems are lifesaving and in no way should be discouraged. However, many adults—including health care workers—are not aware how hot the metal parts of the infant car seat can become when left exposed to direct sunlight in hot weather.

The child care worker must also be aware of unique religious and cultural practices. Called "pseudoabusive" injuries, burns may be incurred within certain folk medicine customs. For example, in Vietnamese or Cambodian cultures the practice of rubbing a coin or alternatively applying a cup, spoon, or shot glass heated in oil to the skin of an ill child's neck, spine, back, or ribs is termed "coining" ("Cao Gio") or cupping, respectively. These cultures believe that this folk medicine treatment will diminish pain, restore appetite, draw out the fever, and strengthen a weak stomach. Managing these situations involves education of the families.

Table 2-2. Heating Units Related to Injury and/or Burns in Children 0 to 4 Years of Age (1989)	
Type of Unit	**Estimated Number of Children Treated in U.S. Hospital Emergency Departments**
Home radiators	8,925
Fireplaces (all types)	7,174
Kerosene or oil heaters	4,151
Heating systems, not specified	3,948
Coal or wood-burning stoves	2,941
Water heaters	347

Table 2-3. Agents Related to Injury and/or Burns in Children 0 to 4 Years of Age (1989)*	
Burn Source	**Estimated Number of Children Treated in U.S. Hospital Emergency Departments**
Irons	11,745
Hair curlers and curling irons	11,362
Hot water	10,495
Cigarettes, pipes, cigars, or tobacco	6,468
Ranges not specified	5,423
Household products, caustics, drain cleaners, ammonia, oven cleaner	3,155
Gasoline and gasoline cans	2,832
Electrical wiring, outlets, receptacles, and extension cords	2,814
All other ovens	2,690
General home or room fires†	1,592
Light bulbs	1,410
Electric and gas ranges	1,116
Fireworks	1,002
Microwave ovens	817
Cigarette or pipe lighters	713
Hairdryers	368
Matches	209

Estimates based on data from the National Electronic Injury Surveillance System, US Consumer Product Safety Commission Product Summary Report, 1989.

†Does not include deaths at the scene that never arrive at emergency departments.

Common infectious or skin disorders should also be investigated. Most physicians should be familiar with the appearance and associated findings of common impetigo, but sometimes cigarette burns become infected and are difficult to differentiate from circular impetigo lesions. Cigarette burns are usually in clusters and in various stages of healing. Impetigo lesions usually do not scar, whereas accidental cigarette burns do. Intentional cigarette burns are usually deeper and scar more extensively.

Staphylococcal scalded skin syndrome may be confused with abusive burning, especially since it often involves the genital area. Scalded skin syndrome is usually widespread rather than limited as is found in an intentional scald. Also, if the child is taken to a doctor and the disorder responds to antibiotics, abuse is not the problem.

If there is blistering or bumps with clear liquid centers, you should question the caregiver about taking the child to a doctor. Some skin disorders produce these findings, but any unusual blistering-type lesions should be investigated.

Adolescents with preexisting psychiatric illness may present with burns that are self-inflicted, although suicide by this means is rare in Western cultures.

◆ PREVENTION

There are several strategies for preventing burn injuries in the community and in the home. When considering an object as a hazard, you must take into account the three factors involved: the host (victim), the vehicle (vector), and the environment. Placing these main points into the context of abusive burns, you would expect fewer bathtub scald burns if there was a maximum water heater temperature of 125°F built into all manufactured units. Antiscald devices are available, which, if installed at the faucet or shower head, will instantly shut off the flow of water if the temperature exceeds a preset value. Liquid crystal thermometers may also be used to check bathtub water temperature in order to prevent scalds. It is not clear whether distributing educational pamphlets and liquid crystal thermometers to families will produce a significant reduction in hot water temperature. The best preventive measure may be to have hot water heaters installed with preset safe temperatures.

Unfortunately, the human host or child victim cannot be modified physically to resist injury, unlike head injury prevention, whereby some host modification occurs by using a bicycle helmet. It is also doubtful that we can change the environment for some burns, as people still cook food and boil water in the kitchen and are unlikely to install barriers around such areas to protect small children. However, parents can be educated to unexpected dangers, such as burns from liquids heated in microwave ovens, from which skin scalds and palatal burns have occurred. Interestingly, water heated in microwaves may not reach a safe temperature until some 10 minutes after water that is heated conventionally.

More importantly, we may and should continue to try to change the vector of the trauma, namely the abusive parent. Obviously, this can be an extremely difficult and complex task. Even though studies show a relationship between socioeconomic status and the incidence of burn injuries, research is needed into effective ways of rehabilitating the abusive parent. Our legal system may successfully remove children from the home of an abusive parent, but this is certainly not ideal. The child then not only struggles with his or her physical imperfections as a result of the burning process but may also suffer further emotional turmoil due to parental separation.

One suggestion is to offer parents anticipating having children a course on child development at a level they can understand. Such classes might also include counseling regarding child temperament characteristics.

Parents should be discouraged from using infant walkers because children have been able to approach hot objects such as oven doors; reach and pull on cords to pots, fryers, and irons; and pull on tablecloths, thereby sustaining serious burns.

In cases of accidental trauma, a child's temperament may determine what he does (the "how" of behavior), his motivation (the "why" of behavior), and his competencies or physical abilities (the "what" of behavior). However, the child's normal patterns, or lack thereof, with regard to sleep, hunger, or elimination functions as well as the quality of his or her mood (i.e., crying or displeasing behavior) may play even greater roles in abuse or nonaccidental injuries.

It has been suggested that high-risk populations should be targeted for abuse prevention strategies. These strategies include education and counseling of parents to achieve realistic expectations for themselves and their children, income supplementation, employment counseling, and provision of day-care services.

Secondary prevention is also important. High-risk parental signals such as teenage pregnancy, unwanted pregnancy, or substance abuse as well as infant prematurity and childhood developmental disorders should be noted. Furthermore, early intervention may be indicated if one notes undue concern over an unborn baby's sex, a mother's denial of pregnancy or severe depression, lack of eye contact or holding of a baby, parental complaints that diapers are messy and repulsive to clean, and numerous emergency department visits. The parent may repeatedly visit the emergency room with seemingly trivial complaints as a way of asking for help. All professionals who come into contact with parents and children should recognize these high-risk signals. When possible, they should intervene with counseling, education, and/or referrals to child protection agencies.

♦ SUGGESTED READINGS

Feldman, KW: Child abuse by burning. In CH Kempe and RE Helfer: *The Battered Child*, University of Chicago Press, Chicago, 1987.

Ludwig, S, and Fleisher, G, eds: *Textbook of Pediatric Emergency Medicine*, The Williams & Wilkins Co, Baltimore, 1983.

National Safety Council: *Accident Facts,* Washington, DC, 1979.

Spear, RM, and Munster, AM: Burns, inhalation injury and electrical injury. In MC Rogers, ed: *Textbook of Pediatric Intensive Care Medicine*, The Williams & Wilkins Co, Baltimore, 1987.

Chapter 3

Sexual Abuse in Children

Vicki McNeese, M.S.
James A. Monteleone, M.D.

A 1-month-old boy was admitted to the nursery. The child had been seen by his private pediatrician because of respiratory distress. A routine chest film revealed that the child had marble bone disease. The child's mother was 14 years old.

Shortly after admission, the hospital social service department received an anonymous phone call stating that the infant was the result of an incestuous relationship. Since marble bone disease is a rare autosomal recessive disorder, consanguinity was definitely a possibility. When the mother was interviewed, she denied the possibility. The Division of Family Services was notified, and it stated that the family had previously been anonymously reported and the allegation had been unsubstantiated.

The infant was scheduled for a bone marrow transplant and, when selecting possible donors, the infant's "grandfather" was found to be a perfect match. The odds of a grandfather being a perfect match are very slim unless he is also the child's father. With that information, the child's mother was removed from the home. While out of the home, with counseling, she acknowledged that she had been sexually abused by her father and the father subsequently admitted that he had abused her.

In recent years, child sexual abuse has captured widespread attention. This is largely due to the highly publicized stories of children sexually molested by the very adults entrusted with their care and well-being. Yet despite our increased awareness and understanding of the dynamics of child sexual abuse, it continues to be a difficult, if not painful, topic for many to contemplate and discuss. Recent attention focused on child sexual abuse clearly depicts the potentially significant effects on and vulnerability of the alleged victim, the perpetrator, and their respective families, as well as evaluators charged with investigating such allegations. It has become increasingly important to develop strict standards for evaluation of sexual abuse allegations. Only through a comprehensive investigation of allegations, which includes objective, thorough, and well-documented interviews, can those involved best be protected.

To conduct objective, reliable, and child-sensitive interviews, the interviewer must be aware of and understand the history and dynamics of sexual abuse as well as have a working knowledge of the evaluation process. Armed with this information, an evaluator can benefit from others' past experiences, positive and negative; assess potential pitfalls and risks to all those involved; and more confidently and comfortably address the challenging task at hand—interviewing the child.

◆ DEFINITION OF SEXUAL ABUSE

Sexual abuse occurs between a child and an adult or older child and is defined as sexual contact or interaction for sexual stimulation and gratification of the adult or older child who is a parent or caregiver and responsible for the child's care. Sexual abuse is a form of child abuse and must be reported to state child protective services. If the perpetrator is not a caregiver, the sexual activity is sexual assault and may not fall into the category of behaviors reportable to state protective services, but must be reported to a local law enforcement sex crimes unit. The sex crimes unit deals with perpetrators of sex crimes who have no role in the child's care but are usually known to the victim or the victim's family. The sex offender often pursues this practice as a career and will abuse many children over the course of time.

The long-term effects of sexual abuse are not clearly known. Some children appear to suffer lasting psychological problems, while others are able to cope effectively. Intrafamilial abuse may be passed from generation to generation.

◆ ABUSIVE OR ASSAULTIVE ACTS

Sexual abusive or assaultive acts include sexual intercourse, sodomy or anal penetration, oral genital contact, fondling, masturbation, digital penetration or manipulation, and exposure. The acts can be reciprocal or one-sided. Of the acts listed, exposure can be the most difficult to define. Some families are comfortable with nudity in the home; they share bathrooms, share bedrooms, or live in small quarters where privacy is at a premium. Exposure becomes sexual abuse when the person exposing is sexually aroused by the event and does it specifically for that purpose.

◆ CLASSIFICATION OF SEXUAL ABUSE

The acts of sexual abuse can be divided into three categories: assault, incest, and exploitation. Assault and incest are somewhat self-explanatory; exploitation includes prostitution and pornography.

ASSAULT

The perpetrator of a sexual assault is usually male. Sexual assault is usually a one-time event in which the perpetrator forces himself on the child. If the child is examined within a short time of the assault, there is generally physical evidence of trauma, such as tears, blood, and bruises, which constitute dramatic, acute findings of abuse. When dealing with an assault case, the child is at greatest risk because the molester is often emotionally unstable. One must make certain that the child is protected and does not return to the situation in which the assault took place; the perpetrator must not have access to the child.

INCEST

Incest is defined as sexual intercourse between persons so closely related that they are forbidden by law to marry. Incestuous abuse usually occurs over a long period of time and often involves a conditioning process. The perpetrator is usually male, although female perpetrators are possible and probably underreported. The abuser may not necessarily be related to the child; he may be a stepfather or paramour but generally is the father figure or provider in the home. Although the classical incestuous relationship involves father and daughter, other common liaisons form between older brother and younger sister, uncle and niece or nephew, and grandfather and granddaughter or grandson.

Classically, there is no evidence of trauma or acute injury. The physical findings are subtle or nonexistent, unless there has been complete penile penetration over a long period. The child usually does not make a disclosure until the abuse has gone on for a number of years, beginning when the child was an infant and continuing with her becoming conditioned and manipulated over many years to accept this as a way of life. Several children in the home may be involved in the abuse.

It is not clear whether the child and the perpetrator should be separated during therapy or the investigation. If possible, the child can remain in the home and hopefully avoid being blamed or blaming herself for the disintegration of the family. She may perceive being removed as punishment. The victim as well as the perpetrator must receive counseling. She often faces alienation, denial, and hostility from the mother, father, and siblings. As a result, she may deny that the abuse took place and retract her disclosure.

If the perpetrator does not admit to the abuse, he should be removed from the home so that he cannot manipulate the child further and convince her to retract her disclosure and allow the abuse to continue. If the other parent does not accept that the child has been abused, the child should be removed from the home, again so that she will not be influenced to change her mind and deny the truth.

EXPLOITATION

Sexual exploitation involving prostitution and pornography is unique in that it often involves a group of participants. It can occur within a family or outside the home, involving several adults and nonrelated children; it is then referred to as a sex ring. In cases involving families, the whole family— mother, father, and children—can be involved, and the children must be protected and removed from the home situation. This is a pathologic situation in which both parents are often sexually involved with the children for prostitution or pornography. Exploited children need the greatest intervention and psychiatric help.

◆ HISTORY

In the late 1970s and early 1980s the growing battle against child sexual abuse, while not without opponents, seemed to be a safe and well-supported endeavor. However, as the momentum to identify and protect alleged victims of child sexual abuse grew, investigatory practices and disposition of such cases were increasingly called into question by critics.

◆ PREVALENCE

The dramatic increase in reports of child sexual abuse in the past decade has caused us to ask if current statistics indicate an epidemic of child molestation or if greater public awareness and acceptance have resulted in increased reporting. Since the victims of child sexual abuse often delay reporting or may never disclose their victimization, the true incidence of child sexual abuse is difficult, if not impossible, to ascertain. Nevertheless, it is likely that increased reporting is the more accurate interpretation of the recent trends we see.

It is estimated that approximately one in four girls will be sexually victimized by age 18. Boys were initially considered to be less at risk for child sexual abuse; however, current studies suggest that the incidence of sexual victimization of male children is notably higher than previously thought, perhaps as high as 16%. This means that one in six boys will experience sexual victimization. It has been proposed that victimization of boys may be comparable to that of girls, although, due to societal and gender expectations, males are less likely to report their victimization experiences. As a result, male victims are often not identified and thus do not receive appropriate intervention services.

It is possible that child sexual abuse is still underreported due to its reliance upon secrecy and lack of physical findings. However, there are also significant problems in the investigatory process, particularly inadequate interviews conducted by evaluators who have not been adequately trained, which leads to an overdiagnosis of child sexual abuse.

◆ EVALUATION PRINCIPLES

A comprehensive, well-documented evaluation by a competent evaluator serves to identify and protect a victimized child as well as safeguard the rights of others involved. It should never be advocated that well-intentioned professionals should knowingly conduct a biased evaluation.

The evaluation of alleged victims of child sexual abuse is rapidly changing. Wherever possible, professionals responsible for assessing alleged victims and their families must be informed of recent findings in the disciplines of medical and mental health care as well as legal practice. Some practitioners responsible for many types of cases may feel ill-prepared to assess allegations of child sexual abuse. Even evaluators who feel confident in their knowledge of child development, as well as their ability to effectively communicate with children, are less confident in assessing the validity and credibility of a child's statement regarding sexual victimization. This is especially true if the alleged victim is a young child, developmentally delayed, and/or in any other way having difficulty in relating experiences and possible trauma.

Evaluators involved in interviewing children about child sexual abuse need to gather accurate information without suggesting particular responses to a child. A well-conducted interview should increase the likelihood that a child will be able to disclose previous abusive experiences and diminish the likelihood of obtaining false or inaccurate information. At the same time, an objective, thorough, and well-documented interview minimizes the likelihood of erroneous conclusions.

Although children recall less information than older children and adults do, what they recall can be accurate. The developing memories of young children are not as proficient at the complex task of free recall, but, if the child understands and is more familiar with a particular event than an adult is, the child may be more accurate. Children are more likely to correctly answer questions about the main actions that took place than those about peripheral details, so it may be difficult for a child to describe the perpetrator, especially if he is an unfamiliar person. Children also have difficulty answering questions requiring abstract conclusions, such as a person's motivations—the "why" questions.

Children's stories often lack consistency, especially young children, principally because children are not sophisticated enough to protect themselves against the appearance of inconsistency. They have difficulty evaluating their reports for possible errors, omissions, inconsistencies, or contradictions. However, it is not the small details (the exact age, the number of incidents, or the time) that are essential, but rather it is the validation of the abuse that is critical. So the question is not whether there are inaccuracies in memory, but whether memory retains essential truths.

Young children do not understand that they can ask for clarification when they do not understand what is being asked. As a result, they will not ask for a question to be repeated or clarified, even if they do not understand what is being asked. Instead, they are apt to give any answer. It is the adults who must be careful to ask questions children can understand, and the adults must also be certain that the child understands and is given the help he or she needs.

The fact that children may not disclose abuse until months or years after the assault increases the chance that they will have forgotten part of what occurred. Whether children's memories fade more quickly than adults' memories is not known. If they do, children are at a relative disadvantage because they are less likely than adults to fill memory gaps with inferred information. Adults who have forgotten part of what happened will attempt to relate a believable coherent story. Because a child may be less able to do so, his or her testimony may appear less coherent, even if it is more accurate than the adult's story.

Are children suggestible? It had been shown that suggestion can alter answers from either children or adults. Children usually say so little in response to questioning that adults are tempted to ask suggestive questions, such as "John taught you that, didn't he?" or "The car was speeding, wasn't it?" These types of questions should be avoided because they can lead to inaccurate answers. In addition, if the questioner is a person of high status as perceived by the child (for example, a policeman in uniform), the child can be suggestible. It should be remembered, however, that it is more difficult to lead a child into making false statements about central information than about relatively peripheral details.

Is there a false memory syndrome? Scientific findings do not support a simplistic explanation that disclosures of childhood abuse are the result of therapist suggestion. This idea may be more indicative of a wish to find another explanation for these terrible stores and a need to locate the problem outside of ourselves. Generally, childhood abuse is confirmed by a constellation of symptoms, including memories, affective fragmentation, flooding and numbness, chronic patterns of denial and dissociation, and current life stresses. These patterns, the hallmarks of childhood trauma, indicate biologic reactions and are not a single memory that might have been suggested.

What about lying? Children's reporting errors are more apt to be acts of omission than of commission, meaning that they are more likely to forget or deny information than to fabricate events that did not occur. Some researchers have determined that children's reports of sexual abuse are true perhaps as often as 90% of the time. However, it is possible that the allegation is a false statement arising in the mind of an adult and imposed on the mind of the child through suggestion, indoctrination, or group contagion. The allegation can also be the result of a delusion or confabulation by the child or involve perpetrator substitution or lying by the child.

It is critical that evaluators responsible for assessing allegations of sexual victimization of a child have knowledge and understanding specific to the field of child sexual abuse. Areas of particular concern include risk factors, the process of victimization, dynamics that may hinder a child's disclosure, and currently accepted techniques for evaluating alleged victims.

◆ RISK FACTORS

While any child is a potential victim of sexual abuse, specific factors may increase the risk for sexual victimization. In general, girls are at greater risk than boys, and children seem to be most vulnerable to sexual victimization during pre-adolescence, particularly between the ages of 8 and 12 years. Other risk factors include family disruptions; parental conflict, absence, or unavailability; and presence of a "nonbiological related father." In recent years the literature concerning child sexual abuse has also started to examine and document the vulnerability of children when a sibling, cousin, or nonrelated child in the home is engaging in sexually reactive or abusive behaviors. Sexual interactions among siblings and cousins are common, and reported cases are usually abusive. Evaluators need to be aware of the potential risk to children who have unsupervised or minimally supervised contact with a child or adolescent who is sexually acting out. A history of sexual victimization in the parents' family of origin and/or a previous sexual abusive experience may also increase a child's risk for sexual victimization.

◆ VICTIMIZATION PROCESS AND FACTORS THAT INHIBIT DISCLOSURE

Most children who are abused recognize that something is wrong, but some lack the maturity to identify what that is or know how to respond to it. In assessing cases of possible sexual abuse, it is important that evaluators recognize and understand the process of victimization, including reasons children don't tell or delay disclosure of abuse. In our experience, virtually all children who disclose a history of sexual abuse later say they wish they had told someone earlier. The victimization process may be seen to involve three overlapping processes: sexualization of the relationship, justification of the sexual contact, and maintenance of the child's cooperation.

FEAR

One of the most common, compelling, and obvious reasons children often don't "tell" is fear. Child victims of sexual abuse not only fear physical repercussions but also fear potential loss of home and/or the love and attention of a nonoffending parent. The offender is usually considerably larger and stronger than the child and wields overt or covert authority. From this perspective, even a vague threat of violence might be sufficient intimidation to leave a child feeling powerless and afraid.

SHAME

Victims of sexual abuse often feel ashamed or guilty and find few safe opportunities to disclose their victimization. Although shame is a powerful factor in maintaining a child's silence, ignorance of personal boundaries and appropriate physical contacts, especially in young children, also contribute to a child's silence or delayed disclosure. Often by the time a child recognizes the abusive nature of a trusted adult's behavior, the child is likely experiencing feelings of responsibility, shame, and/or isolation—feelings that further inhibit disclosure of victimization experiences.

It should be noted that some offenders, rather than using threats, secure a child's compliance and silence through bribes and/or special privileges.

All too often a child's safety depends solely on his or her ability to report the sexually victimizing experience. A frustration for many professionals in the field of child sexual abuse is a child's denial of sexual abuse in the face of overwhelming physical and/or corroborating evidence.

Literature as well as clinical experience emphasizes that a child's disclosure of sexual abuse is a dynamic process. Disclosure often follows a progression that may include denial, tentative disclosure, active disclosure, recantation, and reaffirmation. Denial can be seen as a frequent response when a child is too frightened, threatened, or insecure to acknowledge his or her victimization experience. Recognition of a disclosure progression challenges the common assumption that children can immediately make a disclosure with questioning. Thus evaluation protocols that provide more than a single opportunity for disclosure are most likely to facilitate collection of reliable and accurate information. It should also be noted that while steps in the process of disclosure are identifiable and share common elements, the process for any individual child may be highly idiosyncratic.

◆ BEHAVIORAL INDICATORS

Children may manifest various behavioral changes in response to stress and/or trauma. The particular stress to which a child is reacting may be a divorce, death in the family, the family's relocations (which may necessitate multiple changes in the child's life), a significant illness or injury, physical maltreatment, and/or sexual victimization. Stress-related behaviors often observed in children include, but are not limited to, sleeping and eating disturbances, increased somatic complaints, regressed behaviors, anxiety and/or depression, changes in academic performance, and aggressive behaviors (**Table 3-1**).

Table 3-1. Nonspecific Stress-Related Behaviors Observed in Children and Adolescents

In assessing stress-related behaviors, the abruptness of onset, severity, and chronicity are factors that should be carefully considered. Abrupt and severe behavioral changes may be particularly indicative of emotional distress and/or possible trauma.

1. Sleep disturbances (i.e., nightmares, night terrors, fear of the dark or of sleeping alone, trouble falling asleep and/or frequently awakening during the night, or excessive sleeping).

2. Changes in eating behaviors (i.e., loss of or sudden increase in appetite with resulting weight loss or gain).

3. Regressive behaviors (child's behavior regresses to earlier developmental level, such as clinging and separation difficulties, thumbsucking, and/or diminished bladder and/or bowel control in a child who had been successfully toilet trained).

4. Hyperactivity/hypervigilance/insecure behaviors.

5. Excessive and/or inappropriate fears (i.e., fear of a particular or familiar place, person, or activity not previously noted).

6. Hostile, aggressive, or acting out behaviors/play.

7. Varied and repeated somatic complaints with no known physical etiology.

8. Change/decline in academic performance, school avoidance, or poor peer relations.

9. Behaviors suggestive of or in response to a high level of anxiety and/or depression (i.e., excessive crying, expressed feelings of hopelessness, withdrawal from family and friends, diminished interest in previously anticipated activities, decline in personal appearance, suicidal ideation and/or gesture, and substance abuse).

10. Delinquent and/or runaway behaviors.

Children who have a history of child sexual abuse exhibit more symptoms than children who have no known history of sexual victimization. However, there does not appear to be any significant difference in the presence of stress-related symptoms between child sexual abuse and other types of trauma that children experience. The presence of nonspecific stress-related behaviors is an important factor in the overall evaluation of a child, although evaluators must be cautious when interpreting children's behaviors. Evidence of stress-related behaviors should not be a primary determinant in the belief that a child has been abused. Similarly, the absence of such behavioral reactions should not lead a professional to conclude that a child has not been abused. While most children who have been sexually abused do display some nonspecific stress-related behaviors, other sexually victimized children exhibit no significant observable behavioral reactions. Stress-related behaviors in children should alert a professional to a child's feelings of distress and possible trauma and should be assessed further. Sexually abused children may have an increased prevalence of certain traits, but these traits may also be found in children without histories of abuse.

Specific behavioral reactions in children are often characteristic of that particular child's developmental level. The following outlines some abilities to be expected at specific levels:

PRESCHOOL CHILDREN

Preschool children demonstrate a variety of affective, cognitive, and behavioral symptoms in response to stress. Young children often respond to stress and/or trauma by exhibiting changes in eating and sleeping habits, chronic nightmares, regression, and an increase in fearful and clinging behaviors. Young children may also demonstrate changes in bowel and bladder control, with those who have been previously toilet trained beginning to wet and soil themselves. Preschool children may also demonstrate an increased activity level as well as aggressive behaviors in play activities and their interactions with others.

SCHOOL-AGED CHILDREN

School-aged children may demonstrate various emotional, cognitive, and behavioral changes that can be observed by parents and/or school personnel. These children may display notable moodiness, behaviors indicating a high level of anxiety and/or depression, and diminished academic functioning. These emotional and behavioral reactions may be accompanied by varied and repeated somatic complaints with no known physical cause.

ADOLESCENTS

Adolescents may come to the attention of mental health professionals in response to a crisis or an episode of acting out behavior such as a suicidal gesture, episodes of running away from home, or hostile, aggressive, and/or delinquent behaviors. Adolescents may also respond to personal and family stressors by withdrawing from family or friends, altering academic performance, or changing personal hygiene and appearance. It should be noted that due to the frequent delays in reporting incidents of child sexual abuse, adolescents may present with a history of chronic affective disturbances and behavioral problems. A comprehensive evaluation is indicated to fully assess the extent and origins of presenting problems.

Children may also come to the attention of professionals due to sexually reactive behaviors. Three sexually reactive behaviors likely to be seen in children who have been involved in direct or vicarious sexual experiences are noted in **Table 3-2**. Behaviors that are increased specifically in sexually abused

---

Table 3-2. Behavioral Indicators Specific to Sexual Abuse

1. Excessive masturbation (i.e., at a level which is developmentally inappropriate and not typically responsive to redirection or appropriate behavioral limits established by parent or authority figure).

2. Promiscuity (i.e., preadolescent or adolescent child who demonstrates sexual interactions with peers in frequency and persistence outside the developmental norm).

3. Sexual abuse of others (i.e., child initiates interactive sexual behavior with another child who is vulnerable).

(From Sgroi, 1988.)

children include excessive masturbation, sexual victimization of another child, and promiscuity. Developmentally inappropriate sexualized behaviors in children of all ages who have been sexually abused is one of the most consistent findings.

Children may also demonstrate sexualized behaviors that have not been identified as specific to sexual abuse but are suspicious for developmentally inappropriate sexual knowledge and/or experiences. If observed in a child or reported by a caregiver, such behaviors may warrant further evaluation.

These behaviors include but are not limited to the following:

— Diminished personal boundaries, including indiscriminate kissing, hugging, and/or sexualized touching of other children or adults.

— Developmentally inappropriate "seductive" behavior to solicit attention, acceptance, and/or affection from significant others.

— Curiosity regarding genitalia or behavioral reactions to observed sexual material or situations that is atypical for the child's developmental level.

— Extreme reactions to bathing or toileting.

— Excessive fear or resistance to contact with the opposite sex.

— Strong resistance or refusal to participate in age-appropriate physical or social activities (i.e., physical education classes or sleeping over) where changing clothes or showering is involved.

DIFFERENTIATING NORMAL FROM ABNORMAL SEXUAL BEHAVIOR

Since it has been well documented that children who have a history of child sexual victimization often act out sexually and/or engage in sexual activity with other individuals, it is important that individuals involved in evaluating allegations of abuse understand normal sexual behaviors in children. Normative data regarding sexual behavior of children at different developmental stages can guide an evaluator in differentiating normal sexual behaviors from those indicating sexual abuse experiences.

Children who have a history of trauma, including sexual victimization, may have symptoms associated with a diagnosis of post-traumatic stress disorder (PTSD). Only recently has PTSD been examined as a possible consequence of child sexual abuse. Although now recognized as occurring in children, little is known about the course of PTSD in childhood. There may be PTSD symptom clusters in sexually abused children, including re-experiencing phenomena, avoidance behaviors, and autonomic hyperarousal. Children who develop PTSD may not only suffer from the direct trauma of their abuse but may experience chronic symptoms that can interfere with a child's overall developmental progress.

◆ ADOLESCENT PREGNANCY AND SEXUAL ABUSE

Sexually abused children have delays in cognitive, social, emotional, and psychological functioning that may interfere with overall adaptive functioning. For example, victims of sexual abuse may be at higher risk for mental health and social functioning problems, and young women with a history of sexual abuse may be subject to the long-term negative effects on self-esteem, self-concept, and sexual adjustment. These effects are linked to adolescent pregnancy. Survey data have found that 62% of pregnant and parenting adolescents recruited from school and community programs had experienced contact molestation, attempted rape, or rape before their first pregnancy.

Overall, 55% of the sample had been sexually molested, with the age of the first such experience averaging 9.7 years old. The mean age of the offender was 27.4 years. Half of those who had been raped were raped more than once.

It was noted that young women who had been sexually victimized before their first pregnancy had begun voluntary intercourse earlier and were more likely to have used drugs and alcohol than those not abused. In addition, their sexual partners tended to be older and to use drugs and alcohol, too. Young women who had been abused were less likely to use contraception and more likely to have had an abortion as well as second and third pregnancies. Abused young women were more likely to have been in a violent relationship and reported more emotional abuse and physical mistreatment in childhood. They were also more likely to report that their children had been abused.

◆ SCREENING AND REFERRAL PROCESS

In general, the interview and screening process will be conducted by health care professionals and trained evaluators. It is important that all those involved with the care of children understand the process in order to help in dealing with questions and procedural concerns in these cases.

Due to the complexity and the number of professionals who may be involved in evaluating alleged victims of child sexual abuse, it is necessary to organize initial screening and referral data. This can be accomplished using a standardized format (*see Telephone Referral/Screening Outline, below*). Evaluators must exercise professional judgment when a request is received to interview an alleged victim of child sexual abuse, with an emphasis placed on meeting specific predetermined criteria before initiating any evaluation.

When it is determined that evaluation of an alleged victim of sexual abuse is appropriate, the standardized questionnaire can avoid duplicating services and ease communication among professionals. Similarly, when other action is indicated and/or referral to another agency is made, the information can be easily documented.

The following screening and referral form reflects guidelines for the evaluation of sexual abuse of children proposed by the American Professional Society on the Abuse of Children (1990), the American Academy of Child and Adolescent Psychiatry (1988), and the American Academy of Pediatrics (1991).

TELEPHONE REFERRAL/SCREENING OUTLINE

Date_____Taken by _____

Patient Information:

Caller _____ Relationship to Child_____

Child's Name_____BD_____Age_____Sex: M F

Current Address_____Phone # _____

Parent's Name _____

Living with: Parents__Mother__Father__Relative__Foster Care__Other __

Siblings (Names & Ages)_____

Current/Pending Legal Action: Divorce Y N   Custody Visitation Y N

Other _____

Development Level of Child: Age Appropriate_____Delayed _____

Behavioral Indicators: Y N Sexual Acting Out_____Stress Related ___

Describe _____

Physical Symptoms: Y N Describe _____

Referring Information:

Referred by_____Agency _____

Address_____Phone #_____

Reason for Referral _____

_____

Hotline call made: Y N When_____Reported by_____

Other Agencies Involved: Y N Name, Address, Telephone_____

_____

Is Child Currently Protected: Y N

Alleged Perpetrator(s): Name_____Relationship _____

Male____Female ____Adult_____Child_____(Age)_____(Other) _____

Disclosure: None_____Purposeful_____Accidental_____

Describe_____

Child Disclosed to: Mother___Father___Other Family___Peer___Other __

Reported Incidence: Single_____Multiple_____Last incident _____

Previous Interview(s): Y N By: DFS_____(Date)_____Police ____

                              (Date)_____Other Professional_____(Date) ____

Results of Interview: Disclosed SA_____PA_____Denied____

Previous P.E. : Y N By:_____Date _____

Results of P.E.: _____

Previous allegations of sexual abuse: Y N When _____

Disposition of those allegations _____

Previous sexual abuse evaluation: Y N Location_____Date _____

Is child currently in counseling? Y N Provider _____

Plan:

Notified caller to make hotline report: Y N   NA

Scheduled Appointment: Y N   Interview_____P.E. _____

Parent consult_____ Date _____

Referred child to DFS__Police__Therapist__Attorney__Medical Service ___

(Name)_____Other _____

Comments _____

_____

Additional Telephone Contacts: _____

_____

_____

_____

♦ CAREGIVER INTERVIEW

When abuse is suspected and it has been determined that a child will be interviewed, one interview is generally conducted with the parent(s)/primary caregiver, and/or other appropriate individual(s), in order to obtain applicable information in the following areas: who is in the family and if there is any significant medical or legal history, the child's health history and current health status, the child's developmental level, if there are any behavioral indicators, the family's attitude and practices regarding privacy, nudity, sexuality, and bath time and bedtime patterns, and allegations or suspicion of possible sexual abuse (*see Parent/Caregiver Interview Outline, p. 46*). Detailed information regarding the child's initial disclosure of the event is also obtained. This interview includes the parent or primary caregiver's interpretation of the child's statement and/or behavior regarding possible sexual abuse. This interview should be conducted by the primary evaluator before the child is interviewed, and not with the child present. Statements made by caregivers should be documented specifically and in detail. Caregivers should be aware that the information obtained may be shared with other professionals who are investigating allegations of abuse, as well as those making decisions regarding the appropriateness of legal action.

An information-gathering interview may be conducted with the alleged perpetrator, if he or she is a member of the child's immediate family (parent), when this is deemed appropriate. The purpose of this interview is to gather pertinent data regarding the child's level of functioning and behaviors, the family situation, and the alleged or suspected perpetrator's knowledge of current allegations. The alleged or suspected perpetrator, as well as other family members, may also be referred for further evaluation by an independent assessor.

If information gathered during a parent interview reveals a current pending divorce or custody dispute and the allegations of sexual abuse were first disclosed during legal proceedings, some or all of the parties (parent[s] and child/children) may be referred to a professional able to evaluate all family members.

RELEASE OF INFORMATION
Since review of all relevant information is preferred practice, parents are requested to sign release of information forms. This enables the evaluator to

request information from other sources. Parents may also be requested to sign authorizations permitting the evaluation results to be shared with appropriate child protective, law enforcement, and/or treatment services.

Caregivers are informed that in the case of an open child abuse investigation, investigatory agencies (including child protective services, law enforcement agencies, and court officials) may have access to information gathered during an evaluation. They are also told that reports will be made as mandated by state law to child protective services. Information regarding evaluation procedures will be reviewed with parents at the initial interview.

ASSESSMENT OF FAMILY DYNAMICS

In conducting the parent/caregiver interview, the evaluator carefully assesses family dynamics and possible pathologies. There may be stressors other than sexual abuse that can explain a child's statement or behaviors. Information gathered at the time of the parent/caregiver interview is important, not only to the evaluation process, but also in formulating an appropriate treatment plan.

A behavior rating scale, such as the Achenbach Child Behavior Checklist, may also be used to gather specific information about the types and intensity of a child's problematic behaviors. The rating scale is completed by the child's parent(s) or primary caregiver.

The following is a sample of a parent/caregiver interview that organizes material gathered at the time of the initial contact with the parent or caregiver.

PARENT/CAREGIVER INTERVIEW OUTLINE

Date:_____

Primary Evaluator _____

Parent/Caregiver Interview: (Not to be conducted in presence of the child).

Person(s) Interviewed_____Relationship to Child_____

Family Constellation: (Members in household)

Adult_____Relationship to Child _____

Adult_____Relationship to Child _____

Adult_____Relationship to Child _____

Child_____Relationship _____

Child_____Relationship _____

Child_____Relationship _____

Others_____Relationship _____

Caretakers outside of the home _____

_____

_____

Family History:

Parents are: Married_____Divorced_____Separated_____Single

If parents divorced or never married, does child have visitation with noncustodial parent: Y N Visitation Schedule _____

Date of last visit_____

Child lives with: Parents___Mother___Father___Foster Care___Other ___

Legal Action Pending: Y N Divorce____Custody/Visitation _____

History of child sexual abuse in mother's family of origin. Y N

If Yes - Victim_____Alleged Perpetrator _____

History of child sexual abuse in father's family of origin. Y N

If Yes - Victim_____Alleged Perpetrator _____

History of child sexual abuse of other siblings/children in household. Y N

If Yes - Victim_____Alleged Perpetrator _____

Has child had unsupervised contact with any above named alleged perpetrators? Y N. If Yes, has child ever alleged child sexual abuse by person(s)? Y N - Identify/Describe _____

History of psychiatric illnesses in family Y N _____

History of drug/alcohol abuse in family Y N _____

History of domestic violence in family Y N _____

History of previous child sexual abuse in family Y N _____

Physical abuse in family Y N _____

Previous involvement of Child Protective Services Y N Date _____

Describe _____

Police Involvement Y N Date_____Describe _____

Mother History of: Sexually Transmitted Disease____Genital Warts_____

I.V. Drug Use_____HIV+_____

Father History of: Sexually Transmitted Disease____Genital Warts_____

I.V. Drug Use_____HIV+_____

Has child been exposed to pornographic material? Y N Describe_____

_____

Background Information of Child:

Birth History: Unremarkable_____Remarkable_____Describe_____

Developmental Level: Age Appropriate_____Delayed _____

Language Development: Age Appropriate_____Delayed_____

Toilet Trained: Y N Age: _____

Stress-related Behaviors: Y N Describe _____

_____

_____

Onset and Length of Behaviors:_____

School/Daycare (Name):_____Grade _____

Academic Performance: Average or Above_____Below Average _____

Special Education Services: Y N _____

History of Chronic Health Problems: Y N _____

History of UTI/Bladder Infections: Y N Date: _____

History of Chronic Constipation: Y N _____

History of genital injuries, surgeries, diagnostic procedures: Y N _____

Current Medication: Y N _____

Past or Current Physical Symptoms: _____

Present sleeping arrangements in household: _____

Family Stressors during past year? _____

Has child disclosed history of child sexual abuse? Y N _____

Describe _____

_____

_____

Child Disclosed to: (Name)_____

Relationship_____Date_____

Disclosure: Purposeful_____Accidental_____Spontaneous_____

            Upon Questioning_____By Whom _____

Has child displayed developmentally inappropriate sexual knowledge, sexualized behaviors, and/or excessive masturbation? Y N Explain _____

_____

_____

Alleged Perpetrator(s) (Name): _____

Relationship:_____Location:_____

Last Known Contact (Date): _____

Does child have current contact with named individual? Y N

Describe _____

Hotline Report Made Y N   Date_____Reporter _____

Status of Alleged Perpetrator _____

Other Agencies Involved: (See Referral Form)

Previous interview(s), P.E.(s), and results (See Referral Form)

_____

Does Parent/Caregiver believe child sexual abuse allegations?   Y   N

Uncertain_____

Reason: _____

Collateral Information:

Child reports others present at time of abuse.   Y   N

Describe _____

Others state they observed incident(s) of abuse.   Y   N

Describe _____

Release of Information Signed to Obtain/Release Information To:

Name/Address:

Private Pediatrician   Y   N _____

Hospital   Y   N _____

Division of Family Services   Y   N _____

Law Enforcement   Y   N _____

Therapist   Y   N _____

Other   Y   N _____

◆CHILD INTERVIEW GUIDELINES

The initial child interview is conducted after the caregiver interview has been completed. Ideally, a minimum of two interviews should be conducted with the child. A young child or a child identified as having special needs, such as developmental delay or language impairment, can require additional interviews. At some point in the evaluation process, the child will be questioned directly about sexual abuse. However, repeated questioning of a child regarding sexual abuse, when the child is not reporting or denying abuse, is not done.

Generally, one evaluator conducts both caregiver(s) and child interviews to provide continuity and consistency. Following the collection of all information, the evaluator records impressions regarding the credibility and reliability of a child's statements, the probability that sexual victimization has occurred, and the likelihood of alternative explanations. Based on all available information, conclusions and recommendations can be provided to caregivers and appropriate investigative authorities. Throughout, the content of the interview must be reconciled with other information.

The focus must be on sensitivity to the child's needs at the time of the interview. Children quickly assess the interest, investment, and ease of the evaluator. The evaluator must create a safe and private atmosphere that fosters rapport and trust, diminishes feelings of anxiety, and enables the child to talk openly. This includes securing child-sized furniture and arranging the surroundings in a way that is child friendly. Availability of materials such as paper, pencils, and crayons is suggested to put the child at ease, facilitate nonverbal communication, and help the child clarify verbal statements.

Adequate time should be allotted so that neither the evaluator nor the child feels rushed. The evaluator must be sensitive to the child's pace and emotional responses. If a child is hungry, tired, or needs a bathroom break, the outcome of the interview may be compromised. The evaluation must also be as predictable as possible for the child. The evaluator will explain the purpose and format of the assessment and address the child's expectations and/or fears. While appropriate reassurances can foster rapport and communication, the evaluator is cautioned to not make promises he or she will be unable to keep. Often a child will ask the evaluator, "If I tell you, will you tell my Mom/Dad?" or "If I tell you, will you promise not to tell anyone?" The evaluator needs to be honest and supportive regarding the need to ensure the child's safety. An evaluator can communicate to a child concern by saying, "After we talk, I'll do everything I can to help keep you safe and tell you what I know will happen next." If a child feels betrayed by the evaluator's use of information obtained, it can potentially have negative effects on the child's well-being and on the outcome of the evaluation.

THE DEVELOPMENTALLY APPROPRIATE INTERVIEW
The interviewing approach and the language used by the evaluator should be developmentally appropriate and match the child's age and level of functioning. The evaluator must establish the terminology the child uses for people, things, body parts, and sexual behaviors. The evaluator should ask the child to define words that may be ambiguous before using them in the interview.

Given the importance of communication between the evaluator and child during the interview process, close attention is given to the language exchange. The evaluator should use language sensitive to a child's developmental level. Language should be adapted to fit the child's vocabulary and kept consistent throughout the interview.

It is also helpful to clarify response options for the child before direct questioning. The child should know that he or she is not *required* to answer the question asked by the evaluator; the child has permission to refuse to answer. The child is allowed to say, "I don't want to talk about that now" in response to a direct question rather than give inaccurate information or say, "I don't know" when he or she does in fact know. Also, if a child declines to respond to a specific inquiry, the evaluator may follow up with additional questions, such as, "What do you think might happen if you talk about it?" This helps to clarify how the child is feeling and the source of any reluctance. Hopefully, more than one interview has been scheduled, so the evaluator can return to sensitive questions that a child was unwilling to answer.

If following the initial interview with a child the evaluator is uncertain of the child's cognitive functioning, has doubts about the child's level of language development, or suspects the presence of possibly severe emotional and/or psychiatric disturbance, further assessment by a mental health professional may be suggested as part of the evaluation. A psychological/psychiatric assessment is indicated when the child's delayed development and/or disturbance could significantly interfere with the child's ability to participate in the evaluation. If the child was previously evaluated by a psychiatrist and/or psychologist, the evaluator attempts to secure appropriate records before completing the sexual abuse evaluation.

The following is an example of a form used to conduct an interview with a child.

CHILD INTERVIEW OUTLINE

Child's Name:_____Evaluator _____

Date:_____Others Present _____

General Identifying Information Obtained from Child:

Name   Y N_____Age   Y N_____Birthdate   Y N_____

Home Address   Y N _____School Placement   Y N _____

Identified Members of Household_____

_____

Other: Caretakers/daycare: _____

_____

Developmental Assessment (young children)

Identification of:
Primary Colors   Y N   Letters/Numbers   Y N

Drawings: House Y N   Tree Y N   Person Y N   Other _____

Other Measures_____

_____

_____

Affect/Mood _____

_____

Behavioral Observations/Activity Level _____

_____

Information gathered during initial session (i.e., typical day)

_____

Subsequent Child Interview(s):

Date:_____

Assessment of Possible Sexual Abuse:

Questioning presented to ascertain if child knows purpose of appointment on this date.

Do you know why you are here today? _____

Who brought you (came with you) today? If child gives name(s) only, attempt to establish relationship to child. _____

_____

Ascertain if named person told child to relate any specific information to evaluator on this date.

Did (named person) tell you to say anything to me today? If yes, what?_____

_____

_____

Use of anatomically correct dolls for identification and clarification of general body parts   Y N   Genitalia Y N

Demonstrates knowledge of general body parts   Y N

Identified Private Parts: Male   Y N   Female   Y N

Method of Parts Labeled (Pointing/Verbally Labeled)

Labels male genitalia   Y N _____

Function _____

Labels female genitalia   Y N _____

Function _____

Knowledge of body safety/sexual abuse avoidance skills   N Y

Describe: _____

_____

_____

_____

Explanation given and/or review of sexual abuse avoidance skills with child Y N

_____

_____

Review body safety concept and reassess child's understanding of such.

Adequate understanding demonstrated Y N

Questioning to address possible sexual victimization of child.

If the child discloses sexual victimization, the evaluator should attempt to obtain a narrative of the sexual abuse allegation:

Tell me about that (what happened). Continue to gather information with similar statements.

_____

_____

_____

_____

_____

_____

If child gives a limited statement and/or is unable to give a narrative response, more direct questioning may be necessary to obtain additional identifying information and/or clarification.

If statement of inappropriate touch is given, an attempt should be made to ascertain the following information: (If multiple perpetrators are identified, efforts should be made to gather information on a single individual or abusive experience at a time to avoid confusion.)

Identification of alleged perpetrator(s)

Relationship of alleged perpetrator(s) to child

Sex and age of alleged perpetrator(s)

Type(s) of inappropriate touch

Time, location(s), frequency, and context of alleged abuse

Presence or absence of element of secrecy

Circumstances of initial disclosure including person, time, location, and context

Other children or adults directly or indirectly involved in present allegations of abuse

Physical and/or behavioral response(s) of child at time of abuse (i.e., physical discomfort, actions taken, etc.)

Any prior history or allegations of abuse

Any attempts by adults to instruct child to give inaccurate information

Dolls used in sexual abuse assessment for clarification of child's statements   Y N   Anatomically correct   Y N   Nonspecific   Y N

_____

_____

_____

_____

_____

_____

_____

_____

_____

_____

Drawings

Drawings can be a useful interviewing aid. Drawing is a form of expression that is familiar even to young children. Often a child can communicate ideas and feelings to adults through drawings while achieving a sense of mastery and competence. The use of drawings may be especially helpful with young children, children who are hesitant, and/or those with immature verbal abilities. For further discussion of art therapy, see Chapter 4.

♦ DOCUMENTATION

When an allegation of sexual abuse is assessed, the implications are profound for the child, alleged offender, and their respective families, as well as the evaluator. Accurate recording of information obtained is *critical*. It is common for court proceedings regarding sexual abuse allegations to take place months or even years after allegations were initially presented and evaluated. As a result, detailed written and/or taped documentations regarding evaluation procedures, including statements made by the child, caregiver, alleged offender, and other sources is of utmost importance.

The ability of authorities to protect a child who is alleging sexual abuse frequently depends on the quality and comprehensiveness of the evaluator's records. *Pertinent information to be noted each time a child is seen includes the following:*

1. Individual(s) who accompanied the child to evaluation sessions

2. Persons in the room at the time of the interview

3. The location of the interview

4. The date and time of day the interview took place

5. The length of the interview

6. The use of any interview tools

It is recommended that specific questions regarding possible sexual victimization as well as the exact responses (verbal and behavioral) made by a child be completely, accurately, and objectively documented.

A primary responsibility of the evaluator is to accurately assess and document a child's competence to make a reliable statement. Factors surrounding a child's statement that should be documented include spontaneity in reporting an abuse experience, consistency of core details (over time and with prior statements), child's emotional state, use of age-appropriate language and words to describe sexual contact(s), content of play behaviors or gestures that clarify or demonstrate a child's description of abuse, and evidence of developmentally inappropriate knowledge of sexual acts, anatomy, or vocabulary.

The evaluator should also document any motive expressed by a child or adult to fabricate, deny, or postpone disclosure of sexual abuse. Drawings, handwritten statements, or other materials introduced by the child should be appropriately labeled and maintained as part of the permanent record.

♦ ALLEGATIONS OF SEXUAL ABUSE IN DIVORCE AND CHILD CUSTODY DISPUTES

Sexual abuse allegations that arise during divorce and child custody proceedings present particular challenges. Such allegations are often viewed with immediate skepticism. This may, in part, be due to general public opinion that in the context of a divorce and/or custody dispute, a parent or child may be motivated to deliberately give false information in an attempt to secure a favored legal decision. Professionals disagree on the true incidence of false allegations of sexual abuse that emerge during court litigation involving child custody and visitation rights. Reasons cited for a higher incidence of allegations of sexual abuse in divorcing families include stress, familial dysfunction, and increased opportunities for sexual victimization due to parental separation or divorce. In addition, separation from the abuser may provide the first safe opportunity for a child to disclose that abuse has taken place. It should also be noted that following a parental separation a child's risk for extrafamilial sexual abuse may be higher due to a change in caregivers, including the presence of a nonbiological parental figure in the home.

Allegations of sexual abuse made in the context of parental separation or divorce should not be readily dismissed due to situational factors, but rather given serious consideration and thoroughly evaluated. A complete evaluation of the parents, as well as the child, is indicated to ensure the child's safety and emotional well-being. Allegations of sexual abuse of a child by a parent indicate that a child is at emotional risk even when allegations are unsubstantiated.

◆EVALUATION OF INFORMATION OBTAINED IN INTERVIEWS

The interview with the child is often denoted as the "cornerstone" of a sexual abuse evaluation. Upon completion, the evaluator must assess the reliability and credibility of a child's statement(s) to determine the degree of probability that sexual victimization has occurred.

The use of predetermined criteria to assess a child's statements and behavior in allegations of sexual abuse can assist in minimizing evaluator bias. *The following characteristics of a child's statement and behavior are associated with true allegations of sexual abuse:*

Description and/or knowledge of sexual behavior:
— Description of specific sexual acts
— Description of sexual acts from a child's viewpoint
— Sexual knowledge beyond that expected for the child's developmental stage

Emotional reaction of child to sexual abuse:
— Child's state of mind and affective responses at the time of disclosure
— Child's recollection of feelings at the time of the abuse

Details provided about the context of abusive situations:
— Identity and relationship of alleged offender
— Sex and estimated age of alleged offender
— When and where abuse occurred
— What the victim and alleged offender were wearing
— What clothing was removed and by whom
— Whereabouts of other family members
— How alleged offender induced child to be involved
— Elements of secrecy or coercion
— Other idiosyncratic details/events

Note: Positive findings in the three major areas are not found routinely in every case of sexual victimization.

In evaluating a child's statement for reliability and validity, close attention should be given to the child's language (words), ability to relate core events, and spontaneity. A child's interpretation and subsequent description of sexual victimization depend on the child's cognitive development, verbal abilities, and the extent of his or her life experiences.

Other factors that may corroborate a child's statement and should be considered include statements indicating sexual victimization that are overheard by others, any eyewitness accounts, and the presence of multiple victims with consistent statements of sexual abuse.

◆ CONCLUSIONS

There are few absolutes in the area of child sexual abuse. Exceptions include pregnancy in a child under 12 years of age or medical evidence of specific sexually transmitted disease in young children. *However, after careful consideration of all available information, there can be several possible findings:*

— Reliable history of sexual abuse
— Child gives clear, consistent statements of sexual abuse in age-appropriate language.
— There is no clear evidence of alternative explanations for a child's statement or behaviors, nor motivation for a child or reporting adult to give false information. Corroborating factors may be present, including physical findings or behavioral indicators specific to sexual abuse.
— Suspected sexual abuse
— The presence of physical or behavioral indicators that are consistent with sexual abuse, although child does not make a clear statement or denies sexual victimization.
— Appropriate concern/insufficient information
— A child may demonstrate stress-related behaviors or present vague statements of vulnerability. However, there is no statement or there is denial of inappropriate sexual contact, and supportive evidence is insufficient for finding.
— No evidence of sexual abuse
— Information indicates child or reporting adult made false statement. Presence of alternative explanation for child's statement and/or behaviors, or misinterpretation of initial statement or behavior of child by significant adults.

◆ RECOMMENDATIONS

Following evaluation of all available information and formulation of a conclusion, an interviewer makes recommendations regarding issues of protection, placement, custody and/or visitation, and the appropriateness of additional diagnostic or treatment services. The final disposition of cases regarding allegations of sexual abuse investigated by child protective services or law enforcement agencies is the responsibility of those agencies. However, conclusions and recommendations made by the evaluator may be valuable in making placement and treatment decisions for children and their families.

◆ SUGGESTED READINGS

Boyer, D, and Fine, D: Sexual abuse as a factor in adolescent pregnancy and child maltreatment, *Family Planning Perspective* 24(1):4-11, 1992.

Burns, N, Meyer-Williams, L, and Finkelhor, D: *Victim Impact: Nursery Crimes, Sexual Abuse in Day Care,* Sage Publications, Newbury Park, NJ, 1988, pp. 114-123.

Hechler, D: The battle for acceptance. In *The Battle and the Backlash: The Child Sexual Abuse War,* Lexington Books, Lexington, MA, 1988, pp. 1-12.

Lusk, R, and Waterman, J: Effects of sexual abuse on children. In *Sexual Abuse of Young Children*, The Guilford Press, New York, 1986, pp. 101-118.

Sgroi, S, Bunk, B, and Wabrek, C: Children's sexual behaviors and their relationships to sexual abuse. In *Vulnerable Populations*, Volume 1, Lexington Books, Lexington, MA, 1988, pp. 1-13.

Wakefield, H, and Underwater, R: *Accusations of Child Sexual Abuse*, Charles C Thomas, Publisher, Springfield, IL, 1988.

Chapter 4

ART THERAPY

COLETTE M. RICKERT, LPCC, A.T.R.-BC

Art therapy was established as a human service profession in the United States in 1969 when the American Art Therapy Association was formed. Although many attempts have been made through the years to concisely define art therapy, the intricate blending of the creative process and clinical insights needed to access, diagnose, and treat make this difficult.

Two primary philosophies have existed in the profession. One approach takes the stand that art, by its very nature, is healing and the role of the art therapist is to promote the use of art to facilitate healing. The other approach holds to the belief that doing art is a good beginning, but the role of the art therapist is to companion the client and serve as an assistant in the healing process. This latter philosophy has moved to the forefront during the past few years, and much is being done to create a more clinically compatible profession.

The American Art Therapy Association 1996 defines art therapy as follows:

> Art therapy is a human service profession that utilizes art media, images, the creative art process, and patient/client responses to the created products as reflections of an individual's development, abilities, personality, interests, concerns, and conflicts. Art therapy practice is based on knowledge of human development and psychological theories which are implemented in the full spectrum of models of assessment and treatment including educational, psychodynamic, cognitive, transpersonal, and other therapeutic means of reconciling emotional conflicts, fostering self-awareness, developing social skills, managing behavior, solving problems, reducing anxiety, aiding reality orientation, and increasing self-esteem.

◆EDUCATIONAL REQUIREMENTS
FOR ART THERAPISTS

Art therapists are required to complete a master's degree in art therapy and have between 600 and 1000 hours of supervised practicum experience. After meeting these requirements, the art therapist can apply for registration. A registered art therapist (A.T.R.) is then eligible to take a written certification examination. After successfully passing this, the therapist is qualified as a board-certified art therapist (A.T.R.-BC). This credentialing is maintained by continuing education credits.

♦ MEMBERSHIP

Approximately 4,750 professionals and students are currently members of the American Art Therapy Association. Bi-annual reports are published to illustrate national and international distributions of art therapists. **Figure 4-1** reflects the geographical distribution of art therapists according to the 1994-1995 Membership Survey Report.

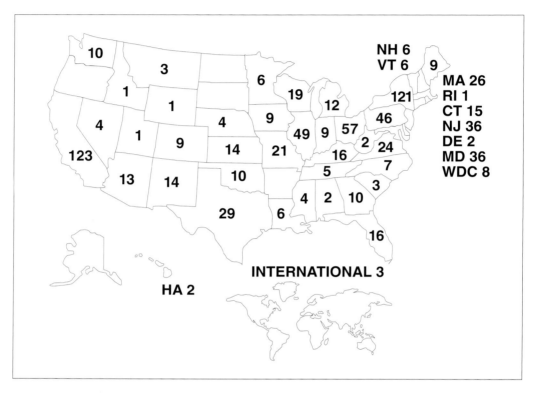

Figure 4-1. *American Art Therapy Association U.S. National Membership. (From Art Therapy: Journal of the American Art Therapy Association, vol 13, #2, 1996.)*

♦ LICENSING OF ART THERAPISTS

Art therapists in each state are exploring options for licensing, while national efforts are made with other organizations and governmental agencies to find the most effective way to achieve licensing. Art therapists are affected by various efforts to change the ways health care is being made available. Governmental, insurance, and licensing issues are evolving as regulatory decisions are explored. New Mexico has had licensing for art therapists since 1993, and Kentucky has just adopted licensing standards. Texas recognizes art therapists as a separate specialty. Art therapists in other states may be eligible for licensing as a counselor based on state requirements.

♦ HISTORY OF ART THERAPY

The field of art therapy evolved from the shared insights of professionals in three main occupations: fine and creative arts, education, and mental health. The people in these fields learned that certain individuals could be reached, could be productive, and could get better when art became a part of their activities.

Artists and writers find that the act of doing art gives them access to their innermost selves. This could be seen as either self-destructive or healing. Artists are often portrayed as people living on the edge of madness, people who cannot function in the "real world" because they are consumed by their art. Vincent Van Gogh certainly represents this stereotyped image—a man so lost in his art and pain that he had to be hospitalized and still succeeded in harming himself. Tennessee Williams, Ernest Hemingway, and many others have struggled with maintaining balance between their art and functioning in real life.

History is also full of people who have used the arts to achieve great successes and solve seemingly impossible dilemmas. Diagnosed as manic-depressive, Winston Churchill struggled with his ups and downs. First, he turned to landscaping his country estate. When he had exhausted those projects, he dreamed about a Muse who brought him brushes and paints and suggested that he might find them useful. In an article about the importance of the arts, he wrote that stress is not reduced by trying to avoid a subject, but is managed and reduced by doing something else. "Change," he said, "is the Master Key." He credited his ability to survive the turmoil and channel the passions that Hitler evoked in him to his use of the arts, painting in particular. Other artists who have certainly paved new paths for mankind by surrendering to their creative process include Pablo Picasso, Norman Rockwell, Robin Williams, and Maya Angelou.

Educators have long struggled with how to teach students effectively. Teaching techniques have mixed success rates, with some students learning no matter what, others benefitting greatly from a teacher's efforts, and some students, despite the best efforts of those around them, unwilling or unable to learn. Yet, it is often this most difficult group of students who respond best to the arts. The student who spends most of his or her time visiting the principal's office, suspended, truant, or in special educational programs for behaviorally challenging students often responds positively to classes or teachers employing or allowing art as part of his or her expression.

In the past when hospitalizations for mentally ill persons were more primitive with regard to understanding what people needed, often those charged with managing clients became frustrated. Mostly by accident and in response to the need to keep these people occupied, workers discovered that patients who drew would sometimes spontaneously stabilize and, in time, recover. Walt Whitman cared for a brother who was mentally unstable and allowed him to use art materials to draw and paint. It was his belief that this was a kinder and more productive healing technique for his brother than any others he knew. As Whitman aged, he explored options for his brother's care should Whitman die before his brother. His belief in the arts led him to an English doctor who was willing to consider the possibility that healing for the mentally ill might require treatments that allowed them to be considered as creative, spiritual beings in pain rather than creatures to be feared. Freud believed in the importance of dreams, which are nothing more than pictures created while sleeping. Jung believed that art was the key that opened the door not only to our unconscious, but also to the collective unconscious of all of mankind. Those who work with children, the ill, and those in pain know that words are not enough.

Today most art therapists see art therapy as an intricate blend of the creative process and clinical interventions. Just as walking can be beneficial and therapeutic, so too can art activities. But walking, by itself, is not therapy. When a person is injured or recovering from an illness or surgery, walking alone will not provide the cure. It may be part of the recovery process but must be under the guidance of a trained professional (doctor, nurse, physical therapist) who will companion that person to the point of recovery. Accessing, diagnosing, and treating an individual using art requires training, education, and experience in how to blend the creative process and clinical theories so that healing and resolution can occur.

At this point, art therapists function in many settings and work with many populations. Art therapy is based on creativity, and where and with whom it is used are limited only by our imaginations. With thoughtfulness and coordination of efforts and needs, it can be applied in most settings and with most populations.

According to the American Art Therapy Association, 1996:

> The art therapist treats a variety of populations in diverse settings, including but not limited to, the emotionally disturbed, the physically disabled, the elderly, the developmentally delayed, both inpatient and outpatient, community mental health centers, family service agencies, rehabilitation centers, medical hospitals, corrections institutions, developmental centers, educational institutions, private practice, and other facilities.

◆ VERBAL VERSUS NONVERBAL COMMUNICATION

Some experts estimate that 65% to 93% of our communication is done through nonverbal means. Art can tap into our nonverbal communication needs and help facilitate a deeper level of relating both with ourselves and with others.

Georgia O'Keefe said,

> I have just been trying to express myself — I just have to say things, you know — Words and I — are not good friends at all except with some people — when I am close to them and I can feel as well as hear their response — I have to say it some way [and so I paint].

The human mind functions much like a computer, and, like a computer, it needs programming. Whereas a computer might operate with a specially designed data entry system, the human mind is programmed with language. An individual gradually learns the language used in the environment and gains access to the mental aspect of personality. As language skills increase, verbalization increases and mental processing skills mature.

There are some basic drawbacks to relying on words to communicate experiences. First, any language has only so many words to describe the world and our experiences in it. For example, English contains about ninety-six words to describe feelings. What words can adequately describe the experience of a person who survives a plane crash, or the experience of a person who has been told that his child was killed in a plane crash? Second, we only have access to the words we already know. If a child goes through an experience that she does not have adequate words to describe, she will only be able to intellectually think of the event with the words she knows at that point in time. If the child is mistreated in utero or as an infant, no words are available to think about that event. This, however, does not mean that the experience is not recorded. Instead of being linguistically recorded in the mind, the computer, or the mental aspect of the child, it is recorded in the emotional, physical, and creative aspects (**Figure 4-2**). Third, abusers often threaten to further harm or kill the child or a pet or another loved one if the child ever tells what happened. In many cases, the ability to put on paper what occurred seems to bypass the inner fears and injunctions not to tell and allows maltreated children to "tell" in another, safer way. Often the pictures by these children reflect some kind of "don't tell" message or handicapping condition that makes it impossible for them to convey the information verbally (**Figure 4-3**). For example, the mouth might be missing from the picture.

It is vital to provide all children with alternative methods of expressing themselves, not only to give them options so that they can "tell," but also so that they can more fully connect with the world around them and learn balance through better integration of their mental, emotional, physical, and creative aspects.

◆ ASPECTS CHART

The mental, emotional, physical, and inspirational aspects of an individual help create a more complete picture of that person. When these aspects are working well together, integration is present. When they are not working well together, disintegration is seen. When people are hurt and the wound is not healed, they move through life in an off-balanced, nondirected way because they are not cohesively connected internally to themselves with respect to mind, heart, body, and spirit.

People with effective inner connections to these aspects can work in a balanced, self-directed way because they are internally cohesive—they are integrated. The Greeks called this being in "timeless time," a term that refers to the experience of being so absorbed in an activity that you forget all sense of time. Integrated individuals have an inherent joy in what is being done and a general lack of stress. The task may be difficult, but the unity within the individual allows him or her to proceed in a controlled, focused, integrated way.

When the four aspects of an individual are considered for assessment, diagnosis, and treatment, a more complete profile can be formulated regarding the actual needs and problems of that individual. Just as a teacher might provide a pretest assessment for the class or a doctor might order a diagnostic test, exploring these four aspects of an individual in visible form creates an opportunity for an art therapist and a client to

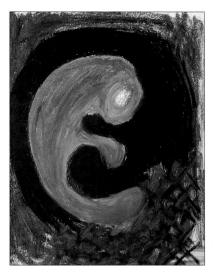

Figure 4-2. This client stated, "The fires hurt the baby. She feels the fires." It represents a prenatal memory.

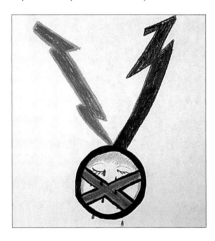

Figure 4-3. This picture was drawn in response to a structured activity asking participants to make a drawing showing why art therapy has been helpful for them. The client said that the red and orange X across the mouth came from her mother's messages to "shut up" and "quit complaining." The mother is shown as the red and orange lightning bolt at the top left of the picture. The brown and black X across the mouth came from her father's message to "never speak to me unless you have something decent to say." He is represented as the black and brown lightning bolt at the top right of the picture.

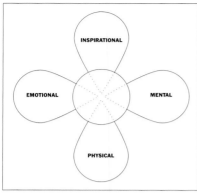

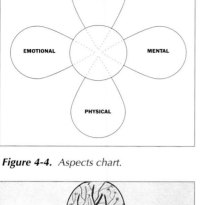

Figure 4-4. *Aspects chart.*

better see what is actually needed—not what the individual thinks he needs based only on mental perceptions. **Figure 4-4** is a shape used to invite individuals to explore themselves from a more holistic point of view.

When individuals have been subjected to abuse, its impact will be reflected in their aspects chart. They will not be able to function in an integrated way because some aspect or aspects of themselves have been injured so that they cannot move forward in a focused, balanced, cohesive way. The aspects of themselves that they are not allowed to use are blocked off or not developed (**Figures 4-5 and 4-6**).

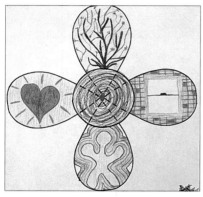

Figure 4-5. *This aspects chart was created by a child, age 12, who has been subjected to emotional abuse due to isolating, rejecting, and overpressuring during visits to a noncustodial parent. Although no overt sexual activities are known, age-inappropriate bathing activities occurred and covert sexual activities have abounded within the home. Note the lack of body-specific features in the physical areas, with colors surrounding the form. Although the mental aspect appears ordered with bricks neatly in place, the window could be broken. This child often dissociates during visits and reports experiencing a see-through barrier. In her words, In the top part of my chart (creative), I drew a plant with buds on it. To me that symbolizes my creative self really growing and full. I feel that at the present time I am trying to work more with that section and make it as big as the other parts have been. In the past I think that it has been smaller than some of the other parts, but now I think it is equal. In the right part of my chart (mental) I drew a clear window, with a brick wall around it. I think that that section is very strong and also very clear. Sometimes my mental side can be "out of it," (i.e., she dissociates) but it seems to always stay clear. In the bottom part of my chart (physical) I drew an outline of a human body with many colors. I think that I am starting to show how great I am on the inside as well as the outside. In the left part of my chart (emotions) I drew a heart with half of the background green and the other half blue. The heart symbolizes that I am starting to be able to show my emotions, but yet they aren't as sad and dreary as they have been in the past. The green and blue is to symbolize how much I love the earth and how happy I feel outside and on the earth. In the center part of my chart (integration) I drew scribbles, but I used all the colors that I used in the loops and I made them flow in a nice even circle that started in the center and worked its way out. I feel that this symbolizes all of them working together and making me "even."*

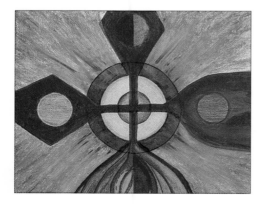

Figure 4-6. *This aspects chart was created by a woman during a deep depression. At the time of the drawing, she was aware of growing up in a home filled with physical violence, high degrees of emotional and verbal abuse, and general neglect. She was not aware of having been sexually abused until she began having recurring nightmares approximately two years later that eventually led her to uncovering abuse memories. Note that the physical area at the bottom is drawn with lines that appear fluid and blood-like. All of the areas contain circles that interrupt their areas. Boundary problems pervaded her home situation. Rectal intrusions were a regular part of her upbringing and "interrupted" her personal spaces and development.*

◆ STAGES OF CHILD DEVELOPMENT AND ART

Children progress through specific developmental stages as they move toward adulthood: learning to trust, becoming an individual, belonging to a group, thinking, identifying with their gender, and developing values. In the same way children must progress through developmental stages with regard to artistic expression. **Table 4-1** is a basic outline of these stages.

Table 4-1. Developmental Stages of Children Related to Their Art	
Age and Stage	*Characteristics*
2 to 4 years—Scribbling	Twenty basic scribbles (see **Figure** 4-7) form the building blocks of art. Generally disordered in approach with controlled, repeated motions, and employing naming, which marks a change from kinesthetic to imaginative thinking. Human figures are not common.
4 to 7 years—Preschematic	Find relationship between drawing, thinking, & environment. Use various symbols in search of a definite concept. For human figures, use circular motion for head, longitudinal for legs and arms.
7 to 9 years—Schematic	Have a definite concept of man and environment; show self-assurance through repeated forms, schemes, symbols; represent the thing itself, with experiences represented as deviances from that scheme; use geometric lines. For human figures, reproduce definite concept of figure.
9 to 11 years—Drawing realism	Removed from geometric lines and from baseline expression; first conscious approach toward decoration. For human figures, attention paid to clothes, emphasizing differences between male and female; more stiffness and emphasis on details; tend to be more realistic.

Table 4-1. Developmental Stages of Children Related to Their Art *(continued)*	
12 to 14 years—Pseudo-naturalistic	Drawings reflect critical awareness of own shortcomings in art, can become shorthand notations; can focus on selected parts of environment; tend not to engage in spontaneous art activity; for some, focus on details such as wrinkles or folds; project nonliteral, personal meaning onto objects and events. For human figures, closer to correct proportions with greater awareness of joints and body actions; facial expressions vary; cartooning; person can be represented by less than complete figure; sexual characteristics overemphasized.
14 to 17 years—Adolescent	Without further instruction, drawings tend to resemble those done at age 12; conscious development of artistic abilities; subjective interpretation to drawings; visually minded may derive pleasure from details such as light and shade; longer attention span with mastery of all art materials; control over purposeful expression. For human figures, some attempt at naturalistic depiction, with awareness of proportion, action, and detail; exaggeration of detail for emphasis; imaginative use of figure for satire.

(Based on Lowenfeld and Brittain, 1987, Plate 26, p. 474-479.)

Scribble 1		Dot	Scribble 2		Single vertical line
Scribble 3		Single horizontal line	Scribble 4		Single diagonal line
Scribble 5		Single curved line	Scribble 6		Multiple vertical line
Scribble 7		Multiple horizontal line	Scribble 8		Multiple diagonal line
Scribble 9		Multiple curved line	Scribble 10		Roving open line
Scribble 11		Roving enclosing line	Scribble 12		Zigzag or waving line
Scribble 13		Single loop line	Scribble 14		Multiple loop line
Scribble 15		Spiral line	Scribble 16		Multiple-line overlaid circle
Scribble 17		Multiple-line circumference circle	Scribble 18		Circular line spread out
Scribble 19		Single crossed circle	Scribble 20		Imperfect circle

Figure 4-7. *The basic scribbles. (From Kellogg, R: Analyzing Children's Art, Mayfield Publishing Co., Palo Alto, CA, 1970. Copyright© 1969, 1970 by Rhoda Kellogg. Reprinted by permission of the publisher.)*

Maltreatment affects creative development as well as other aspects of the child's well-being, making it difficult to move through the stages correctly. Often children become stuck at the stage where the abuse predominantly occurred, or they regress consistently to that age when they try to make representational art. Creative development for the well-treated child flows from stage to stage, always moving toward a more complete and mature expression of the self (**Figure 4-8**). Because art accesses their nonverbal communication areas, when victims of maltreatment try to create, they create from what they see, who they are, and where they have been, which is founded on a baseline of injury rather than good health. Children who are not mistreated and can explore their mental, emotional, physical, and inspirational aspects without fear learn to integrate themselves internally and then integrate with their external world. Children who have to disintegrate themselves to survive cannot explore integration because they must use their energy to brace, dissociate, protect, and defend themselves. These efforts to survive are reflected in their art.

♦ ART MATERIALS

Caretakers of children and professionals who interact with children, although not art therapists, can have available various art materials so that a child can easily access them. It is natural for children to want to explore and play with art materials, and this helps to create an environment that allows them to express themselves, even when words may not be known or permitted. Art activities not only foster integration of the individual, but also allow children to express the many complicated experiences they go through on their way to adulthood.

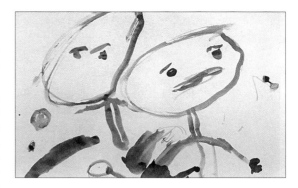

Figure 4-8a. *"Mommy and Daddy" painted by a 4-year-old child who had just left the scribbling stage.*

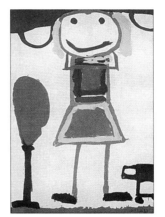

Figure 4-8b. *"I am Standing in My Back Yard," painted by a 6 1/2-year-old girl. Note the developing signs of the child's awareness of the relationship between objects and color. She has painted herself as much larger than the tree, showing the egocentrism at this stage of development.*

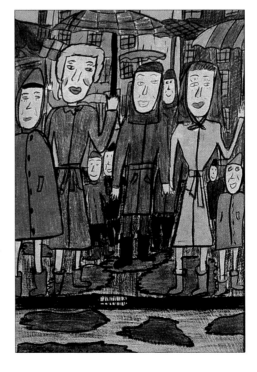

Figure 4-8c. *"Standing in the Rain," drawn by an 11-year-old girl. Color, use of space, and wealth of detail combine to give an aesthetically pleasing whole. The artist's growing visual awareness is coupled with her directness and freshness. (From Lowenfeld, V, and Brittain, WL: Creative and Mental Growth, ed. 7, Macmillan Publishing Co., Inc., New York, 1982.)*

Each person develops his or her own way of thinking, speaking, walking, and dressing, and these individual characteristics eventually come to be the way we know that person. The same is true of a child's creative expressions. When permitted, each child will develop a nonverbal symbolic system of expression. His or her dreams, feelings, thoughts, and experiences will be expressed in his or her own personal style. Over time, caretakers and professionals can learn to understand and communicate with a child on his or her creative level in much the same way that we learn to communicate with a child verbally. If children do not feel "spied on" or criticized, they continue to express themselves in their academic, personal, and creative efforts. Caretakers who observe the drawings and creations with sensitivity to the child's feelings will find a way of "hearing" what the child is saying. If a problem exists or is developing, the caretaker who has learned to listen to the child's creative voice will hear and see what is happening. If they expect children to communicate with them at this very deep and personal level, it is crucial that caretakers and professionals resist the urge to define themselves as responsible by exerting control over children. It is much more effective to focus on providing a safe, structured, and protective environment within which children can grow and evolve their own ability to control themselves. The freedom to explore oneself is too often a luxury not afforded to children. Instead they are forced to use their creative energies to construct defenses against forces that are bigger and stronger than them physically, psychologically, mentally, and emotionally. This kind of environment does not allow for creative and honest exploration or development.

Table 4-2 lists various art materials that can be made readily available for children to use. It is important to provide materials appropriate for childrens ages, interests, and ability levels.

Table 4-2. Art Materials	
Paper—all shapes, sizes, types	Traditional 8½ X 11 or 11 X 14 sheets
Old wallpaper books	Used wrapping paper
Tissue from inside shoe boxes	"Stuff"—anything that is interesting to touch or see
Pencils	Clay
Shoulder pads	Pens
Popsicle sticks	Construction paper
Colored pencils	Small tree branches
Flour and water	Crayons
Pipe cleaners	Food coloring
Cray Pas	Stickers

Table 4-2. Art Materials *(continued)*	
Pastels	Beans
Markers	Beads
Oil crayons	Nuts and bolts
Plastic crayons	Tape of all sizes and shapes
Water pencils	Old holiday cards
Water crayons	Magazines and catalogs
Water colors	Paper towel or toilet paper rolls
Tempera paints	Styrofoam boards (from food packages)
Finger paints	Rubberbands
Brushes	Scissors
Newspapers	Buttons
Boxes	Glues of all colors and styles
Fabrics	Thread and yarn
Plasticine	Scrap fabrics

◆ SYMBOLIC INDICATORS
OF POTENTIAL ABUSE

Although every individual has a personal style of creative expression, no matter how primitive or practiced they may be, certain symbols seem to reappear in the creations of individuals who have been maltreated. However, even if a person's artwork does incorporate these symbols repeatedly, it does not necessarily mean that the person has been abused.

Symbolic communication is subjective. It is vital that caretakers and professionals remember that indicators of abuse are exactly that—indicators. Abuse cannot be determined on the basis of one picture, not even many pictures. Symbolic language must be looked at in the context of the individual's overall life, circumstances, and intent.

Dr. Spring's research with known adult survivors of abuse, found the trends and symbols obtained in **Table 4-3** occur more frequently than in the artwork of people not identified as victims of abuse. I also see these in the artwork of adults abused as childen. Many of these indicators also appear in the artwork of abused children. The understanding of symbolic communication is not intended to intrude on people and their art. Art therapists are trained to evaluate art and yet must continually receive both supervision and education to maintain their objectivity in regard to their clients' artwork. It is with somber and serious warnings to view children's artwork as a whole and as an expression of their entire self that these possible indicators are presented.

Table 4-3. Trends and Indicators Related to Abuse Found in Children's Art

This list is based on Dr. Spring's conclusions after studying 8,000 drawings and completing her empirical research in 1988.

- Contain noticeable use of disembodied eyes (adults) and wedges (adults and children)

- Display extremes in both color and content; may be more intense, may be avoided

- Exhibit an overall fragmented, separated, and confused quality showing degrees of incongruity

- Lean more toward abstraction than realism or representation (adults); fantasy and stories (children)

- Expose more angular properties in the compositions, but also include many circles that are not eye shaped

- Style tends to be inconsistent, fluctuating from passive to aggressive use of materials and forms

- Express intense feelings that focus on rage and sadness, depression and confusion, helplessness and inescapability, threat and fear, as well as lack of control

- Show an absence of the future and an enjoyment of life, as well as an inability to solve problems

- Reveal a confusion about life, suicidal ideation, detachment, and an inability to concentrate or understand their emotional state, which is expressed verbally as an inadequacy in attempting to solve problems

- Have an explosive and/or scattered quality

- Reveal fragmented bodies, disembodied eyes and genitalia, stick figures, and other forms that suggest regression to an earlier developmental stage

- Victims tend to direct their drawings toward the past and feelings about their traumatic experiences whether remembered or not; children focus on uncomfortable relationships

- Victims consistently use red or black or combined red and black in the same drawing in varying degrees and patterns. They use yellowish green colors less than nonvictims but use yellow at about the same frequency

Repetitive symbolic forms chosen by victims include the following:

1. Circles: circular pattern of crisis cycle, depression, obsessive thinking, circular behavior, "can't break the chain," and addictions

2. Chains: trapped, helpless, chained to abuse (adults)

3. Chains with penises or female genitalia: chained to sexuality, sex, and sexual abuse (adults)

4. Floating or detached objects: dissociation

5. Yellow sun with wedge rays: "it is threatening to hope"; hope disguised with magical thinking

6. Encapsulation and compartmentalization: withdrawal, isolation, protection, and addictions

7. Concentric circles: depression and suicidal ideation

8. Ears, no mouth: heard, cannot tell

9. Closed eyes: "don't see," "don't tell"

(Spring, 1993, p.54,55.)

◆The Role of Art Therapists
in the Legal System

The art therapy profession is playing a greater role in the assessment, diagnosis, and treatment of child abuse. With this expanded role, art therapists are now being called into court cases to provide expert testimony. Because of the demands placed on witnesses and the role of art in this process, careful study and in-depth preparation are required. Publications are available for review before testifying.

◆Summary

Art therapy is a human service profession that focuses on the process involved in healing. Each time a person creates a work of art, he or she moves a piece of himself or herself outside for the world to see. The individual is looking at the inner self and seeing a reflection of their true self in the artwork. Art therapy can benefit almost anyone if the person is willing to more fully express inner feelings and thoughts.

An art therapist can and should be consulted when a child's or an adult's drawings consistently and significantly deviate from developmental norms. Issues that may be resistant to traditional therapy or those that are too difficult to talk about can be quite responsive to art therapy. Art therapy bypasses the criticism of technique and focuses on helping the client move toward integration by helping him or her express how they experience themselves, others, and events in a more complete way.

The rest of this chapter will present case studies showing how, through art therapy, abused individuals were able to communicate about their abuse. These studies also illustrate the thoughts and feelings of persons who have experienced abuse or neglect.

Case Study 1

This client attended group therapy sessions for a number of years and spoke very rarely in the group. When asked specifically if she preferred to discontinue therapy or be moved to another group, she stated that she wanted to stay. Eventually an art activity was suggested that she responded to with noticeable interest. When asked to make an object that would represent her siblings, she created these masks (**Figures 4-9 and 4-10**). Her therapeutic journey became more fluid after these masks were done. She was raised in a family where children were never to speak unless spoken to first by an adult.

She was supposed to sit still and not move whenever she was at home, and if she did express herself or move, her brothers verbally assaulted her. She was isolated from other children and rejected and ignored by other members of her family. She cannot recall if she was physically or sexually assaulted.

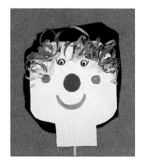

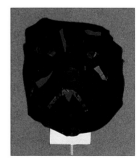

Figure 4-9a,b. Front and back of mask on a stick. This mask is of a brother she considered "two-faced."

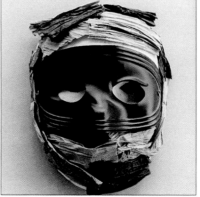

Figure 4-10. Mask of brother who never spoke to the client.

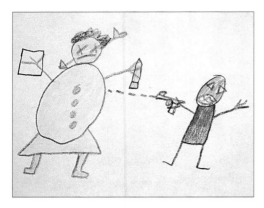

Figure 4-11. *The client drew what he wishes he could do—kill his teacher.*

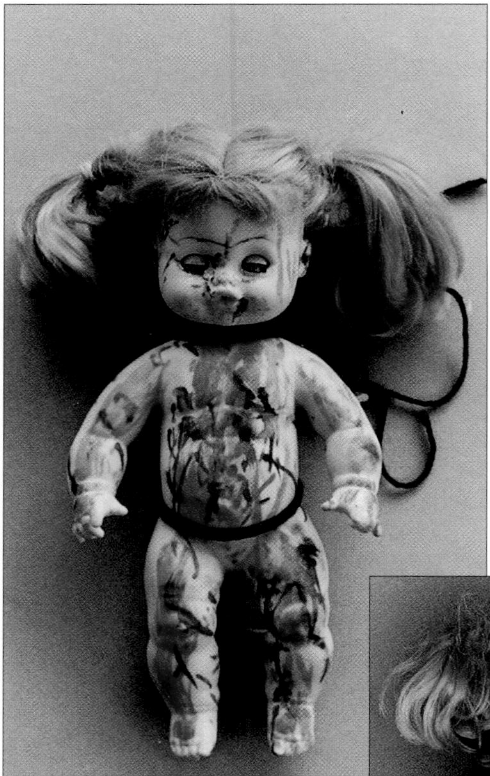

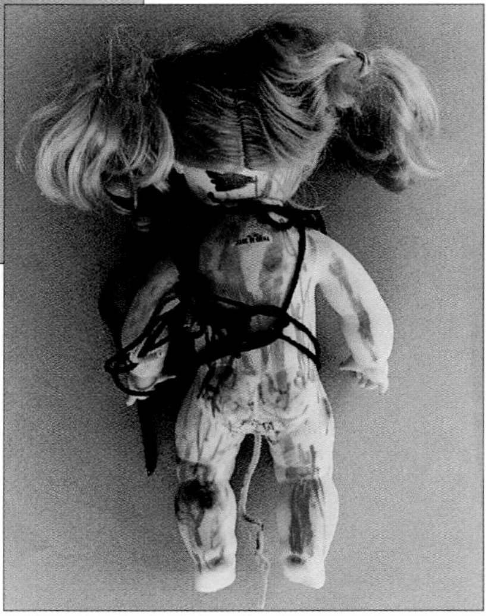

CASE STUDY 2

This child was first brought to therapy because of behavioral problems at school. He appeared to have Attention-deficit Hyperactivity Disorder with moderate indications of a learning disability in the area of reading comprehension. After initial resistance to coming to therapy, when he said "There's nothing wrong with me. It's everybody else!" he became comfortable in the therapy setting and began doing art activities that were a blend of topics suggested by the therapist for assessment and diagnostic purposes (for example, **Figure 4-11**) and spontaneous drawings he created based on the things that seemed to be worrying him at that time. During the process of treatment, a prior sexual assault was depicted (**Figure 4-12**). The mother had known about it and proper authorities had been involved, so everyone thought that the experience had been resolved and the child was simply a "behavior problem" at school. During treatment he received medication for depression and difficulty paying attention at school. After therapy, moving to a new house in a different neighborhood, and beginning a different school, he was no longer considered a behavior problem. He adjusted well (**Figure 4-13**), and medications were reduced significantly.

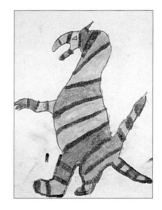

Figure 4-13. *Final drawing presented to his therapist as a going-away present, indicating that he was done with counseling. He stated that the therapist "no longer needed to know his private business" and that he did not need to come to therapy any more. This final picture shows a full-figured and colorful character, depicting the client when he chose to leave therapy— having set boundaries, full-figured, and richly colored.*

Figure 4-12a,b. *Spontaneous creation of an abused child wherein he replicated the rectal sexual abuse that he had experienced. The experience was confirmed by his mother. At the time of the abuse, counseling had been sought and all of the proper steps had been taken so that the issue seemed resolved.*

CASE STUDY 3

This young adult male murdered his father. Therapeutically this case is of note because his artwork had been saved by his mother from the time he was very young, so that samples exist from most of the stages of his life. Legally it is of interest because it explores the impact of sexual abuse, post-traumatic stress disorder, and dissociative states in relation to a crime where the client admitted killing his father and was able to verbally address, during the trial, his experience as a child and a man.

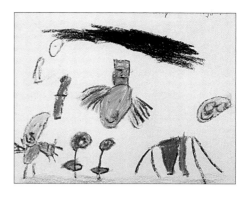

Figure 4-14a. Indications of abuse. Partial figures rather than whole.

The art was first reviewed without the therapist being aware of the criminal case, the events connected with the case, or the person's prior history. Yet the art is filled with commonly seen indicators of possible abuse. The symbolic language the client developed and expressed in art shows probable sexual abuse by sodomy. The abuser seems to be male and the creator of the art seemed to have nonspecific tensions with a female, probably his mother. Indicators of possible abuse that exist throughout his artwork include the following:

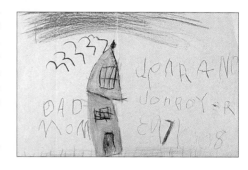

Figure 4-14b. Phallic depiction of house.

- Partial rather than whole figures (**Figure** 4-14a)

- Phallic symbols exaggerated beyond common levels of developmental sexual concerns (**Figure** 4-14b)

- Secret or "hidden" pictures (many were drawn on the back of another picture) (**Figure** 4-14c)

- Indicators of disintegration (**Figure** 4-14d,e)

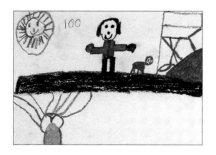

Figure 4-14d. Here the client is showing himself as the dog between a man with a blue shirt and a huge pair of red pants; there is a spider coming up from the ground that is also threatening him.

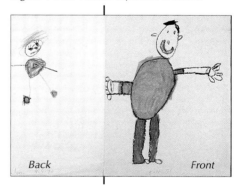

Figure 4-14c. "Hidden" pictures-one drawn on the back of another.

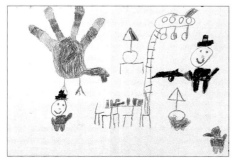

Figure 4-14e. This picture is an example of disintegration. The client is "telling" his story at a young age. The abuse by sodomy and enemas done by his father with a turkey baster are depicted here as a dark man with a phallically projected gun, wedged lamps, a space ship that he wants to take him away, and a turkey hovering over him.

Figure 4-15a. *Drawing to show something the client's father would like. Note the anal shape of the buckeye.*

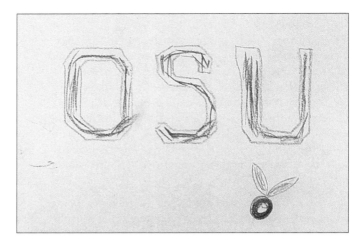

Figure 4-15b. *Drawing to show something the client's mother would not like—blood dripping out of a Coke bottle.*

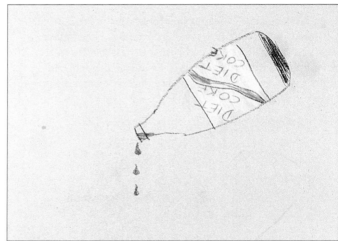

Figure 4-15c. *Drawing of what everyone saw when they looked at this family— proper, church-going people.*

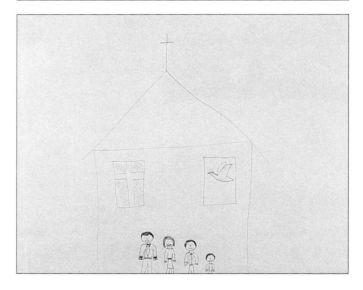

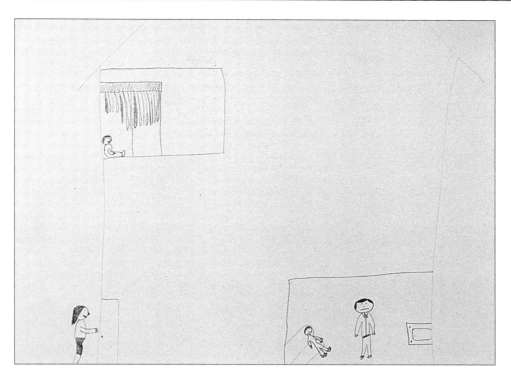

Figure 4-15d. *Drawing of what went on when his mother was gone. His mother is outside the house, ready to return. His father is downstairs playing with his brother and the client (as a child) is hiding up in his closet.*

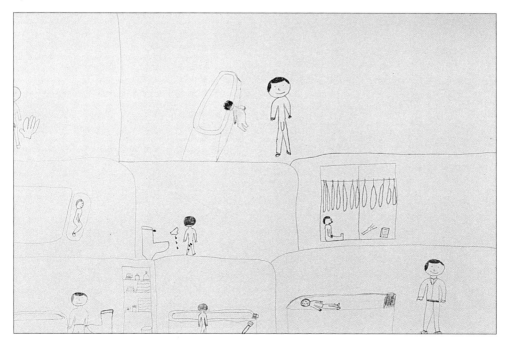

Figure 4-15e. *After the client had killed his father, this picture was drawn in response to the art therapist's request to describe what happened to him while he was growing up. He drew and described these scenes. He told of being sodomized, hiding near his mother's bed to be safe, hiding in the closet to be safe, bleeding from rectal intrusions, fearing his father, and keeping silent, never telling about these events.*

As the client went from drawing to drawing, he verbally and nonverbally depicted the abuse he had experienced. When the assessment was complete, it became apparent that the client had "told" his story at a much earlier time in his life. The sodomy and the enemas administered by his father using a turkey baster can be seen in a number of the pictures. Of particular interest is the similarity of the art in **Figure 4-16, a and b**, which were done many years apart. The positioning of the shovel in his father's hand is paralled, and these pictures essentially tell the same story.

Figure 4-16a,b. *Parallel pictures drawn many years apart.*

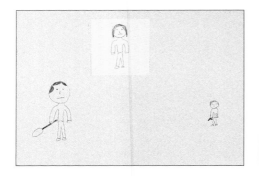

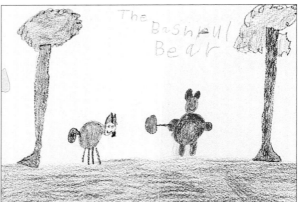

Figure 4-17a. *Hopeful aspects are seen in these two pictures. The client is small and everyone is basically drawn the same.*

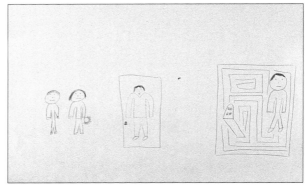

Figure 4-17b. *He draws himself as still encapsulated, but bigger. Dad (in the maze) is not as rigid and not as large. Mom and her husband are matched in color and are shown as different from the others.*

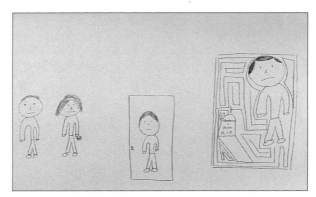

CASE STUDY 4

This client grew up in a house with a violent and sexually abusive mother. Many times during therapy, she was completely unable to speak, aware that she was unable to speak, and frustrated with this condition. A person of extremely high intelligence, she was deeply distressed with her inability to understand why she drew seemingly inexplicable pictures of violence, enemas, sexual trauma, and cruelty (**Figures 4-18 to 4-23**).

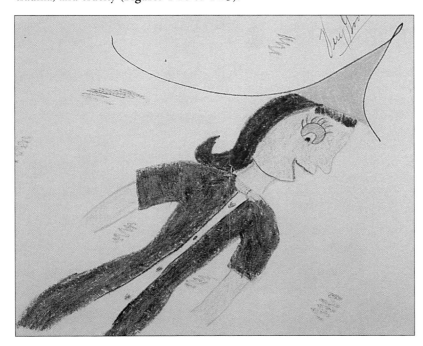

Figure 4-18. *Picture created during elementary school years.*

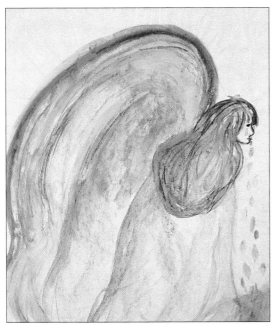

Figure 4-19. *After continued and repeated physical and sexual abuse, the client became aware of the presence of an angel who would watch over her. This painting reflects the client's sense of the angel weeping about what this woman was experiencing as a child. It was done 4 years before the client had any conscious memories of having been sexually assaulted.*

Figure 4-20a. *These drawings depict a lack of boundaries or protective images; transparencies; X's; and distorted or missing body parts. They were done 5 years apart and reflect abuse memories the client is still trying to sort out. Shows the client at the age of 5 years.*

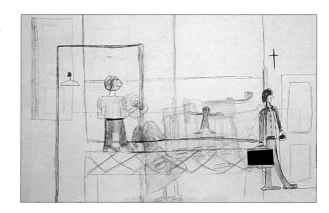

Figure 4-20b. *Shows the client at about the age of 1 year.*

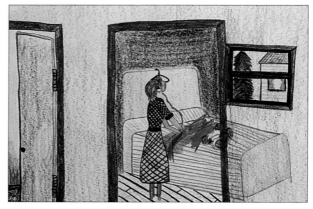

Figure 4-21a-c. *These three drawings reflect the client's relationship with her mother and the abusive behaviors she experienced that led to her eventual dissociation at the age of 4 years. The client saw herself as having an evil companion who would deal with the mother while the client went to sleep crying.*

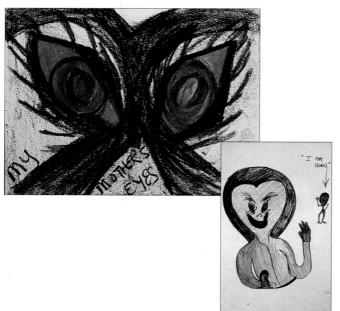

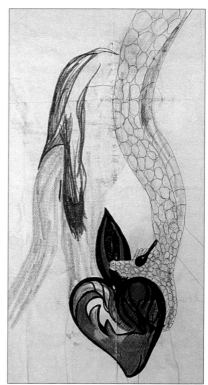

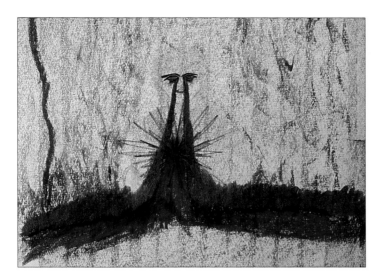

Figure 4-22. *Shows client feeling sad and locked in behind a glass wall as a child.*

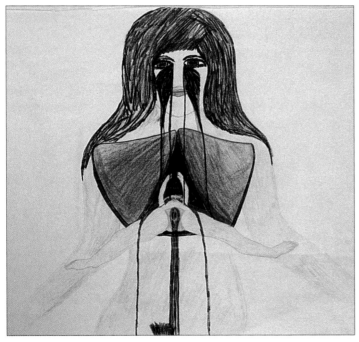

Figure 4-23. *This drawing is an integration and awareness picture. It was done during a time when the client was first aware that she had been sexually assaulted both vaginally and rectally by her mother. She depicts her "child self" being taken into her own heart to love and protect. Although the tears of the woman flow down on the "child self," the client expressed an awareness that these were cleansing tears and that, in time, she was certain that the wounds would be washed clean.*

◆ SUGGESTED READINGS

Anderson, FE: *Art for All the Children: A Creative Sourcebook for the Impaired Child,* Charles C Thomas, Publisher, Springfield, IL, 1978.

Cohen-Liebman, MS: The art therapist as expert witness in child sexual abuse litigation, *Art Therapy* 11(4):260-265, 1994.

Gardner, H: *Artful Scribbles: The Significance of Children's Drawings,* Basic Books, Inc., Publisher, New York, 1980.

Kaufman, B, and Wohl, A: *Casualties of Childhood: A Developmental Perspective on Sexual Abuse Using Projective Drawings,* Brunner/Mazel, Inc., Publisher, New York, 1992.

Kellogg, R: *Analyzing Children's Art,* Mayfield Publishing Co., Publisher, Palo Alto, CA, 1970.

Landgarten, HB: *Clinical Art Therapy: A Comprehensive Guide,* Brunner/Mazel, Inc., Publisher, New York, 1981.

Levick, MR: *They Could Not Talk and So They Drew: Children's Styles of Coping and Thinking,* Charles C Thomas, Publisher, Springfield, IL, 1983.

Liebmann, M: *Art Therapy with Offenders,* Jessica Kingsley, Publisher, London, 1994.

Lowenfeld, V, and Brittain, WL: *Creative and Mental Growth,* Prentice-Hall, Inc., Publisher, New Jersey, 1987.

Malchiodi, C: *Breaking the Silence: Art Therapy with Children from Violent Homes,* Brunner/Mazel, Inc., Publisher, New York, 1990.

Malchiodi, CA: Introduction to special section on sexual abuse dissociative disorder, *Art Therapy* 11(1):34-36, 1994.

Rankin, A: Tree drawings and trauma indicators: A comparison of past research with current findings from the diagnostic drawing series, *Art Therapy* 11(2):127-130, 1994.

Rubin JA: *Child Art Therapy: Understanding and Helping Children Grow Through Art,* Van Nostrand Reinhold Co., Publisher, New York, 1978.

Spring, D: *Sexual Abuse and Post-Traumatic Stress Reflected in Artistic Symbolic Language,* Ann Arbor, MI, 1988, UMI Dissertation Information Service, Publication No. 9002893.

Spring, D: *Shattered Images: Phenomenological Language of Sexual Trauma,* Magnolia Street Publishers, Chicago, IL, 1993.

Wadeson, H: *Art Psychotherapy,* John Wiley & Sons, New York, 1980.

Wohl, A, and Kaufman, B: *Silent Screams and Hidden Cries: An Interpretation of Artwork by Children from Violent Homes,* Brunner/Mazel, Inc., Publisher, New York, 1985.

Chapter 5

ORAL INJURIES OF CHILD ABUSE

LYNN DOUGLAS MOUDEN, DDS, MPH, PICD, FACD

Injuries of the head and facial regions are the most common of all physical child abuse injuries. In particular, injuries to the mouth and oral structures are a common factor in child abuse cases. Assault on the commicative "self" of the child is often the compelling reason behind abuse directed at the mouth, along with the adult's easy access to the child's head. Furthermore, any physical or emotional discomfort the child experiences, such as injuries to other parts of his or her body, may cause crying. Efforts to silence a crying child often result in injuries to the mouth. While treatment of oral injuries is usually referred to the general dentist or oral surgeon, proper evaluation of an abused child cannot be complete without a thorough visual oral examination.

The types of oral injuries that may be encountered in child abuse include trauma to the teeth, to supporting structures, and to surrounding tissues. The principal oral injuries of child abuse include missing and fractured teeth, oral contusions, oral lacerations, jaw fractures, and oral burns.

◆ ORAL INJURIES TO INFANTS

Abuse injuries to oral structures of the infant should be considered separately from those of older children. Infants generally do not have teeth before 4 to 6 months of age. The pattern of eruption of primary teeth varies widely and is usually not important in deciding whether or not child abuse is present. However, delayed eruption of primary teeth may indicate a pattern of child neglect resulting from poor nutrition either for the child or for the mother during pregnancy.

The difficulties and frustrations surrounding an infant's feeding may lead to abuse. Intra-oral lacerations have long been recognized as possible indicators of forced feeding. The injury occurs when excessive pressure is used while feeding with a nursing bottle or when a utensil is misdirected during feeding. If the adult feels that the child is uncooperative during bottle feeding, he or she may use excessive force to introduce the nipple into the child's mouth or press too firmly against oral structures. This can cause bruises or contusions. Pushing the bottle against the infant's mouth can also tear the lip tissues. Forced feeding with a utensil can lacerate the tongue, the floor of the mouth, or the lip (**Figure 5-1**).

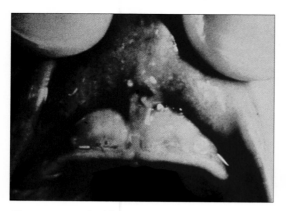

Figure 5-1. *Result of forced feeding.*

◆INJURIES TO TEETH

All injuries to teeth and supporting structures should be referred to a dentist as soon as possible. The injuries to teeth can include movement within the tooth socket, fracture, or loss of the tooth. Any trauma to a tooth that does not result in loss of the tooth may, however, result in loss of the tooth's vitality. Even relatively minor trauma may disrupt the nerve supply to the tooth and the tooth dies. Immediately after trauma to the tooth, no evidence of the tooth's lack of nerve supply may be seen, but, after several weeks, a nonvital tooth appears discolored or markedly darker than surrounding teeth.

MOVEMENT OF TEETH

A tooth that has been moved within its socket often causes tears in the periodontal ligament and may bleed. Such teeth may also be much more mobile than normal. A traumatized tooth can also be displaced in any direction. This happens with accidental injuries as well as in abuse. Contact directly on the tooth or a blow to the face that transmits force to the tooth can cause the displacement. Either the abuser's hand or an object can deliver enough force to displace one or several teeth.

In severe cases, the entire tooth can be forcefully expelled from the alveolar bone. The tendency for any tooth to react in this way during trauma is related to the force and direction of the trauma as well as the anatomy of the root(s). Expelled teeth caused by abusive injuries are almost exclusively limited to front teeth because they are supported by a single root. Multirooted teeth are less susceptible, both because of their location in the back part of the mouth and because of the physics of forcing the tooth out bodily. Because the root anatomy of a primary tooth is likely to be less cone-like than that of a permanent tooth, expulsion of teeth during physical violence is less common in children with primary dentition.

At least two cases have been reported of children abused by having permanent teeth "extracted" by the parents. In these cases, one adult held the child while another removed the intact teeth without any form of anesthesia.

Traumatic tooth expulsion requires immediate dental consultation. The tooth must be kept moist using isotonic saline solution or even milk. The chances for successful reimplantation are best if the procedure is accomplished within 30 minutes of the avulsion. No effort should be made to cleanse the tooth or to remove any tissue fragments before the dentist reimplants it. Attempts to clean the tooth may result in the loss of tissue important to periodontal tissue regeneration. Reimplanted teeth must be stabilized for a minimum of 7 to 10 days.

TOOTH FRACTURES

Fractures of teeth can involve the crown, the root, or both. While tooth fractures are sometimes seen in abusive injuries, they are more likely to result from accidental injury. Fractures occur either when the tooth is struck with a hard object or when the tooth comes into contact with a hard surface.

Fractures can involve only the enamel, extend into the dentin layer, or involve the tooth's pulp. Timely referral to a dentist is mandatory for treatment of tooth fractures. Modern restorative materials and bonding procedures can save teeth with fractures that only a decade ago would have required full crowns or even extraction.

◆ ABUSE INJURIES TO ORAL SOFT TISSUES

GINGIVA

Trauma that affects teeth is also likely to affect the surrounding gingiva. In addition, trauma from a hard object striking the child can produce contusions or lacerations of the gingiva without apparent trauma to adjacent teeth. X-ray examinations are needed in all cases of gingival trauma to properly diagnose any damage to the teeth or bone.

ATTACHMENT TISSUES FOR TONGUE AND LIPS

Abuse trauma can cause mild to extensive damage of the attachment tissues of the tongue and lips. Along with lacerations caused by forced feeding discussed previously, many forms of abusive trauma can tear these tissues. Blows to the face can displace the lip far enough to stretch the lip's attachment tissue beyond its limit, causing laceration of the attachment tissue. Forcing a hard or sharp object into the mouth can also lacerate these areas.

LIPS

Any force to the mouth can cause contusions and lacerations of the upper or lower lip. Abuse injuries to the lips are evidenced by marks either from the offending object or from the child's own teeth. When a blow is directed at the face or lips, the oral tissues can come into forceful contact with the child's teeth. The lips may show "bite marks" from the child's own teeth. In addition, if the child is wearing either fixed or removal orthodontic appliances, these appliances can damage the lips during trauma. You must exercise caution when examining the child's mouth if orthodontic appliances are in place because the lips can become trapped in the wires or brackets, a very painful situation. Bruising or laceration at the corners of the lips can also result from the use of a rope or other material to gag and silence the child.

TONGUE

Although laceration of the tongue occurs with abuse involving a sharp or hard object in the mouth, most abusive injuries of the tongue are caused by biting it. Any blow to the jaw can trap the tongue between the upper and lower teeth. These injuries usually involve the sides of the tongue and resemble the jagged indentations seen with a bite mark in soft tissue. If the bite involves the back part of the tongue, the marks may appear like an area of crushed tissue.

Bite marks to the tongue inflicted by the child's own teeth are likely to show a curvature consistent with the child's own arch. A bite mark on the tongue from an abuser may show a curve in the direction opposite to the child's dental arch (**Figure 5-2**).

HARD AND SOFT PALATE

The palate is often injured in accidents, such as when the child falls with an object in the mouth. Abusive injuries to the hard and soft palate generally occur when a foreign object is introduced into the mouth or when the child is struck while an object is already there.

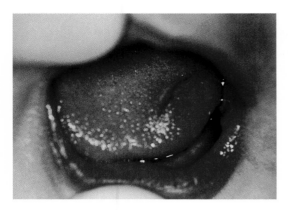

Figure 5-2. Bite mark on child's tongue from the abuser.

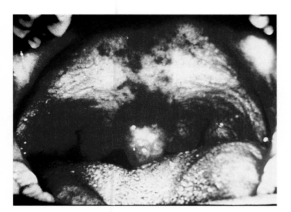

Figure 5-3. Palatal contusions from forced oral sex.

Forced oral sex can also bruise the palate (**Figure 5-3**). Repeated forced oral sex has been destructive enough to erode away the palate and expose underlying bone.

BURNS

Any oral soft tissue can be burned. Abusive burns result from the introduction of a hot object into the mouth, forced feeding of a food or liquid that is too hot, or the use of caustic or acidic fluids (chemical burns).

◆ DENTAL IMPLICATIONS OF CHILD NEGLECT

Generally, dental neglect is usually just one manifestation in the overall neglect of a child. It has been defined as lack of care that (1) makes routine eating impossible, (2) causes chronic pain, (3) delays or retards a child's growth, or (4) makes it difficult or impossible for a child to perform daily activities. Untreated dental problems are as serious as an untreated wound in any other part of the body because neglecting dental treatment can lead to complications that affect the entire body.

The American Academy of Pediatric Dentistry has defined dental neglect as the caregiver's failure to seek treatment for untreated rampant caries, trauma, pain, infection, or bleeding. Rampant caries is generally defined as decay involving every tooth, including the lower front teeth, which are typically the most resistant to decay. Because gross decay of these front teeth is so obvious, rampant caries is easily discernible to everyone who sees the child's smile.

Also included in the Academy's definition of dental neglect is the failure to follow up on treatment needs once the caregiver has been informed that these conditions exist. Many parents have told practitioners that they were totally unaware of the conditions in their child's mouth before receiving the dentist's diagnosis. Therefore parents' failure to follow through with treatment is probably more important in determining dental neglect than is their lack of knowledge. Also, most practitioners would agree that no neglect may exist if parents are providing for their children's needs in a manner consistent with their own financial situation or available economic assistance.

The Academy's definition serves as neither a law nor a standard of practice. It is merely a guideline for those practitioners evaluating a patient's oral health in light of societal norms. It is up to the health care professional to weigh the guidelines and legal definitions against regional or local norms and access-to-care issues.

The most common form of dental neglect is failure to provide treatment for teeth with caries. Multiple carious teeth can debilitate an otherwise healthy child, while caries that have led to more serious problems cause not only pain, but also fever, malaise, and lethargy. Infection can penetrate alveolar bone and enter the gingiva, usually near the tooth's apex.

Baby bottle tooth decay (BBTD) is a severe form of rampant caries resulting from the habit of putting a child to bed with a nursing bottle. If the milk or another sugar-containing liquid remains in contact with the teeth for extended periods, serious tooth decay can result. In BBTD, all teeth may be affected and amputation of the tooth crowns may occur. While failure to provide treatment for such severe involvement can be considered neglect, some Native American tribal councils have considered BBTD as a form of child abuse, not child neglect, because it is a direct result of actions taken by the adult.

Other conditions may constitute dental neglect if left untreated. These include severe malocclusions, abnormal tongue positions, cleft palate or lip, missing teeth, or other malformations that may lead to speech or eating disorders.

◆ DENTISTRY'S INVOLVEMENT IN PREVENTING CHILD MALTREATMENT

The American Dental Association (ADA) added the required recognition and reporting of suspected child abuse to their *Principles of Ethics and Code of Professional Conduct.* Official ADA policy further states that dentists should "become familiar with all physical signs of child abuse that are observable in the course of the normal dental visit."

In an effort to address prevention issues, the Prevent Abuse and Neglect through Dental Awareness (P.A.N.D.A.) Coalition has been established in Missouri. The P.A.N.D.A. Coalition is a public-private partnership between the dental community, social service agencies, and a dental insurance company. The success of the program is evidenced by dentists' increased reporting of child abuse cases since the program's inception in 1992, leading to its replication in 29 additional states in the United States and two coalitions in Romania. Interested individuals and organizations from each remaining state of the United States, from Canada, and from Israel are also working toward forming P.A.N.D.A. coalitions.

◆ SUGGESTED READINGS

Council on Dental Practice: *The Dentist's Responsibility in Identifying and Reporting Child Abuse and Neglect*, ed. 3 American Dental Association, Chicago, 1995.

da Fenesca, MA, Feigal RJ, and ten Besel, RW: Dental aspects of 1248 cases of child maltreatment on file at a major county hospital, *Pediatr Dent* 14: 152-157, 1992.

Larkin, S: Child abuse on the rise, *MO Dent J* 72:18-31, 1992.

Mouden, LD, and Bross, DC: Legal issues affecting dentistry's role in preventing child abuse and neglect, *JADA* 126: 1173-1180, 1995.

Schmitt, BD: Types of child abuse and neglect: an overview for dentists, *Pediatr Dent* 8 (special issue): 67-71, 1986.

Chapter 6

Multiple Personalities and Dissociative Disorders

Barbara Y. Whitman, Ph.D.
Pasquale J. Accardo, M.D.

Sheryl, a 12-year-old seventh grader, was referred to a multidisciplinary clinic for evaluation of continuing learning problems which had become more problematic after she entered a departmentalized learning situation with multiple teachers. She was noted to be behind in reading, had severe spelling and other sequential processing difficulties, and displayed attentional and comprehension problems. She was described as chronically withdrawn, asocial, and moody, and her parents would frequently find her sitting in the family room and staring for hours, particularly when upset. It was also reported that she exhibited occasional flashes of rage. However, it was noted that she seemed to display episodes of brilliance and talent. She occasionally wrote sophisticated and spellbinding poetry and sometimes produced astonishingly talented artwork. She was unable to explain what enabled her to perform so brilliantly or prevented her from regularly producing work of this calibre. Although socially withdrawn and inept most of the

time, it appeared that if she wanted to reach a goal she would single-mindedly pursue it. For example, once she managed to get herself elected class president, and she succeeded at track and field events. She was described by both of her physician parents as a misfit in the family, unable to relate to or get along with her three highly successful siblings. After extensive psychoeducational and psychological testing, she was diagnosed as having a neurologically based specific learning disability, a dysthymic disorder, and an overanxious disorder of childhood. Appropriate therapies were recommended.

Sheryl made an emergency return to the clinic when she was a senior in high school. She was talking of suicide, and her parents wanted additional evaluation. During this emergency visit, it was reported that psychotherapy had never been pursued because her parents felt her behavioral problems were related to stubbornness; they did not believe a child could be "depressed." This episode of suicidal ideation was actually her second. Her first episode had occurred 2 years previously, and

Sheryl had been referred to her pastor for counseling. This second episode concluded with an immediate referral to a psychiatrist for medication and therapy.

The following September Sheryl enrolled as a freshman at a local private college. Within 6 weeks she was exhibiting major vegetative symptoms so noticeable that college personnel contacted Sheryl's therapist. She was hospitalized for 4 weeks. After the first week she was allowed to leave the hospital during the day to attend classes. After being admitted to the hospital there was an instant stabilization of mood, occurring within 48 hours. During hospitalization it was noted that she had a shallow level of understanding of the need to explore how she got there, how to cope when leaving, and a generally oppositional demeanor toward any subject other than how she could "get out of here." After discharge she exhibited no engagement or effort during her weekly therapy sessions. Before she left college for winter break, she reported being afraid to go home because "she didn't want the voices to start again."

After she returned from the school break, the subject of voices was vigorously pursued during therapy. Simultaneously reports from a consulting psychiatrist noted that she was presenting an "entirely different" young lady to him than was reported as being presented to the primary therapist. A confrontation of these discrepancies with Sheryl ultimately led to discussions of incidents such as memory loss, articles appearing that she didn't remember buying, and people telling her she had a good time at a movie she didn't remember attending. Ultimately the therapist invited the source of the "voices" to emerge. To date, 33 personalities have been identified. Etiology appears to have been chronic and sadistic sexual abuse from age 3 to age 10 by her maternal grandfather. Both Sheryl and her family indicated that "she was his special grandchild," and they further emphatically reported that "she was devastated when he died." She has, as yet, not divulged the facts of the abuse to her family.

Sheryl is typical of the difficulty of diagnosing multiple personality disorder (MPD) in children. For her, there was never any indication of any sort of abuse, which is the major cause of this disorder. Her "host" personality is indeed "learning disabled," although several of her other personalities are artisans. She was so scared of the "voices" that she never divulged their presence until moving to her college dorm. This move so greatly altered her external environment that she was unable to continue to function and hospitalization was required. Even with this episode, it was not until she was going home for a month and would be unable to see her therapist that she "let it slip" that she heard voices. Her age when this symptom was revealed, combined with her history, was compatible with a schizophrenic process. However, enough contradictory data were present that shortly thereafter the MPD diagnosis was confirmed.

♦ DEFINITION

MPD can be a devastating and hard-to-treat psychiatric disorder whose origins tend to lie in childhood. Over 90% of all cases are directly attributable to severe abuse in early childhood, so current theories interpret MPD as one form of childhood post-traumatic stress disorder.

MPD is characterized by the existence within an individual of two or more distinct personalities or personality states. Each personality is fully integrated, having his or her own unique memories, behavior patterns, and social relationships. When the personality is dominant, it determines the host individual's behavior. Transition from one personality to another is usually sudden (within seconds to minutes) and is most often precipitated by stress, reflecting a complex psychophysiologic process termed *dissociation*.

PREDISPOSING FACTORS

Two predisposing factors for MPD are currently recognized: (1) exposure to severe and overwhelming trauma, particularly during childhood, such as frequent and inconsistent alternating abuse and love, and (2) an innate and probably genetically determined psychophysiologic tendency to dissociate. Both factors—exposure and genetic tendency—are necessary; neither factor alone is sufficient to produce the disorder.

♦ EPIDEMIOLOGY AND HISTORY

Determining the incidence and prevalence of MPD has been hampered by two difficulties: (1) diagnosing the disorder and (2) dealing with the sociopolitical and professional context in which diagnoses are formulated. A brief understanding of the history of this disorder in psychiatric thinking is needed to understand the current state of knowledge regarding how widely this disorder occurs and who is at risk.

MPD is not a new psychiatric entity. Recognizable case histories of MPD in both adults and children were reported as early as 1817. In the last major pre-Freudian psychology textbook, cases of MPD were given extensive coverage. The disorder was then lost in psychiatric controversy for a number of years and has only recently resurfaced as a "legitimate" psychiatric entity. Since 1980, a number of investigators have begun to clarify the epidemiology and consequences of this disorder.

In the earliest reports, MPD was described as the splitting of the total consciousness into complementary parts that coexist and mutually ignore each other, yet can share objects between or among themselves. The primary self often needs to invent "hallucinations" to mask and hide from itself the strange incidents and incongruous deeds of the secondary personalities. Each personality, nevertheless, has a conscious unity, continuous memory, habits, a name, and a sense of its own identity. This phenomenon was considered rare, associated with hysterical anesthesia, and discussed in conjunction with hypnotism, spiritualism, and the question of the location of the seat of the soul.

Although trauma similar to what might produce amnesia was considered a possible precipitating factor, the model used to explain the phenomenon was posthypnotic suggestion. Descriptions of these dissociative processes have been subjected to conflicting theoretical interpretations. Unfortunately, the recommended use of a planchette to facilitate communication with these alter egos tended to link the entire MPD phenomenon with hysteroepilepsy as a product of suggestion, if not fraud. Freud's theory of repression was chosen over Janet's theory of dissociation, resulting in a 60-year hiatus (circa 1920-1980) in the study of dissociative disorders. At the same time that interest in dissociation was declining, Bleuler introduced the diagnostic entity misnamed "schizophrenia." Subsequently, many MPD patients were misdiagnosed as schizophrenic.

Accurate statistical evaluation of MPD also relates to its relationship with severe abuse. Only recently have we recognized the widespread incidence of child abuse and child sexual abuse.

> *In 1980 in the brief section of the Comprehensive Textbook of Psychiatry dealing with incest, the only epidemiological comment is a reference to a 1955 paper estimating that incest affects one family out of a million in North America. This estimate was low by four orders of magnitude. . . . Child abuse underwent a ten thousand fold shift in prevalence in a very short time, and was transformed from a vanishingly rare curiosity to a major public health problem. (From Ross, C: Epidemiology of multiple personality disorder and dissociation, Psychiatric Clin North Am 14(3):503-517, 1991.)*

A shift in the incidence and prevalence estimates of MPD is only now beginning to follow the earlier shift in its major causative factor. Current prevalence estimates range from a very conservative 0.5% of the general population to a high of 10%. In a population of individuals who have come for counseling and been referred to psychologists and psychiatrists, prevalence rates may reach 25%.

♦ETIOLOGY AND PATHOPHYSIOLOGY

MPD is usually associated with maltreatment beginning in early childhood and frequently extending throughout adolescence. The abuse, which can be sexual, physical, emotional, or often some combination of these, is usually "unprovoked" and often exhibits "marked deviance." "Unprovoked" implies that the abuse is not excessive discipline in response to child misbehavior, but is rather purposefully imposed, unusually severe, and often exhibiting both bizarre form and sadistic methods. This extreme end of the abuse spectrum is exemplified by satanic cult practices, which can include witnessed child sacrifice. Finally, the abuse is usually inflicted by the parent or another primary caregiver.

The last two decades have forced us to recognize the reality that the sexual abuse of children is common. Simultaneously, mental health professionals have acquired a new and deeper understanding of the psychological impact of traumatic events. This knowledge is both derived from and focused by the post-traumatic stress disorders resulting from the Vietnam combat experience. Research has yielded better understandings of the nature of trauma and the trauma response mechanisms that define these disorders. Research has also highlighted the potential for long-term consequences following traumatic events, particularly when appropriate psychological intervention is unavailable. Such knowledge has contributed to the evolution of procedures such as routine "crisis debriefing" and supportive therapy following major traumatic events, for example, earthquakes, hurricanes, riots, and other natural or man-made disasters.

While much of the progress in this area evolved from post-trauma work with adults, children have not escaped attention. Events such as the Chauchilla bus incident, firearm tragedies in schools, and similar events where children were the primary targeted victims have all broadened our understanding of both the immediate impact and the long-term results of such trauma in children. While emotional health cannot be guaranteed through immediate and competent intervention, emotional devastation and long-term illness are highly likely when intervention is lacking. The prevalence of severe child abuse and child sexual abuse as well as the increased knowledge regarding the long-term consequences of such trauma allow the recognition and identification of MPD as the most severe form of post-trauma consequence.

DISSOCIATION

Since physical escape from abuse or trauma is often impossible for children, a frequent coping mechanism that allows a form of escape is dissociation, or a psychological distancing of self from the event. In MPD the dissociation is so complete that a discontinuity of "self" and "memory" results. Escape by dissociation, while psychologically creative, is also a psychologically devastating solution to an evil situation. The solution is creative in that the child maintains his or her love for the perpetrator in one personality, the memory of the painful experience and feelings in another, and frequently the angry and aggressive emotions and behaviors in yet another. Unfortunately once that route of defense has been chosen, external stimuli unrelated to the original stress can precipitate dissociative episodes and create additional personalities.

Not all dissociation is found in victims of severe child abuse or child sexual abuse. Many authors note that some forms of dissociation are normal developmentally. Even among a severely abused population, many children and adults dissociate emotionally as a coping strategy. This dissociation, however, is limited to the emotional sphere with no loss of continuity of self or memory. Thus many victims will describe severe abuse in great detail, with no apparent demonstration of affect. They often note companion depersonalization and out-of-body phenomena such as "there was a spot on the wall where I routinely went and watched as he raped me." For these victims, therapy involves a reintegration of the feelings and the experiences along with a working through of the feelings.

The ongoing puzzle of MPD is that the dissociation is so complete that the multiple personalities can continue to coexist. Each personality is either unaware of the others or there is an internal system of personalities who are aware of each other but who operate outside the conscious awareness of the host personality. Frequently one or several of these personalities will emerge, engage in behavior not compatible with the host personality, and then retreat, leaving the host personality "holding the bag." Thus the prevailing personality, unaware of the existence of the others, must often manage the consequences of another personality's actions, such as meeting the demands of the promises made by these other selves. All the while, the host personality remains unclear as to why he or she does not remember either the interactions described or the periods of time during which they occurred. People with MPD become masters at covering up these perceived deficiencies. Their lives are a constant balancing and disguising act for what each personality perceives as its "terrible memory," if not its "craziness," and which must be kept secret from other people.

◆ WHEN IS IT MPD?

Despite clear-cut and readily identifiable risk factors, the diagnosis of MPD in high-risk pediatric populations remains the exception rather than the rule. In addition to the factors already discussed, underdiagnosis is also due, in part, to the nature of the disorder itself.

DIAGNOSTIC CRITERIA

There are two diagnostic criteria for MPD:

1. The existence within an individual of two or more distinct personalities or personality states, each with its own relatively enduring pattern of perceiving, relating to, and thinking about the self and the environment.

2. The recurrent assumption of full control of the person's behavior by at least two of these personalities.

These criteria are deceptively straightforward. Conceptually, confirming the diagnosis of MPD, particularly in children, is complex, as illustrated by the reported 6.8-year average interval between the first mental health contact and an accurate diagnosis made in adults. Studies also indicate that the MPD child receives an average of 2.7 other psychiatric diagnoses before an accurate diagnosis of MPD is made.

What is it about this disorder that makes diagnosis so difficult? Unlike the diagnosis of depression, where a clearly defined symptom list can be used to make systematic inquiry for critical findings, MPD presents the examiner with multiple personalities who frequently are not consciously aware of one another. Since dissociative processes occur, by definition, out of consciousness, one cannot merely ask, "Do you dissociate?" Unless an episode of dissociation is witnessed and recognized, diagnostic data must be pursued through more indirect approaches.

Diagnosing childhood MPD is doubly difficult. The array of emotional symptoms, post-traumatic indicators, conduct disorders, hallucinatory signs, attention discrepancies, and school difficulties parallels the signs representative of dissociative disorders in adults. The investigation of these symptoms in children, however, is more often performed through physical or developmental channels rather than psychiatric services. Thus, many MPD children are referred to neurologic services for possible seizure disorders presenting as "staring episodes," or to developmental clinics for evaluation of inconsistent attention and learning problems. Even when a child psychiatric evaluation is obtained, a number of developmental factors make it difficult to determine if a given child's dissociative behavior is normal or pathological. Even when clearly pathological, some personalities can be nonverbal or preverbal. These personalities can exhibit marked acting out that is diagnostic, but the children still could be unable to understand or respond to diagnostically useful questions.

For the diagnosis of children, the data collection starts from the diagnostic red flag of possible abuse and obtains information from both the child and caregivers. The diagnostic process precisely parallels that of adult MPD but seeks signs that are exhibited within the child's developmental sphere of action. An MPD screening checklist to score pediatric behavioral signs may be useful in dealing with these at-risk children.

A family history of MPD represents a significant and heavily weighted risk factor. To the extent that such a history is present, it is necessary to rule out MPD rather than to rule it in.

The diagnosis of MPD in both children and adults requires a different perceptual filter for the "third ear"; the usual clues and cues regarding truthfulness or defensiveness can be missing. A host personality asked about certain behaviors could truthfully deny their presence because that personality can be completely unaware of events that were engaged in by another of the subject's personalities. The evaluator's usual "lie detection" parameters, such as eye gaze, body posture, nervous gestures, and defensive voice tones, are of little use for the simple reason that the particular personality is not "lying." This phenomenon is of special importance to professionals investigating the possibility of multigenerational child sexual abuse.

◆ WHAT DOES MPD LOOK LIKE?

MPD is depicted in the popular media as a flamboyant, rare female disorder. The cinematic presentations of *The Three Faces of Eve* and *Sybil* compellingly depicted the complexity, devastation, and totality of this disorder. MPD, however, in fact, is neither rare nor, in most affected individuals, flamboyant. Unlike most psychiatric disorders, where the problem that is present usually indicates a specific differential diagnostic decision tree, the chief complaint in MPD rarely suggests an MPD diagnosis. The most frequently described presentation of MPD is depression in the host personality. A typical MPD history will be vague and unclear. There are many "I can't remember for sure" answers or clever and subtle redefining of the questions by the MPD patient through oblique or tangential responses aimed at covering up half-realized memory gaps. Facts stated at one time may be "forgotten" or denied by another personality at another time. A useful diagnostic clue is presented when the evaluator begins to wonder who is more forgetful—the evaluator or the patient. When this occurs it should raise the question of need for a major reorganization of the presenting data to account for this "forgetfulness." That perspective should lead to consideration of MPD as a possible diagnosis, particularly in the presence of a previous history of abuse.

INVESTIGATING MPD

Once adult MPD is suspected, confirmation requires two levels of investigation. A conclusive diagnosis will usually need to evolve over several sessions and involve sources of information other than the patient.

FIRST LEVEL

During the first level of investigation adult victims of child abuse are questioned about the presence of extreme, unexplainable, and bothersome forgetfulness that causes them to have a sense of always being on edge and needing to constantly conceal and check their behavior. *Other areas to be investigated are as follows:*

1. Flashbacks or broken threads of memory

2. Unexplained periods of lost time, both minutes and days, sometimes viewed by the patient as "walking blackouts," but unrelated to alcohol use

3. Waking up and not knowing how they got where they were or what they were doing in the recent past

4. People they do not know frequently calling them by other names and seeming to know them

5. A childhood reputation for being a "liar" that remains puzzling to the host personality

6. The appearance of items of clothing, jewelry, books, or other personal goods in their possession that they cannot recall buying or, conversely, the unexplained disappearance of such items

7. Frequent and troublesome "dreamlike" states including sleepwalking

8. Marked differences in handwriting from time to time

SECOND LEVEL

When several of these symptoms have been documented, the evaluator can then probe more deeply for the presence of the occurrence of voices (other personalities) that argue in the patient's head but that are not psychotic in character; an awareness of sometimes being unable to control personal behavior; long periods of lost time such as several childhood years in succession; and unexplained severe mood swings and dichotomous behavior states (such as impulsive and dangerous risk-taking alternating with cautious or phobic states) as reported to them by friends.

When a diagnosis of MPD becomes almost certain and other personalities have not yet spontaneously revealed themselves, the therapist may issue a direct invitation for them to come forward. Thus the diagnosis proceeds from a suspicion to an investigation of possible external signs that in turn point the way to internal signs. Such signs sometimes are confirmed by the affected individual and lead to validation of the therapist's suspicions and finally to the appearance of alternate personalities.

◆ IS MPD REAL?

Despite substantial corroborative research, the persistent, overriding question surrounding MPD continues to be "Is it real?" This has remained unchanged for most professional mental health care workers over the past century. Recognition and acceptance of this disorder have been slow. For many, MPD is deemed the product of hypnotic suggestion, hysteria or malingering, or a variant of other personality disorders. Indeed, many assign MPD to a "false memory syndrome" phenomenon. However, when abuse and the functional status of many MPD victims are evaluated, clear evidence exists that this disorder is very real and very debilitating to those affected. In many case reports the therapist makes no use of hypnotism nor has the patient ever been subject to hypnotism. Clearly, the recognition of childhood MPD has lagged even further behind in acceptance than has adult MPD.

◆ THE FUTURE

When these abused children are appropriately identified and adequately treated, outcomes and prognoses are positive. When, however, children with MPD remain undiagnosed and untreated until adulthood, the course of therapy is long, stormy, and prognostically uncertain. In contrast to many other psychiatric disorders, the causative factors of this disorder along with the psychological efficacy and cost-effectiveness of early identification and treatment can be documented.

The past decade has seen a re-emergence in the study of this disorder and the stark realization that unless this disorder is recognized and treated at its point of origin, early childhood, a public health problem of epidemic proportions can be created that can have impact on succeeding generations.

MPD is currently recognized as a creative psychophysiologic defensive response to a specific set of inescapable and uncontrollable experiences occurring within a specific developmental time frame. Effective treatment requires an understanding of the developmental factors and the initial adaptations to cope with the overwhelming trauma while it is occurring. More importantly, both effective treatment and primary prevention require that professionals identify MPD in its incubation phase, those childhood years following identified abuse incidents.

FORENSIC QUAGMIRE

MPD presents us with several forensic issues that are, as yet, unresolved. From the point of view of the person with MPD as a victim, recent court rulings have suggested that when one personality is seductive, promiscuous, and cooperative in getting into a compromising situation, another personality then emerges to stop. Continued forceful sexual interaction constitutes rape. This decision suggests that the person with MPD may be incapable of fully informed consent.

The more difficult ethical and legal complexities occur when one (or more) personalities have perpetrated abuse or murder. Incarceration or long-term institutionalization for these offenses accompanied by treatment for the "insanity or incompetency" may yield an integrated person who no longer has MPD. Does one then release this person, or does the person remain in care or custody based on the actions of a "person" who no longer exists?

MPD challenges our most basic beliefs and assumptions concerning the workings of the mind and leaves us with questions we are currently ill equipped to answer. Perhaps this also contributed to its loss of stature in the psychiatric literature for a number of years: What we don't see doesn't haunt us. Current evidence regarding the prevalence and destructiveness of this disorder strips us of the luxury of this blindness.

♦ SUGGESTED READINGS

James, W: *Principles of Psychology*, Volumes 1 and 2, Henry Holt, New York, 1890.

Kluft, R: Childhood multiple personality: Predictors, clinical findings, and treatment results. In R Kluft, ed: *Childhood Antecedents of Multiple Personality*, American Psychiatric Press, Inc, Washington, DC, 1985.

Putnam, F: *Diagnosis and Treatment of Multiple Personality Disorder*, The Guilford Press, New York, 1989.

Schreiber, FR: *Sybil*, Regnery, Chicago, 1973.

Thigpen, C, and Checkley, H: *The Three Faces of Eve*, McGraw-Hill Book Co, New York, 1957.

Chapter 7

MUNCHAUSEN SYNDROME BY PROXY

JAMES A. MONTELEONE, M.D.

John's case was followed from birth in the hemophiliac clinic. His mother was a known carrier of hemophilia. She had two brothers with a bleeding disorder. John was found to have only a mild case, with only two episodes of bleeding that required special attention in the emergency room in the first 2 years. The bleeding was controlled easily and required only short periods of hospitalization. When he was 2, his mother asked to be taught home care to manage his future bleeding episodes. She was an eager and excellent student. Soon she was calling every day, stating that John had sustained a fall or that she had noticed blood in his stool. This was followed by her appearing in the clinic on a daily basis stating that John had fallen or that she had noticed blood in his stool. No one had witnessed the falls. He was hospitalized 37 times and while in the hospital was found to have unexplained drops in his hemoglobin levels. The child was placed in foster care and experienced no bleeding episodes over an extended period of time. The mother was ordered by the court to see a counselor. The child was returned to his mother's care with supervision. He continues to do well.

Baron Von Munchausen was a teller of outrageous tales who lived in the 18th century. Some of his tales, authored by one of his friends, Rudolph Raspe, were published in a children's book entitled *Baron Munchausen's Narrative of His Marvelous Travels and Campaigns in Russia* (1936).

In 1951 one researcher described an unusual group of patients who went from physician to physician fabricating stories of illness; they were willing to subject themselves to numerous tests and needless surgery. He called this syndrome the von Munchausen's (or Munchausen) Syndrome. A variant of the syndrome was described in a case report of two hospitalized children. Unlike the original Munchausen Syndrome, in this case the parent fabricated the illness in the child and presented the child to a physician for treatment. This variant was dubbed the "Munchausen Syndrome by Proxy." Among the incidents reported that fall in this category of disorder are instances in which several mothers deliberately poisoned their children and then tried to convince their physicians that the child was ill.

Naturally, such falsification of medical illness can cause emotional harm by propagating a self-image in the child as chronically ill and can cause physical injury with unnecessary medical testing and possible pointless use of medications to treat false symptoms. In some cases, it has led to the child's death.

◆ WHO IS INVOLVED?

Munchausen Syndrome by Proxy (MSBP) affects children of widely varying ages. Children have presented with factitious illness by proxy from as young as neonates to as old as 21 years. Perpetrators of MSBP are found in all socioeconomic groups; some deceptions are unsophisticated while others are complex, requiring complicated investigative techniques to unravel. In general, the child appears to have a persistent or recurrent condition or illness that cannot be explained. There may be abnormal laboratory studies without strong evidence of underlying disease, or, conversely, there may be normal laboratory results that do not support the illness reported. For example, a child may develop a rash but is unable to tolerate prescribed drug treatments because of reported vomiting or other untoward reactions. The parent, usually the mother, is willing to have the child undergo diagnostic procedures and medical treatments even if they are invasive. If the child is hospitalized the situation may go from bad to worse, with the child becoming febrile or lapsing into a coma, or the illness may disappear and the child appear well again. Presenting complaints can vary widely, with the parent complaining that the child is tired all the time, the child stops breathing and turns blue, or the child convulses. Deliberate poisoning may be seen, sometimes involving prescription medicines. Children have also been injected with medications, such as insulin, to produce coma and with foreign substances, such as feces, to produce infection.

◆ WHAT SHOULD YOU LOOK FOR?

As you review the child's medical history, you may note that there have been numerous visits to the doctor and numerous hospitalizations. In addition, the child usually has undergone many diagnostic procedures, frequently involving several different hospitals and a variety of physicians. Many times a rare disease has been diagnosed or strongly considered. Experienced specialists often remark that they have never seen a case like this before.

Most of the mothers seem loving. They do not appear cruel, negligent, or uncaring. If the mother has other children, they are rarely discussed. All the mother's energy is focused on the sick child. She usually denies any knowledge about how the child came to be ill. The mother spends an excessive amount of time on the hospital ward with the child and refuses to leave the child alone in the hospital, even for an hour. She often insists that she is the only one the child can relate to and accept food, drink, or medicine from. The mother, despite her child's problems, does not seem as worried about her child as are the medical and nursing staff. In fact, she may be very conciliatory about the child's condition with the hospital staff. The mother may be familiar with medical terminology and procedures. Often she has had nursing training or worked in a medical setting. In addition, the mother may have had other children with these symptoms or may have herself complained of them. Often the mother becomes overly friendly with hospital staff. There is often conflict among medical professionals in the case, some believing the child is ill and some holding that the diagnosis should be MSBP. The father is usually distant and minimally involved.

The child may talk about his or her death, taking an active part in the pretense. However, he or she usually improves when separated from the parent. Interesting, the symptoms often stop and the child improves when the charade is exposed and the parent confronted.

APPEARANCES ARE DECEIVING

Mothers are able to pull off the deception in a number of ways. Bleeding can result from the mother adding her blood to the child's vomit, urine, or feces. Sometimes blood is smeared on the child's face or genital area. The blood is usually obtained by the mother pricking herself. One mother used blood from an open thigh wound; another stirred a vaginal tampon in the child's urine specimen. A few mothers have simulated blood in a specimen from the child by adding paint, cocoa, or phenolphthalein. One mother produced feculent vomitus by adding soft feces, which she stored in a container in her room, to the child's vomit.

Fevers have been produced by rubbing thermometers or immersing them in hot liquid. Biochemical abnormalities are simulated by adding chemicals, such as salt, to a specimen. Various tricks have been used to distract the person who is taking the specimen.

Rashes have been fabricated by rubbing the skin repetitively with a fingernail or a sharp object to obtain a bullous lesion, by applying caustic solutions to areas of skin, and by painting with a dye such as phenolphthalein.

Neurological symptoms can be produced when the mother gives the child a sedative or tranquilizer prescribed for herself. Usually the mother gives the medications in doses greater than those prescribed for herself. One mother applied pressure to the child's neck to induce seizures.

Seizures are a common presenting complaint in the MSBP syndrome. The best way to rule out a convulsive disorder is by taking a careful history. Commonly, when children are said to have had a seizure at school or a similar place, in the presence of a third party or parties, questioning the party or others present at the time of the reported seizure reveals that no seizure was witnessed.

CATEGORIES OF MSBP

Various researchers have suggested a spectrum of categories for MSBP:

— Perceived Illness   — Help Seeker

— Doctor Shopping   — Active Inducer

— Enforced Invalidism   — Doctor Addict

— Fabricated Illness

As with all forms of child abuse, it is the degree of abuse that matters. This will influence actions taken by social agencies.

PERCEIVED ILLNESS

Perceived illness is described as the mother who is anxious, inexperienced, under stress, lonely, and needlessly worrying that her healthy child is ill. She perceives symptoms in her child that others do not observe. The child is taken to the doctor on many occasions because she cannot be reassured. Therefore the child is forced to undergo unpleasant investigations and treatments. This process would not be classified as child abuse, unless the mother's persistence and refusal to accept normal results were excessive and the quality of the child's life was seriously impaired.

DOCTOR SHOPPING

This parent seeks help from a succession of different doctors, claiming that her healthy child is ill. As each doctor in turn refuses further investigation, she consults yet another doctor. She tells none of the chain of doctors that she has seen anyone before. The result for the child is a series of the same investigations. When the parent's convictions about illness reach these proportions, it is child abuse.

ENFORCED INVALIDISM

Enforced invalidism is seen when a parent with an ill or disabled child seeks to keep the child ill or increase the degree of disability, or, if the child has no disability, to ensure that the child is regarded as incapacitated and in need of special attention or assistance.

FABRICATED ILLNESS

Fabricated illness results when the parent lies to the doctor about a child's health, giving a convincing history of illness, and fabricates physical signs or alters health records. This causes the doctor to perform detailed investigations and prescribe treatment. The parent invents the illness while the child is young and continues and intensifies the story as the years pass. When they are older, some children participate in the deception. Some have become dependent illness addicts and have grown up to have the Munchausen Syndrome.

HELP SEEKER

The help seeker, comparable to the category of perceived illness, fabricates illness in a child on a limited basis, but a desperate request for help with parenting is the clear motivation. These mothers respond well to psychiatric intervention. They are at one end of the spectrum.

ACTIVE INDUCER

At the other extreme of the MSBP is the active inducer, who will make life-threatening assaults on very young children.

DOCTOR ADDICT

The category of doctor addict, similar to the doctor shopper, represents the other major class of cases. Neither as dramatic as active inducers in symptoms and danger nor as blatant as help seekers in their request for intervention, doctor addict mothers are frequently written off as cranks or overanxious and their children as psychosomatic or depressed. They are less likely to be identified than the active inducer cases, since doctor addiction can evade resolution for longer than cases in which the victim is hospitalized with an acute condition.

◆ FAMILY DYNAMICS

In one study, at the time the fabrication was discovered, 15 of the 17 pairs of parents were living together. Their mean age was 29 years, ranging from 24 to 37 years of age. Most of the mothers lived in the hospital with the child or visited the child for long periods each day. The fathers kept a low profile; 10 of 15 rarely visited the child in the hospital. This was particularly noteworthy in view of the perceived severity of the child's illness. Six of 11 husbands had jobs which required them to be away from home for long periods or in the evenings, and 2 others were considered extremely unsupportive of their wives. The fathers did not appear to know of the fabrication and had difficulty in believing it when told. In 10 of 15 families, there was a discrepancy between the social and the intellectual level of the parents. In each the wife either came from a higher social background or seemed much more intelligent than her husband. In 15 of 17 families there were other children. In 5 families a second child incurred the syndrome or died of suspicious circumstances. In 10 families there was nothing to suggest involvement of older or younger siblings.

◆ EVENTUAL OUTCOME

The following consequences may be in store for children who are falsely labeled as ill:

1. They will receive needless and possibly harmful treatments.
2. They may develop a genuine disease.
3. They may die.
4. They may develop chronic invalidism.
5. They may develop Munchausen Syndrome as an adult.

If the diagnosis of MSBP is made, you must remember that sometimes a story is false. A small degree of suspicion should be maintained at all times.

MUNCHAUSEN SYNDROME BY PROXY AND APNEA

There is a high prevalence of MSBP in the subgroup of apnea patients who have had two or more episodes of apnea terminated after mouth-to-mouth resuscitation. The beginning of the episode is only in the presence of the parent, but the episode is witnessed by other persons called for assistance. When these infants die, the presumptive cause of death is sudden infant death syndrome (SIDS), but no autopsy is done. Since it is impossible to distinguish between SIDS and other causes of death without an autopsy, it is essential that all infants whose deaths are not explained have an autopsy.

PRESENCE OF OTHER ORGANIC DISEASE

Sometimes the evaluation is complicated because, in addition to the fabricated illness, the child may actually have a legitimate illness, such as hemophilia, asthma, or a convulsive disorder. The mother uses this genuine illness as a basis for her complaints. For example, she precipitates problems by causing bleeding in the hemophilia patient or by withholding or increasing the prescribed medications in children with asthma or a convulsive disorder.

◆GUIDELINES WHEN MSBP IS SUSPECTED

If you suspect MSBP, you should take the following steps:

1. **The child's safety is the primary concern. These children are at risk— 10% of them will die, and another 8% will have long-term morbidity.** You must continue to behave as if the mother's story of her child's illness is accurate, because it may be.

2. Social service and child protective services must be notified immediately.

3. The child should be separated from the mother for a sufficient length of time to determine if the symptoms and signs occur in her absence. Try to get the mother to voluntarily leave. If she will not, this action may require legal enforcement and a court order.

4. The possibilities of simulating or producing illness are endless and as diverse as the human imagination. Nothing is farfetched, especially when one suspects poisoning. Consider all sources, food, syringes, and intravenous bottles as possible evidence. Save all specimens for toxicological assay. Check the reliability of the signs; for example, test whether the rash washes off with water or alcohol and whether the blood is actually blood.

5. The medical team, social service, and protective agencies must work out a plan of action. It is wise for the child protection team to have a protocol outlining the procedures to follow. **Remember, the child is not free of risk because he is in the hospital.** If the mother is producing illness, there is a 70% chance she will produce it in the hospital. The protective plan may include video monitoring of the child. As in any other child abuse case, the plan should include whether the child should be removed from the home or can remain there under supervision.

6. If the child is verbal, interview him or her alone. An experienced counselor is recommended.

7. Check with physicians, hospitals, employers, and schools for details of the history relating to the child, the family, the mother, and her life. It is common for the mother to fabricate details of her life, such as schooling, employment, illnesses, and hospitalizations. Check out the mother's witnesses to illness in the child and interview them about the facts they have allegedly seen. Check past medical records. Do not allow the mother to talk you out of the search. Look for unusual illnesses in siblings of the patient or unusual illnesses in the parents. Check out the social and work histories as well.

8. Pay careful attention to documentation.

9. Be supportive, not accusing, when dealing with the family. State the case clearly and simply. Tell the parents that the case has been reported to protective services. Be prepared to immediately protect the child. Protective services and the court should be on notice so that a court

holding order on the child may be obtained if necessary. The object of confronting the parents is not to persuade them that it is true or to obtain a confession. Rather, it is to tell them that someone knows and will take steps to protect the child.

Note that no food, drink, or medicines may be brought in by the family. **The child should never be left alone with the parent, and the person in attendance should be aware that the mother may try to harm the child while she is there.** *The parent must be watched at all times while she is with the child.*

Because the mother may be suicidal, psychiatric care should be made available to the mother and father immediately after disclosure of the diagnosis. In addition, the child should have a psychiatric and/or psychological evaluation.

CONFRONTATION

In general it is the responsibility of the physician to confront the parents immediately if he or she suspects the charade. Usually, the fabrication ends following confrontation. When confronted, most perpetrators do not acknowledge the abuse but do stop the actions.

CHILD SURVEILLANCE

Video surveillance has been effective as a means of confirming the diagnosis of MSBP. In answer to the critics of video surveillance who believe that it is not ethical, it should be pointed out that it is the child who is being watched secretly by the camera, not the mother. Videotaping is performed for the child's protection and is therefore ethical. There is no entrapment since the presence of the surveillance apparatus does not increase the likelihood that the illegal act will be committed. The method is legal, and the information obtained has been used as evidence in a legal proceeding.

◆ SUGGESTED READINGS

Asher, R: Munchausen Syndrome, *Lancet* 1:339-341, 1951.

Meadow, R: Munchausen Syndrome by Proxy: The hinterland of child abuse, *Lancet* 2:343-345, 1977.

Meadow, R: Munchausen Syndrome by Proxy, *Br Med J* 299:248-250, 1989.

Rosenberg, DA: Web of deceit: A literature review of Munchausen Syndrome by Proxy, *Child Abuse Negl* 11:547-563, 1987.

Chapter 8

NEGLECT AND ABANDONMENT

WAYNE I. MUNKEL, M.S.W., L.C.S.W.

This chapter cannot begin to explain the complex issue of neglect but can only look at the outcomes. Usually, if there is no unfortunate outcome, neglect goes undetected and unreported. It takes a death or shocking evidence before many cases of neglect are brought to light.

A severely malnourished 7-year-old boy was taken to the emergency room by ambulance. The child's mother found him unresponsive in bed and not breathing. The mother stated that the child had had a cold for the past few days and appeared to be recovering.

He was emaciated and dirty, he had bedsores on his buttocks and hips, and the soles of his feet were crusted with dirt that had to be scraped off. Under the dirt were several infected wounds, one looking like a cigarette burn. Attempts at resuscitation were successful, and he was intubated and given fluids and antibiotics. He had severe bilateral pneumonia. After several hours in the hospital he suffered cardiac arrest. Attempts at resuscitation were futile.

There were three other children in the family. All, although poorly clothed, were well nourished and healthy. The mother was single, and none of the children had the same father. The mother was receiving public aid and had been reported for abuse and neglect several times in the past. She was regularly visited by state child protection services, the last visit the week before the child's admission. The worker did not see the child during the visit, although he was supposedly sick and in bed at that time.

The school was contacted. The three siblings had been to school regularly. The dead child had missed a number of days in the past and had been absent for the previous 2 weeks. One of the teachers stated that on several occasions the child had come to school in obvious distress. He was dirty, malnourished, and unable to work on his school assignments. On one occasion, the child was so weak he had to crawl up the stairs. His teacher had suggested they report the child to the Division of Family Services. The school principal

decided that since the other children seemed to be doing well, he would just send the child home.

The media caught wind of the story and took pictures of the home, which should have been condemned. But as we review the case it is clear that the media had chosen this family as a scapegoat for the child protection system itself. In truest perspective, the system was the cause of the child's death. Had the mother received better services, the child would have survived and thrived. The school's role in the tragedy, although understandable, compounded the situation.

Given this history, typical of so many cases, it is easy to see that neglect resulted in death. But too often the causative responsibility is shared among several factors that can be difficult to define. Furthermore, neglect is often difficult to prevent. This chapter will attempt to identify the various forms of neglect and abandonment, just touching on the "who" and the "why," which constitute a social problem beyond the scope of this chapter.

As is true with most problems, there is a spectrum of neglect that ranges from mild to severe. It is easy to agree on what constitutes severe neglect and what should be done about it. Beyond that, unless an obviously bad outcome is brought to light, nothing is done or, in most cases, can be done. The following case illustrates this point:

A 2-month-old child was found dead in his crib by his mother. The cause of death was suffocation. The child shared the crib with a 2-year-old and a 4-year-old sibling. The medical examiner decided that the cause of death was accidental. One of the siblings, while sleeping, probably laid on the child and caused the suffocation.

Was neglect involved here? Who was neglectful? The mother? No one told her the child would be in danger if he slept with others. If the mother had had more money, she could have afforded beds for each child. If she had been better educated she would, hopefully, have known better.

A mother leaves seven children in the home while she goes on a date. The eldest is 8 years old. He has been told not to play with matches and has been reprimanded for this very thing. While the mother is gone, there is a fire and all of the children are killed. It is declared an accident caused by a child playing with matches. The neighbors and firemen had trouble reaching the children because the windows were barred and the door had a deadman board against it. The family was known to the state protective services.

This case certainly illustrates neglect and shows that the neglect must be shared by the mother, the landlord, the neighbors who were aware that the mother often left the children alone, the fire inspector, and the state protective system.

Some feel that the consideration of neglect should be simplified. Missouri law defines neglect as **"reckless failure to provide, by those responsible for the care, custody, and control of the child, the proper or necessary support, education as required by law, nutrition or medical, surgical, or any other care necessary for his well-being; and food, clothing or shelter sufficient for life or essential medical and surgical care."** This definition in the law clearly allows for broad interpretation by the courts.

◆ INCIDENCE AND DEFINITIONS

In 1980, neglect reports accounted for almost half of all child maltreatment reports. Neglect is also often noted as a component in other forms of abuse, but the concept of neglect as a separate entity is poorly defined. This is still true as we see the challenge of preventing neglect growing even greater in a climate of uncertain economic conditions and changing political realities.

Simply stated, neglect is the failure of caregivers to provide for the basic needs of their children. Failure to meet these needs may vary in degree from mild to severe and can be acute or chronic. No workable definition that quantifies the degree of neglect has yet been found. While there is general agreement on what constitutes extreme neglect, little agreement has been reached concerning what constitutes milder forms of neglect and the harm caused by neglect.

DEVELOPING CRITERIA TO DEFINE NEGLECT OBJECTIVELY

The degree of harm suffered by the child was the impetus for the first national study on the incidence of child neglect. The National Study of the Incidence and Severity of Child Abuse and Neglect defined neglect as a situation in which it could be shown that, as a result of caregiver inattention to the child's basic needs for care, protection, or control, the child experienced predictable injury or impairment of serious or greater severity.

In addition, an affirmative answer had to be obtained to the following questions:

1. Had the caregiver been informed of the child's need or problem by a competent professional, or under the circumstances of the situation, would the child's need have been apparent to most reasonably caring and attentive adults?

2. Was the caregiver physically and financially able to obtain or provide the needed care, protection, or supervision?

The Department of Health and Human Services has added a category titled "endangered." This new category allowed for reporting children who had no present evidence of abuse through neglect but for whom it was reasonable to suspect there was the risk of injury due to neglect. This change added a substantial number of children who were considered to be neglected. While the risk of harm or endangerment is a category of neglected children that may need intervention to prevent future neglect, the lack of sufficient resources available to child protective services (CPS) and other human services leaves this category of neglect unserved in many states. Although we have seen a dramatic increase in child abuse and neglect reports between 1980 and 1986, there has only been a meager 4% increase in funding.

Overreporting, which is defined as reported cases that are investigated and closed without services being provided, has led some parent groups to advocate changes in laws to redefine abuse and neglect and to protect parental rights. Others feel that rather than redefine abuse and neglect, children and parents would be better served by expanding the support and resources of the child protection system and the training of child protection workers.

◆ TYPES OF NEGLECT

When a child exhibits an injury or other signs that could result from neglect, it is the responsibility of the child care professional to look for a mechanism to explain the physical signs. For example, a child who falls and is seriously injured may reasonably appear to have suffered an accident. When you have suspicions about the cause of a child's condition, a good social history is necessary to determine if it was, in fact, an accident or if neglect or intent played a role in the event.

It is not uncommon to hear or read accounts of children found living in squalid conditions. These reports have common themes: children who aren't fed or bathed, extremes of temperatures, and a building filled with debris and contaminated with urine, feces, and vermin. The conditions found are generally described by investigators as the worst they have encountered. In the following sections, conditions that constitute or contribute to the neglect of children are discussed. These conditions may be seen first-hand by workers going into the home or may be inferred when the children are examined outside their home environment. The neglect they suffer may be revealed through their physical appearance, by their health status or injuries, or, in some cases, by their death.

PHYSICAL ENVIRONMENT
INADEQUATE SHELTER

Frequently a house where neglect exists is overcrowded with people, furnishings, trash, or garbage; for example, 25 persons may live in a four-bedroom house. The children simply get lost in the house because of the adults' inattention. They are not supervised because each adult assumes that someone else is managing the child's care.

INADEQUATE SLEEPING ARRANGEMENTS

When a child does not get adequate sleep, he or she may appear as chronically fatigued or listless, particularly as noted by schoolteachers or neighbors. The child's need for sleep may not be met because there are too many people living in the house, too much noise, too many people sleeping in one bed, or no beds available. The practice of allowing or forcing children to sleep with adults can contribute to sexual abuse of the child. This is frequently exacerbated by the lack of consideration for personal boundaries and/or poor self-control (often as a result of drug or alcohol use). Another problem involves bedding that is inadequate for cold weather or soiled with feces or urine. Furthermore, the child may be denied privacy from opposite-sex children or adults, contributing to a sense of shame that can lead to a lack of sleep. Another source of anxiety results from fear when different people are free to roam the premises, posing a threat to the child's security.

UNSANITARY CONDITIONS

As noted, frequently in neglect cases the house is filled with an accumulation of garbage and trash. Toilets are unusable, and there may be animal and/or human feces on the floors. Often uncontrolled vermin—rats, spiders, cockroaches—are present. Food preparation under these circumstances is unhealthy and can cause ongoing illness in the child as well as others in the house.

STRUCTURAL HAZARDS

Not uncommonly, the house or dwelling has partially collapsed. Stairs may have broken steps, and railings are missing on stairways, porches, or balconies. Windows and doors are in poor repair, with broken or jagged glass. The doors and windows are without screens, and floors and ceilings have holes. Badly worn floors may be covered with large splinters.

HOUSEKEEPING PROBLEMS

The condition of the house and furniture indicates the lack of even minimal care. Dirt and filth cover the surfaces, especially in the kitchen and bathroom. Clutter and trash are everywhere, obviously having accumulated over a long period of time.

ENVIRONMENTAL HAZARDS
FIRE HAZARDS

Exposed or frayed wiring is frequently found in the home. Fuel containers are stored in living areas, and combustible materials are placed near heat sources. Beds are too close to heat sources, which could result in burns of unaware children, as well as fires. Metal bars on windows and "deadman" props against doors impede evacuation should a fire occur in the house.

SUBSTANCE ACCESSIBILITY AND USE

Chemicals or drugs may be within reach or easy accessibility of children who can climb up to storage areas. Illicit drugs in the house or the use of the house in drug traffic are particularly hazardous to children and often accompany neglect.

EXCESSIVE HOT WATER TEMPERATURE

In houses where neglect is practiced, the temperature of the hot water available at the tap may be greater than 130°F. The time required to burn skin with water at this temperature is less than 30 seconds; if the water is at 140°F a burn can occur in 3 seconds; at 147°F it only takes 1 second for a burn to be inflicted. Thus if an unsupervised child accidentally turns on the hot water tap a serious burn can result in as short a time as 1 second.

INADEQUATE CARE STANDARDS

NUTRITION

The food may be of poor quality and lacking in nutritional value. The diet is inadequate with regard to the basic food groups and does not offer any variety, indicating a lack of meal planning or haphazard planning. Often no adult caregiver prepares meals on a consistent basis. The food provided may also be inappropriate for the child's age and developmental abilities. Food found stored in either a cupboard or in a refrigerator may be spoiled. Unfortunately, in many cases no food is available. The mealtime itself may be marked by chaos or unpleasant routines for the child, further adversely affecting his or her nutritional status.

CLOTHING

Clothing for neglected children is inadequate and inappropriate for the weather and season. It may also be dirty, ill-fitting, or in a poor state of repair. The child's footwear may be inadequate for the season, too small, too large, or in poor repair.

PERSONAL HYGIENE

Neglected children often show evidence of not having bathed for a lengthy period of time, smelling of urine, feces, or sweat, covered with crusted dirt, and hair unkempt. The child often states that he or she has not bathed. Poor dental hygiene is evident by severe dental caries and mouth odor. When asked, children may state that they do not brush their teeth. Furthermore, neglect is evident when there is the persistent presence of lice.

HEALTH CARE

Neglect implies that even minimal health care is not obtained and the child lacks immunizations. The adult either overuses emergency services, going to the hospital for even slight problems, or does not use them at all, even with severe injury and illness. When medicine or rehabilitative equipment is prescribed, the prescription goes unfilled. Dental caries and other dental needs remain untreated. Regimens recommended for the treatment of chronic illness are not followed or compliance is poor. Prescribed psychological help is not obtained.

SUPERVISION

The lack of supervision by the parent and/or caregiver can lead to injuries that could have been avoided and to repeated injuries. The key question to be answered is whether the behavior of the parent and/or caregiver contributed significantly to the child's injury.

DEVELOPMENTAL NEGLECT

EDUCATION

Neglected children are often not enrolled in school after the state-required age. The adult caregiver permits chronic truancy and fails to provide encouragement for the educational process. The adult caregiver also fails to provide the necessary control, discipline, or role model for learning, socialization, and responsible behavior.

EMOTIONAL GROWTH

When there is emotional neglect, the child's needs for emotional support and encouragement are not provided by the adult caregiver. The adult caregiver is unavailable emotionally, is indifferent, or rejects the child. Because there is inadequate supervision, the child engages in dangerous behaviors for long periods of time. The child's need for emotional security is not met.

◆ATTACHMENT DISORDERS

Attachment disorders are defined as the caregiver's rejection of the child and the parental role. Abandonment can occur because attachment to the child, or bonding, which normally develops during the prenatal or immediate antenatal period, fails to occur. Because the parent fails to develop feelings of attachment to the child, the sense of responsibility for providing for the child's basic needs also does not occur.

ABANDONMENT

In general, abandonment is a legal term with legal implications that refers to the physical aspects of neglect and fulfills certain rigid criteria. However, in addition to physical abandonment, which frequently results from an attachment disorder, there is emotional abandonment, which, in the long run, is potentially more devastating. In emotional abandonment the parent, usually the mother, in one way or another completely withdraws from nurturing and meeting the child's needs for security. This parallels the general aspects of abandonment, where the caregiver does not meet the child's needs for physical security. The child's needs are either not met or are provided for by others.

Parental characteristics, rather than those associated with the child, and environmental factors are the best predictors of the potential for abandonment. Among the predisposing characteristics are sexual promiscuity with or without alcoholism, financial problems, and relatively poor state of health. Depression, especially when severe, also can be a factor in causing abandonment.

The circumstances and conditions associated with abandonment can be categorized into the following six types:

1. Fatal or near-fatal abandonment
2. Abandonment with physical needs provided by others
3. Throwaways
4. Parental custody refusal

5. Lack of supervision

6. Emotional abandonment

FATAL OR NEAR-FATAL ABANDONMENT

Children abandoned with the intent to kill either die or are saved by fortuitous circumstances. Children can be abandoned in places where they are likely to be found and subsequently cared for. Sometimes, however, they are not found in time to prevent serious health problems or death. A set of twins was put in trash bags and placed in a dumpster by the mother who then called the father and told him where they were. A young mother placed her child in a gangway in subzero weather where the baby would be found by a passerby. A 2-year-old child was found, bound hand and foot, in a suitcase under a hospital dumpster by a security guard. The child's gag had been slipped off her mouth and the zipper of the suitcase was left open so that the child's cries could be heard. A newborn infant was found by an alert security guard in a gym bag on an icy street in a public park. Abandonment at its worst is abandonment infanticide. In these instances the child is left to die or is left in conditions likely to result in his or her death.

These children and their parent(s) obviously had great need of protective services. Fortunately most children are found in time to prevent serious health problems or death.

ABANDONMENT WITH PHYSICAL NEEDS PROVIDED BY OTHERS

Children can be abandoned under conditions that result in the child's physical needs being met by others. These children are left at hospitals, sitters, relatives, friends, neighbors, licensed providers, or extended care facilities. Children who are not picked up 2 days after the agreed upon or arranged pickup are considered abandoned. (NOTE: This time may vary from state to state.) In other cases, hospitals and extended care facilities care for children for various periods of time and the caregiver has little responsibility, if any, for providing basic needs. These interludes initiate separations between parent and child and provide an opportunity for parents to abandon the child. Handicapped children are especially susceptible. Prematurely born children often have serious health problems that require lengthy hospitalizations in high-technology environments. In some cases, no attachment is formed between the parent and child. Temporary abandonments by parents because of incarceration or emergency hospitalization without care plans are not considered legal abandonment unless there is a previous history of physical abandonment.

THROWAWAYS

Some children, particularly adolescents, are thrown out of their homes by their parents or caregivers. They may be physically thrown out, locked out, or refused admittance to the home upon their return after having run away or after delinquent behavior. In some cases the parents or caregivers relinquish parenting and turn legal custody of the child over to juvenile authorities. The child's delinquent or incorrigible behavior is often cited as the reason for this action rather than the parents' inability to parent. These children are emancipated prematurely and abandoned with regard to care. They are vulnerable to exploitation, often wander the streets, and are totally left to their own resources to provide for their survival.

PARENTAL CUSTODY REFUSAL

Some parents are unable or unwilling to accept custody responsibilities for their children. The children in these circumstances live an uncertain existence. They spend days or weeks with different relatives, parents' friends, or even total strangers. The shuffling of children from one caregiver to another is a chronic situation and is usually based on the parents' unwillingness to parent rather than an acute financial or housing problem. The child's need for a stable environment is not met. Financial and housing difficulties, however, do occur among these families and can play a significant role. Each case must be investigated individually.

LACK OF SUPERVISION

Children who are unsupervised for long periods of time, who engage in dangerous activities, who stay away from home overnight—and the caregiver does not know where they are and makes no attempt to locate them—are in a sense abandoned. They may become throwaways later in life, or their parents or caregivers may refuse custody when these children get into predelinquent or delinquent activities. It should be noted that the problem did not begin at adolescence; the seeds were sown at birth.

EMOTIONAL ABANDONMENT

Emotional abandonment has been described in the backgrounds of many adults. As children, they did not form secure attachments. The parent may have been physically present but emotionally absent or unavailable to the child. Often these are severely dysfunctional families in which these individuals describe periods of emotional abandonment and overcontrol. Some experienced physical abandonment in conjunction with the emotional absence. Often these adults were sexually victimized as children and later by others, even their therapists. The dynamics present in these emotionally scarred adults can be found in members of other severely dysfunctional families where physical abuse and neglect occur.

The effects of the parents' behavior, through abandonment, leave the child in a confused, emotionally stressed state. The child's sense of trust in an adult's availability to meet his or her needs is severely shaken. This lack of trust may have lifelong consequences in relationships with others. As adults these victims may exhibit no understanding of what is right and what is wrong. They often experience difficulty bonding to their own offspring and may have marital problems. If their youth included juvenile delinquency, this can be carried into adulthood as antisocial behavior. Unless they receive treatment, a cycle of emotional and/or physical abandonment can continue.

◆ FAILURE TO THRIVE

Nonorganic failure to thrive is an interactional disorder in which parental expectations, parental skills, and the resulting home environment are intertwined with the child's developmental capabilities. An effective approach to this syndrome must consider the multiple etiologic factors involved.

Nonorganic failure to thrive in some instances relates to child abuse or neglect. This syndrome can be associated with maternal deprivation or emotional abuse and for that reason has also been referred to as psychosocial dwarfism. Nonorganic failure to thrive is characterized by physical and developmental retardation associated with a disturbed mother-infant relationship.

A high percentage of failure-to-thrive cases, where children are slow to develop or learn, involve victims of deprivation and neglect. Pediatricians must evaluate the psychosocial environment of children who are not growing properly. Often the reason given is that the parents were also small, but in many instances the parents were small for the same psychosocial reasons. It has been found that in children with failure to thrive without organic cause, the typical child's height is below the third percentile for his age and birth weight. He is thin and even emaciated. Pot belly, hypotonia, episodes of diarrhea, tension, misery, and cold, dull, pale and mottled skin are characteristic. These children are apathetic and withdrawn, avoid personal contact, and are emotionally and verbally unresponsive, often avoiding eye contact. They may have temper tantrums. Many appear to be insensitive to pain and have self-inflicted injuries. Some are encopretic and enuretic. Insomnia and disrupted sleep are common, with the result that they often roam the house at night, probably searching for food. Some eat and drink inappropriate substances from the garbage can, toilet bowl, or a dog's or cat's dish. Questions regarding their behavior in the home must be evaluated cautiously, because families usually hide any psychological harassment and physical abuse of children. These findings are summarized in **Table 8-1**.

With nutritional neglect or deprivation, the child does not consume enough calories and other nutrients to grow and develop at the expected rates. In failure to thrive the child is found to be below the third percentile on standardized growth grids and is not growing at the expected rate; he may, in fact, actually lose weight and show no change in length or height. In some cases the child may receive sufficient calories, but because of emotional deprivation he still does not thrive. This phenomenon has been called maternal deprivation or psychosocial dwarfism.

FAMILY DYNAMICS

Family dynamics have been researched in an attempt to understand failure to thrive. Although stress, parental skill and education, and personality each play a role in failure to thrive, parental interaction with the child, the family support system, and parental relationships are more basic to

---

Table 8-1. Findings in Dwarfism

The Child's Appearance
- Short stature
- Usually thin
- Infantile proportions
- Pot belly (with episodes of diarrhea)
- Skin dull, pale, and cold
- Limbs pink or purple, cold and mottled
- Edema of the feet, legs, hands, and forearms
- Poor skin care, excoriations, abrasion, and ulcers
- Sparse, dry hair with patches of alopecia
- Dejection and apathy
- May have bruises, small cuts, burns, or scars

The Child's Behavior
- Passive with or without catatonia
- Rocking or head-banging
- Retarded speech and language
- Delayed development
- Solitary and unable to play
- Easily bullied
- Gorging food and scavenging from wastebaskets, etc.
- Particularly notable—during their convalescent stay in a hospital they have marked growth spurts that relapse as soon as they return to their home environment.

The Child's Progress in the Hospital
- Rapid recovery of growth and liveliness
- Slower progress with speech and language
- Affection seeking, but may be shallow or even promiscuous
- Attention seeking
- Severe tantrums at the slightest frustration
- Rocking and head-banging when upset
- Remain greedy and scavenge food

The Child's Later Behavior
- Speech and language immaturity
- Gorging of food that may last 6 months or more
- Restlessness with short attention span
- Rocking and head-banging if stressed
- Difficulties with peer group and learning in school
- Soiling and wetting
- Stealing and lying
- Tantrums and aggression

the problem. Nonorganic failure to thrive has been found in families whose interactional style could be described as disengagement. These families have poor communication among all members, and there is minimal interaction between family members. The preexisting disengaged style is responsible for the lack of parental bonding. The pervasive lack of nurturing and attachment by the parents causes the child to respond similarly. The child develops a feeding and behavioral problem. Infants in these families adopt the disengaged style by becoming withdrawn, undemanding, and unresponsive. Thus the failure-to-thrive infant is viewed as the symptom of a breakdown in the family system.

Parental denial of the physical and behavior problems in failure-to-thrive children is significant. The more severe the family dynamics problem, the more likely the child will have an attachment disorder.

CHILDREN AT RISK

Children begin an interactive role at age 4 months. The mother-child interactional roles are defined when the child is between 5 and 12 months of age. It is during this first year of life that most children with nonorganic failure to thrive are initially admitted to hospitals, with 25% admitted during the first month of the child's life. These children are most vulnerable at this time, at the highest risk for morbidity and mortality.

Failure-to-thrive children can also be targeted for abuse if the family situation is left untreated. Failure to thrive requires close follow-up with the entire family by the physician, child protective services, and other health agencies to ensure the child's recovery and to prevent further nutritional and emotional neglect or possible abuse.

◆ FETAL NEGLECT

Included in good prenatal care are instruction in nutrition management, medical checkups to monitor fetal development and the mother's health, and education regarding the avoidance of toxins harmful to the developing fetus. Poor nutrition and cigarette smoking are well known to cause lower birth weights. In addition, fetal alcohol syndrome is a recognized result of alcohol abuse by the mother during her pregnancy. Heavy metal intoxication causes brain damage and adversely involves other systems of the developing fetus. Rubella is known to cause birth defects. The effects of illicit drugs, e.g., heroin, marijuana, amphetamines, cocaine, and crack cocaine, have been documented for harm caused to the developing fetus as well as contributing to inadequate parenting skills and interest on the part of the mother. Cocaine use during pregnancy specifically results in newborn infants with growth retardation and small brain size; increased rates of anomalies of the genitourinary, cardiac, and central nervous system; renal malformation; and cerebral cortical atrophy, among numerous other harmful effects.

Two issues emerge regarding neglect in the prenatal period of development. First, what level of responsibility does a mother have toward her developing fetus? Second, what should society do about mothers who ingest harmful toxins and injure their developing child? These questions are especially pertinent when the majority of infants exposed to drugs or alcohol are discharged to addicted families where they are at risk for further abuse and/or neglect. Opinions differ as to the rights of the fetus and the rights of the pregnant woman. The debate over this topic is unlikely to conclude soon.

114

The emotional relationship between parent and child begins before the child is born and is particularly malleable throughout pregnancy and during the first year of life. Research has shown that prevention efforts are effective at these early stages. Prenatal testing of pregnant women could accurately predict which women are at risk for neglecting their yet unborn child. Mothers whose children avoid them give descriptions of their own childhood experiences that have had cognitive distortions of their relations with their mothers. Mothers who have been rejected by their mothers may, in turn, reject their own children.

♦ DRUGS AND ALCOHOL

In addition to the physical effects in the developing fetus, drug and alcohol use is a significant contributing factor in the maltreatment of children. Parents and/or caregivers under the influence of these toxins commit thousands of neglectful and abusive acts each year. Drugs and alcohol facilitate the sexual abuse of children by lowering inhibitions in both the adult and the child. Their contribution to the problem of neglect is considerable. The purchase of drugs and alcohol by a parent or caregiver diverts financial resources, often a scarce commodity, from providing for the basic needs of the family—food, shelter, and warmth. Under the influence of these substances, the parent or caregiver cannot provide optimum care for the children. The level of care declines; for infants, the lack of care can be catastrophic.

The use of drugs in the home or trafficking in drugs has demoralizing effects on the child. Values in the home conflict with societal values, and this discrepancy can leave the child confused and unable to resolve the dilemma. The child may also be exposed to criminal behaviors or victimized by persons coming and going from the house.

The presence of illicit drugs in a child's environment produces the risk of serious harm. Children and infants may become intoxicated themselves through deliberate poisoning, passive inhalation, accidental ingestion of drugs or alcohol, or accepting drugs proffered by an adult or older child. Cases involving children who have been healthy but who seek medical attention with unexplained neurologic symptoms or seizures, children who apparently fall victim to SIDS, or those who die unexpectedly in other situations should be screened for the presence of alcohol or drug intoxication.

♦ THE EFFECTS AND OUTCOMES OF CHILD NEGLECT

Neglected children suffer hurts in their bodies, their minds, their emotions, and their spirits. The hurts in their bodies mend and heal, but the hurts in their minds, emotions, and spirits have far-reaching ramifications. Neglect of their bodies can be recognized through delayed intellectual development that affects performance in preschool and school. Emotional hurts can be exhibited by aggression and depression. When the spirit is hurt, the child no longer tries to succeed, instead withdrawing from life. The joy of childhood is lost.

DEVELOPMENTAL EFFECTS

The early years of life are critical periods of development for the child. Neglect during this time can cause development to stop, freeze permanently, or even fail to occur. The body, mind, and emotions of children operate on a developmental timetable that is individually determined. These developments cannot be put in an emotional deep-freeze or placed on hold while parents work through problems sufficiently to make it safe for the child to live in the home. Some families are untreatable or cannot be treated in time to meet the developmental needs of the child.

Each neglected or maltreated child needs an individual treatment plan to meet his or her needs and to heal the hurting parts of his or her life. All too often the treatment services provided by child protective services are parent oriented rather than child oriented. Services are dropped when the crisis appears to have resolved. But some children need help from the day they are born and still others may need a lifetime of treatment services. Unless we meet these needs, we will be failing our children.

LONG-TERM EFFECTS OF NEGLECT

The long-term effects of neglect reveal extreme variations in the child's behavior or illness. Extreme neglect can result in child fatalities. One-fifth of unexpected child deaths (defined as those occurring before arrival at the hospital or within 10 days of being hospitalized) are suspicious for abuse or neglect. Children who do not die from abuse or neglect may suffer long-term sequelae. The effects of malnutrition, for example, include lower intelligence, slowed growth, poor teeth, deformities, and life-long poor health.

Children who have been neglected have an increased incidence of psychopathology. They tend to be slow and cognitively impaired, have difficulty relating to others, and have an increased frequency of unsocialized conduct disorders. Adults who were neglected as children may be unable to trust others, develop problems with anger, suffer feelings of low self-esteem, have a decreased ability to form enduring, satisfying relationships, and exhibit impaired social skills. Mothers who neglect their children seem unable or unwilling to provide for the health, safety, or well-being of their children. In turn, their children have difficulty mustering the energy or resources to deal with various tasks. As preschoolers they are dependent, have poor ego controls, are negativistic, and frequently are noncompliant.

Another widely studied effect of physical abuse and neglect is the link to delinquency and adult criminality. Most studies link abuse and neglect in some combination. Victimization in childhood has demonstrable consequences in adult criminal behavior. While there is a clear relationship between childhood victimization and later adult criminal behavior, the majority of subjects do not demonstrate extreme behavioral problems or damage. There is a need to look for more subtle forms of damage in evaluating these cases.

Among the outcomes in those with subtle forms of damage, we see the developmentally frozen child or the untreated, neglected child becoming the neglecting parent in the next generation of the cycle of neglect. Whether extreme or subtle, the effects of neglect create unhappy, unproductive, and sometimes violent adults. The cycle can be broken through the treatment of neglected children and neglecting families as well as the prevention of neglect.

◆ PREVENTION

It is possible to break the intergenerational cycle of neglect. Primary prevention of neglect involves finding those at risk and connecting them with resources that provide supportive programs aimed at preventive measures. However, currently, most efforts in preventing neglect involve secondary prevention. Thus the system waits until a neglected child is recognized before efforts are made to prevent further neglect and to treat the harm already done to the child. Prenatal and perinatal predictors of neglect have been identified that could form the basis of primary prevention programs. Early diagnosis of attachment disorders, problem parenting, family stress, failure to thrive, and parental rejection of the current parent point to areas where preventive efforts may be directed to help both the infant and the family.

Truly effective programs addressing primary prevention of neglect are generations away even if we start now. However, if we treat the victims of neglect today we can be accomplishing primary prevention for a future generation. Treatment of the neglecting parent or caregiver can also decrease the damage at the present time.

Families are only one context in which neglect occurs. These families live in a society that neglects children. The social welfare infrastructure developed to offer support for families has been reduced or dismantled over the last decade. Many of these services reduced stress factors known to be associated with neglect, such as insufficient income, inadequate housing, social isolation, family discord, and use of drugs and alcohol. The loss of these supportive services has stressed families even more. Cuts in funding for education, mental health, and public medical care as well as limited access to this medical care have exacerbated the neglect of children. As stated earlier, the drug problem and associated crime have led to the deaths of children and extreme physical neglect. In addition, the economic changes noted have led to neglect in families involved with traditionally secure professions, such as farming and manufacturing.

The child protection system was designed to evaluate families and to provide services to aid in correcting conditions known to produce neglect and abuse. Yet it has not met the increasing demands for investigation, treatment, and prevention services that we have seen over the past decade. The result has been the loss of trained clinically oriented workers, decreased treatment capabilities, and poor general ability to perform the functions mandated by statutes. The impact of the cocaine and crack epidemic has overwhelmed child protection services as well as the foster care system. There is a crisis in the child protection system that now represents a national emergency.

During the last decade the issue of prevention gained legislative attention. Forty-nine states now have trust funds for prevention programs. In 1988 the funds for prevention programs totaled $32 million.

Treating and preventing chronic neglect consume both time and resources. It is frustrating to work with neglectful families, and success comes slowly, if at all. As stated earlier, some families are untreatable. Focusing prevention or treatment on the individual neglected child or neglecting parent will not guarantee that neglect will not occur.

◆ REGIONAL CENTERS

Programs or regional centers have been developed to address the unique needs posed by premature infants, genetic disorders, hemophilia, and learning disabilities. Many child protection workers feel that regional child abuse centers could concentrate resources and expertise to manage and treat child abuse and neglect more effectively. These centers can gather research data and information for prevention and treatment programs. Regional centers could be located in medical facilities or be free standing. A multidisciplinary center can bring together all the agencies involved in the investigation, coordination, treatment, and prevention of child abuse and neglect. In view of the current lack of funding in numerous fields, the regional center concept may be the most cost-effective means to manage the existing problem of child abuse and neglect and to further advance the knowledge base related to the problem.

◆COMMUNITY FAMILY SUPPORT CENTERS

Another approach that shows promise in providing the integration and coordination of services is the development of community family support centers. Several authors have urged the development of a single site for services delivery. Family support centers can be found in a number of states. Legislation in the state of Missouri has enabled the Division of Family Services to pilot a number of such projects throughout the state, and models will be selected for state-wide implementation at a later date.

◆SUGGESTED READINGS

Bays, J: The care of alcohol- and drug-affected infants, *Pediatric Annals* 218:485-495,1992.

Brazelton, T: Why is America failing its children? *New York Times Magazine*, September 9, 1990.

Cicchetti, D, and Toth, SL: A developmental psychopathological perspective on child abuse and neglect, *J Am Acad Child Adoles Psychiatry* 34:51,1995.

Helfer, RE: The neglect of our children, *Pediatr Clin North Am* 37:923, 1990.

Martin, H, and Kempe, CH, eds: *The Abused Child: A Multidisciplinary Approach to Developmental Issues and Treatment*, Ballinger Publishing Co, Cambridge, MA, 1976, XI-XIII.

Mayhall, PD, and Norgard, KE: *Child Abuse and Neglect: Sharing Responsibility*, John Wiley & Sons, New York, 1983.

Tower, CC: The neglect of children. In *Understanding Child Abuse and Neglect*, Allyn and Bacon, 1989.

Chapter 9

PSYCHOLOGICAL ABUSE

PEGGY S. PEARL, ED.D.

As far back as anyone can remember, Carol has regularly told Mary how lazy and stupid she is. Everywhere they go, Carol is heard telling Mary what she is doing wrong. Carol routinely tells Mary, as well as anyone else who will listen, that all of Carol's problems began when Mary was born. Carol has long complained that she couldn't keep a job because Mary was so demanding. When Mary entered school, she was behind her age mates, wouldn't attempt new assignments, and did not appear to enjoy any activity. At the first parent conference, Carol told the teacher that she had always recognized that Mary was lazy, stupid, and a troublemaker. Mary had a very short attention span. In third grade, Mary was referred to the school psychologist for depression. Later that year she was found sitting on the playground in below-zero temperatures without a coat, gloves, or hat. When asked what was wrong she said, "Nothing...," without looking at the teacher. Although Mary never complained to anyone, another student called the teacher's attention to the fact that Mary's hands "looked weird." The school nurse referred Mary to a pediatrician. Mary had frostbite.

Emotional abuse is the core issue and major destructive factor in the broader topic of child abuse maltreatment and, therefore, exists in all types of neglect, physical abuse, and sexual abuse. Psychological maltreatment of children and youth consists of acts of omission (such as ignoring the child) and commission (such as repeatedly telling the child that she is stupid), both of which are psychologically damaging. Psychological abuse involves the presence of hostile behavior as well as the absence of positive parenting techniques. Such acts damage immediately or ultimately the behavioral, cognitive, affective, or physical functioning of the child. Emotional abuse is a concerted attack on a child's development of self and social competence. It may or may not be a conscious act by the parents or other caregivers. Emotional abuse damages the child's psychological development and emerging personal identity. Emotions are primary to cognition and precede the development of cognitive processing skills. Hence, the assessment of cognition can yield evidence of psychological abuse. Emotional neglect can take place anywhere and may be relatively more prevalent in wealthier countries.

Psychological abuse is the most elusive and damaging of the types of maltreatment for a child. Emotional abuse interrupts the process of attachment, affective development, and the evolution of empathetic capacities. As a result of the failure to develop empathy, the child is impaired in his or her ability to appropriately receive and transmit emotional information. Some researchers feel that the lack of attachment, continual attack on the child's sense of worth, and failure to provide emotional nurturance, coupled with neglect and perhaps early physical abuse, impair the child's total capacity to respond emotionally. Alexithymia, an inability to consciously experience and communicate feelings, appears to be linked to human maternal deprivation. Because affective development precedes cognitive and physical development, early diagnosis and treatment are needed to minimize damage to the individual's development and maturation. This will hopefully reduce the societal costs of emotional abuse and increase the likelihood that the victim will live a full and productive life.

◆ FORMS OF EMOTIONAL ABUSE

Psychological abuse can take many forms. It is always involved in the adult's struggle for absolute control of the child. The younger the child and the less developed the child's sense of self and identity, the more serious the physical, social, and emotional consequences. Emotional abuse of older children with a well-established sense of self may have less impact than the same action on a younger child or a previously maltreated child.

When a child experiences the emotion of fear or feels distress, a parent normally responds with compassion and love as well as physical comforting. Such emotionally interactive responses are appropriate and form a core component of "attachment." When parents do not respond in this way but repeatedly respond with anger and rejection, attachment does not develop and the child experiences psychological maltreatment.

Psychological abuse varies in intensity from occasional to mild to extreme over a sustained period of time. Categories of psychological abuse are listed in **Table 9-1**.

In most dysfunctional families, children experience many types of maltreatment. In some families, all children are treated or mistreated similarly, while in others each child is treated uniquely and affected individually. The child's developmental stage influences both the parent-child interaction and the impact of the interaction on the child. The more nurtured the child has been before the maltreatment and the more secure the child's attachment to his or her caregiver(s) early in life, the less impact the maltreatment will have on the child.

Table 9-1. Categories of Psychological Abuse

1. *Ignoring* the child and failing to provide necessary stimulation, responsiveness, and validation of the child's worth in normal family routine.

2. *Rejecting* the child's value, needs, and requests for adult validation and nurturance.

3. *Isolating* the child from the family and community; denying the child normal human contact.

4. *Terrorizing* the child with continual verbal assaults; creating a climate of fear, hostility, and anxiety, thus preventing the child from gaining feelings of safety and security.

5. *Corrupting* the child by encouraging and reinforcing destructive, antisocial behavior until the child is so impaired in socioemotional development that interaction in normal social environments is not possible.

6. *Verbally assaulting* the child with constant name calling, harsh threats, and sarcastic putdowns that continually "beat down" the child's self-esteem with humiliation.

7. *Overpressuring* the child with subtle but consistent pressure to grow up fast and to achieve too early in the areas of academics, physical/motor skills, and social interaction that leaves the child feeling that he or she is never quite good enough.

IGNORING

Ignoring parents or other caregivers fail to acknowledge the child's presence or needs (**Table 9-2**). The ignoring parent is neither physically nor psychologically available for the child, either consistently or on an unpredictable basis. Ignoring is often part of serious physical neglect in which the child is not fed, clothed, sheltered, bathed, supervised, or acknowledged as being in need of these basics.

Case Example

Martha seldom if ever calls any of her children by name. She neither talks to them nor looks at them. Martha's house is spotlessly clean but meals are rarely prepared and seldom is there food that the children can readily prepare for themselves. Following a visit with her daughter, Martha's mother brought the youngest child to the emergency room, concerned about the child's lack of appetite. He was diagnosed as nonorganic failure to thrive. On examination of the other children, each child was found to be in the lowest percentile on growth charts, with abnormally short limbs, poor skin coloring, and extreme delays in muscle development. A visit to the school found that the oldest child was barely passing, had poor social skills, and was withdrawn and passive. Discussion with Martha revealed that her husband, Tom, is a workaholic, a very successful lawyer who spends long hours at the

Table 9-2. Parental Ignoring Behaviors
Does not respond to child's needs
Fails to stimulate child in appropriate manner
Does not look at child
Does not call child by name
Does not attach or bond to child
Fails to recognize child's presence
Shows no affection for child
Psychologically unavailable for child on consistent basis
Fails to allow child normal and appropriate privacy

Table 9-3. Substances and Maneuvers Creating or Simulating Illness in Victims of Munchausen Syndrome by Proxy

Psychoactive Drugs

Phenothiazines	Chloral hydrate
Methaqualone	Imipramine
Amphetamines	Amitriptyline
Barbiturates	Codeine

Drugs/Substances Altering Fluid and Electrolyte Balance

Excessive table salt	Phenformin
Excessive water	Salicylates
Insulin	Theophylline
Furosemide	Chlorthalidone

Miscellaneous Toxins

Pepper	Laxatives
Naphtha	Lye
Warfarin	

Other Mechanisms

Starvation

Suffocation

Fabricated history of previous diagnosis of serious illness, e.g., operable cardiac disease, epilepsy, various conditions

Inflicted vaginal/rectal injury to produce bleeding

Altered laboratory studies, e.g., simulation of cystic fibrosis by altering sputum samples, putting salt in collection for sweat test, adding fat to stool collection

Injection of contaminated material into intravenous lines

Putting parent's blood into child's urine

Removal of blood from child's central venous line

(From Wissow, 1991.)

office. His income is one of the highest in the community, from which he generously provides for his family. However, he spends little time at home and little of that time with his children. Even from cursory observation of Martha, she appears depressed and merely says that she misses her husband's company.

Studies of ignored children in institutions describe socioemotional deprivation so severe as to cause infant mortality of more than 33%. Most maternal deprivation cases involving infants do not result in death because of medical intervention. However, each year the number of failure-to-thrive cases is growing.

Case Example

Jane is a 21-year-old single mother of three children. She has had normal pregnancies, and each child was observed as normal at birth. However, each child now appears developmentally delayed and malnourished. Their skin is dry with little resiliency and a pale color. Their hair is dull, dry, and brittle. Their scalp is very dry. The children appear lethargic, as if drugged. The oldest child, 3 years, 6 months old, lacks language. In the doctor's waiting room, nurses observed the eldest child feeding the 6-month-old infant. The mother sat nearby, ignoring the children and their activities.

RESULTING CHARACTERISTICS

Once treated, failure-to-thrive infants remain apathetic and lethargic. They are developmentally delayed, both physically and behaviorally. After they begin to look normal physically, behavioral problems remain for children who were failure-to-thrive infants. They experience a higher frequency of temper tantrums at all ages, isolation, and socioemotional delay, and they commit more petty theft. They have been described as engaging in attention-seeking behavior, superficial displays of affection, selfishness, and spiteful actions.

Other physical conditions are linked to severe emotional neglect during childhood, including psychosocial and deprivation dwarfisms, sleep and eating disorders, and motor abnormalities. Studies of psychologically unavailable parents find that the children fail to thrive and develop normally. These children are both emotionally and cognitively delayed. One extreme form of parental ignoring is Munchausen Syndrome by Proxy (*see Chapter 7*). The child's needs are ignored as the parent attempts to meet her own needs. In this syndrome, a parent, usually the mother, fabricates symptoms for the child, or actually causes illnesses, that result in unnecessary medical procedures (**Table 9-3**). Extreme lack of concern for the needs of the child is also seen in the behaviors of the caregiver obsessed with the sexual maltreatment of her child, which is now termed "contemporary-type Munchausen Syndrome by Proxy." The caregiver, usually the mother, allows or requires that the child go through multiple unnecessary sexual abuse evaluations and pelvic examinations.

In addition to the physical harm, the child learns to live under the absolute control of adults who cannot be trusted. Children of depressed mothers, who were emotionally unavailable to their children on a consistent basis, show both emotional and cognitive developmental delay. The schizophrenic parent or character disorder parent also is in such need emotionally that she or he is consistently unavailable to the child. Ignoring is an act of omission, passive and neglectful, as compared to rejecting, which is an act of commission, active and abusing.

REJECTING

Rejecting parents refuse to touch or show affection to their child and/or do not acknowledge the child's presence or accomplishments as well as constantly "rejecting and demeaning" age-appropriate behaviors. **Table 9-4** lists parental rejecting behaviors.

Table 9-4. Parental Rejecting Behaviors
Refusing to allow child to get needed psychological or medical treatment or educational services
Belittling and ridiculing child
Purposefully and continually embarrassing child
Singling child out for criticism and punishment
Failing to allow child to develop autonomy or independence
Confusing child's sexual identity
Undermining attachment of child with others
Routinely rejecting child's ideas
Ridiculing or punishing age-appropriate behaviors as too immature
Routinely calling child "dumb," "stupid," "freak," "nerd"
Privately and publicly routinely putting child down
Inappropriately attributing undesirable characteristics to child
Continuing to treat adolescent as young child
Denying child's needs and making child meet adult needs
Making child perform household tasks because the parent finds the task undesirable

With an infant, the parent refuses to form an attachment. The parent does not respond to the child's behaviors to have basic needs met, such as when the child cries for food or with a wet diaper. Nor does the parent respond to the child's smiles and vocalizations of pleasure. As the child grows, the parent does not talk with the child or become involved in the preschooler's activities. The child is not included in family activities. The child may spend long periods of time in solitary play, often in another room with the door closed. As the child develops, the parent consistently communicates a negative definition of self to the child. The parent belittles the child and his or her accomplishments, both privately and publicly calling the child "dummy," "clumsy," "dunce," "nerd," and/or "freak." The parent has very low expectations of the child in school, telling the child that he or she can't expect to pass or do well in school, "because you are too dumb." The school-aged child or adolescent is treated like a small child and not allowed to act in age-appropriate ways. The parent does not acknowledge, or openly rejects, the changes associated with adolescence, including social roles, physical size, sexual development, or increased cognitive ability. The child is told of his failures and seldom if ever included as a valued individual within the family. The parent commonly fails to have empathy for the child's needs.

Rejecting parents generally appear overwhelmed by the convergence of social and economic hardships. Commonly, rejecting parents are reacting to large families, limited material resources, limited education and job skills, and few emotional and social supports, all of which stress the parents and limit their ability to nurture their children (**Table 9-5**). These parents feel materially and psychologically unable to move beyond concern for themselves to concern about their role as caregivers, teachers, and providers of emotional support for their children.

Table 9-5. Family Circumstances Associated with Increased Risk for Rejection
Unwanted pregnancies
No opportunity for caregiver to spend time alone
Lack of involvement by father in child rearing
Marital discord
Social and instrumental isolation of family from the community

Case Example

Jane feeds her son regularly on schedule but seldom if ever holds him while she gives him his bottle. She lays him on the sofa and props the bottle, telling him and others how much of her time he takes and what better things she could be doing than taking care of him. When she feeds him baby food she fails to make eye contact or talk to him. When she changes his diaper the only comments she makes are in disgust at how terrible it smells and what a mess he has made that she must clean up. She is seldom in the same room as the child and does not talk to him or play with him when they are physically near each other. She describes him as a "troublesome baby." However, other family members comment that he is a good baby since they never hear him cry.

RESULTING CHARACTERISTICS

Children who have been psychologically and/or physically rejected by parents or other primary caregivers are hostile and aggressive, have impaired self-esteem, and show either excessive dependency on parents and/or other adults or "defensive independence." These children and teens appear emotionally unstable and unresponsive, eventually perceiving the world in negativistic terms. They see themselves as having few strengths and skills. They view the world as being hostile and unwilling to assist them. They feel isolated and in turn reject others, including their own children.

ISOLATING

Isolation of children can come from a variety of parental motivations, but the resulting behavior prevents children from having normal opportunities for social relations with both adults and peers. **Table 9-6** lists parental isolating behaviors. Some isolating parents are themselves fearful of the outside world and want to

Table 9-6. Parental Isolating Behaviors
Not allowing child to participate in normal family routine
Not allowing child normal contact with peers
Physically separating child from family unit
Failing to allow child to participate in the social aspects of school
Avoiding physical contact with child, e.g., hugging, touching, holding
Routinely teaching child to avoid and distrust peers
Locking child in room, basement, attic
Punishing requests for interaction with family or others
Binding or gagging child to prevent interaction
Refusing, without justifiable reason, to allow child contact with noncustodial parent, grandparent, or siblings
Hiding child from outside world

protect their children from the dangers they believe exist from contact with others. These families usually have a very limited amount of social contact, which deprives the children of learning social skills with a variety of individuals.

Isolation is also present in sexually abusive families and in families in which ritualistic abuse occurs. The isolation is to keep what happens in the family a secret and to keep the children from learning that there is any other way of life. Other isolating parents are themselves without social skills and merely lack social contacts and/or supports and do not provide the opportunity for their children to acquire these.

Case Example
   Neither Maria, 14, nor Christine, 10, are allowed to have friends over to play or go to other homes to play. Their mother believes that other children will introduce her girls to drugs and other "evils of the world." The girls were taught at home until recently, when their mother had to go to work to help pay off some medical and home repair bills. Since entering the public schools the girls have not made friends. Christine has had problems doing group social studies and language arts. Both girls are excessively anxious about trying new experiences at school. They worry about someone taking advantage of them, and as a result peers tease them.

RESULTING CHARACTERISTICS
Isolating families often directly teach their children that contact outside the family is undesirable. School-aged children are not allowed to participate in co-curricular school activities, youth activities, or neighborhood play groups. Adolescent children are given home responsibilities and are prohibited from participation in school activities. Some families even remove children from school or do not encourage school attendance. Frequently children who have been isolated for long periods of time lack the social competence to experience success or enjoyment at school and therefore do not like to attend.

TERRORIZING

Terrorizing involves threatening the child with extreme or frightening punishment. **Table 9-7** lists parental terrorizing behaviors. The parent intentionally stimulates intense fear, creates a climate of unpredictable threat, or sets unattainable expectations and punishes the child for not attaining them. The discipline techniques are often arbitrary or beyond the child's ability to understand. The parent may tease or scare a young child in the name of humor, but the results terrorize and confuse the child. The parent disciplines the child by playing on fears that are normal for that age, such as loud noises or the dark. The terrorizing parent uses the feared situation "to scare the child into behaving." Parents may tell preschool children that if they don't behave the "monsters will drag them away in the night," or the night-light is "watching and if you're not good, the night-light will zap you." One of the normal fears of adolescents is that their peers will see them as different or that they will not fit into social settings. The terrorizing parent threatens the adolescent with "public humiliation."

Table 9-7. Parental Terrorizing Behaviors
Excessive threats and psychological punishment
Threatening and frightening child with guns, knives, whips, etc.
Bizarre means of discipline
Excessive use of guilt-producing activity
Chaotic behavior as to frighten child
Laughing at or ridiculing child when frightened, or putting child down for expressing normal fears
Punishing child by playing on normal childhood fears
Refusing to comfort infant in distress
Inconsistent and capricious disciplining of child
Continually threatening suicide or to leave child
Threatening to harm others in child's presence
Knowingly permitting child to view or be involved in violent behavior
Routinely engaging in fights and frightening behavior in front of child
Binding and/or gagging child
Permitting others to terrorize child
Failing to provide shelter, consistency, and safety for child

Case Example

Sam repeatedly has had his dad threaten him and other family members with a gun, a bullwhip, and a switchblade. He has never seen them used on a family member but regularly hides so that he cannot be found in case his dad comes home mad.

Resulting Characteristics

Terrorizing parents play mind games with older children. These games are designed to be no-win, where the child becomes very anxious, fearing the consequences. When parents place the child in the middle of arguments, as often happens in divorces, the child also becomes terrorized by the no-win situations. A child may be blamed for everything that goes wrong in the family, regardless of whose behavior is inappropriate. Constant criticism often leaves children so traumatized that they will not act because they fear they will be criticized.

Ritualistic Abuse

Ritualistic or multiple-victim, multiple-perpetrator abuse is the most damaging form of abuse. It is the systematic, bizarre misuse of the child physically, socially, sexually, and emotionally that includes some supernatural and/or religious activities by a group of adults. Ritualistic abuse is ". . . carefully integrated and linked with a symbol of overriding power, authority, and purpose. . ." such as a religion or pseudoreligion. In this type of abuse, children are routinely involved in ceremonial sexual activity with adults, with other children, and to a lesser extent with animals. Use of bondage, excessive threats, and force can be present. This activity is usually performed in front of other adults and children. Children are physically tortured, drugged, and forced to ingest drugs, human and/or animal feces, urine, blood, and flesh. They are buried alive in boxes and bound to crosses, and some stories are told of sacrificing children to the devil.

The children, as well as the adults involved in this activity, are removed from normal social interaction and activity and are taught a very antisocial value system. The "family" environment is one of absolute control by one individual. The children are told that what is happening to them is because of their bad behavior or sin and that they must be punished or they must cleanse themselves during the ceremonies. Children are constantly told that they are of no value except for how they can be used by the "all-powerful one," the group leader.

In ritualistic abuse cases, children are systematically terrorized into participation and silence. Initially the victim appears normal and denies any ritualistic involvement or multiple-perpetrator activity. Over time, when the child feels safe, the child is able to recall memories and begins to describe experiences to a therapist or other trusted individual.

The following are commonly used methods of terrorizing children to silence in ritualistic abuse:

> *Preschool children are given a "mock operation." The child is laid blindfolded and nude on a table. The stomach is brushed with either a local antiseptic or a very cold liquid. Then a sharp pointed object is used to draw an outline on the child's stomach. The child is told that an animal is being placed in his stomach, and if he tells anything that has happened to him the animal or demon will eat the child up to protect the secret. The child may be drugged to drowsiness before the "operation" and then given additional drugs to induce sleep. On waking, the child is asked what has just happened to check for effectiveness and to begin the terrorizing.*

> *Children of any age can be systematically programmed so that when they see a specific thing or hear a specific word they will "forget everything" they know or they will remember specific bizarre threats of what can happen to*

them if they tell. The word or object is usually something that the child frequently hears or sees, such as a postal truck or the word "light."

Children are taught to believe that others can "read" their minds to know what they are thinking. They are also taught to believe that "good is bad and bad is good, hate is smart and love is dumb."

SEXUAL ABUSE

Sexual abuse of children involves different types of psychological abuse. Commonly, children are terrorized with extreme threats and the excessive use of power and control. The adult uses extreme methods to both gain and maintain control over the child's mind. The child is told that if he or she tells anyone about the abusive events, the parent or perpetrator will go to jail, the child will be taken away and never be allowed to see family members again, the child will become very ill and die, or some family member or beloved pet will die. Victims experience psychological trauma from shame, guilt, uncertainty, and fear of breaking up the family. Not only do the role changes in the incestuous family not conform with societal norms, but the common use of sexual exploitation within the family teaches the child socially inappropriate interpersonal communication skills. Corrupting also occurs in incestuous families as the child is taught inappropriate adult and child behaviors that do not conform with community standards.

CORRUPTING

Parental corrupting behaviors (**Table 9-8**) teach and reinforce antisocial or deviant patterns that tend to make the child unable to function in a normal social setting. In milder forms, the parents convey approval of or encourage the child's precocious interest and/or behavior in the area of sexuality, aggression, violence, or substance abuse. In the more serious forms, the parents continue to encourage and reinforce as the child's antisocial behavior grows more intense and destructive to self, others, or property. Reinforcing or ignoring delinquent behavior is parental corrupting behavior.

Corrupting can begin with rewarding the infant for oral sexual contact, creating drug dependence, encouraging violence toward peers, laughing at antisocial behaviors, and continuing to encourage these behaviors as they grow more habitual and serious. Common parental corrupting behaviors include allowing adults to use their children for sexual activity including prostitution and child pornography, allowing children to

Table 9-8. Parental Corrupting Behaviors
Allowing and/or forcing child to watch pornographic materials
Teaching child sexually exploitative behaviors
Teaching child illegal activity
Knowingly allowing others to teach illegal activity to child
Praising child for antisocial/delinquent behavior
Positively responding to child's antisocial behavior
Instructing child in antisocial/illegal activity
Assisting child in delinquent behavior
Failing to discipline child for delinquent behavior
Teaching child that "bad is good and good is bad"
Giving drugs or other contraband to child
Exposing child to harmful influences or situations
Using child as a spy, ally, or confidant in parent's romantic relationships or marital or divorce problems

sell and deliver drugs, and encouraging drug use. In ritualistic abuse cases, often children reveal, after they feel very safe, that they were encouraged to have sex with younger children.

Parents who knowingly allow children to engage in any illegal activity are corrupting those children. Corruption is also occurring, however, when parents merely fail to teach their children the social skills necessary for successful interaction in the world around them and leave them vulnerable to learn inappropriate behaviors from those who would take advantage of them.

In families where parents are corrupting their children, the parents could be repeating the parenting cycle. They pass on the type of parenting they received. Parents who themselves have antisocial behaviors commonly transmit those values, actions, and attitudes to their children. These parental behaviors result from some events or series of events in their own lives. Research suggests that most antisocial and criminal behavior is a consequence of child maltreatment.

Case Example

Sixteen-year-old Katrina's mother has had a series of boyfriends living in the home for many years, most of whom have had substance abuse problems. Both alcohol and drugs are common in the home. Katrina tells her friends that she can supply them with almost any drug they want anytime they want them. She has her own car and no curfew. This year her school attendance record has been poor, but she has notes from her pediatrician, who is her grandfather, to "excuse" each absence.

RESULTING CHARACTERISTICS

Children who are mistreated during the first year of life fail to develop a basic sense of trust and therefore see the world around them as negative. They believe that people are not to be trusted or valued. These children frequently are taught that you have to take care of yourself—"take or get taken." This lack of respect for others leads them to have no respect for themselves. The consequence of corrupting children is that from an early age the children demonstrate antisocial behavior. These children have a pseudo-mature behavior, unlike normal behavior of age mates. They are "street-smart kids." From a very young age, they demonstrate few positive emotions and are unable to play in an age-appropriate manner. They often are rewarded for stealing and assaulting peers. As a result they are unaware that their behavior is inappropriate. Commonly these families devalue formal public education and fail to send their children to school on a regular basis or fail to discourage school absences, further isolating the children from learning appropriate social skills, values, and attitudes.

VERBAL ASSAULTING

Verbally assaulting the child with constant name calling, harsh threats, and sarcastic putdowns that continually "beat down" the child's sense of worth with humiliation is a type of emotional abuse. **Table 9-9** lists parental verbally assaulting behaviors. In the verbally assaultive family, words are used to humiliate and control. Repeatedly the child is told of the things that he is doing wrong without regard for what he does well. The child is often unfavorably compared with other family members or with downcast individuals. The child is regularly called derogatory names. The verbal putdowns and attacks can occur in the privacy of the home. Frequently, however, the child is publicly told what he has failed to do and how worthless he is. The verbally assaultive behavior is so pervasive in the family's functioning that child care professionals routinely hear the verbal assaults. These verbal assaults are usually delivered in a loud voice, which further accents their negativity.

Case Example

Phil is 3 years old. He had been developing normal language, but a radical change has occurred. The neighbor is worried; she hears Phil's dad continually telling Phil to shut up all of that chattering and not to talk when the television is on. "No one wants to hear you talk, we want to listen to the television." Phil's mom is telling all her friends, in front of Phil and whomever else is around, that he's "just retarded, can't talk, and the most awkward child she has ever seen."

RESULTING CHARACTERISTICS

As a consequence of verbal battering, children have a flat or negative affect, low self-esteem, and often self-mutilating behavior. These children are withdrawn and shy and have no sense of initiative. The children feel they are incapable of any achievements. They are unable to recognize positive social feedback when it is given to them. In some families, one child is scapegoated and routinely verbally assaulted or the brunt of routine family sarcasm while other children receive no emotional abuse. The scapegoated children are a high risk for failure to thrive, psychological dwarfism, childhood depression, and suicide. Usually, the child's physical appearance is one of poor posture and flat affect or excessive acting behavior.

OVERPRESSURING

Primarily a middle class phenomenon, overpressuring parents consistently have inappropriately high expectations for their children. As David Elkind described in *The Hurried Child: Growing Up Too Fast Too Soon,* many parents today tend to be more concerned about a child's intellectual achievements than his or her psychological well-being. Children are expected to perform intellectual tasks early to prevent being labeled "normal or average" as compared to peers. Instead of facilitating cognitive development as intended by the parent(s), this parental behavior actually impairs both cognitive and emotional development. **Table 9-10** lists parental overpressuring behaviors. Overpressuring begins when parents toilet train too early or attempt to teach 3- and 4-year-old children to read, count, and work on computers and continues with inappropriate "pressuring and hurrying" throughout the child's life. Graduating tenth rather than first in the high school class or earning an ACT score of 25 is seen as failure by the parent. The parent views the child's consistently coming in second in a swimming meet or a golf tournament as

Table 9-9. Parental Verbally Assaulting Behaviors

Continuous verbal attacks, especially in loud voice

Failing to protect child from verbal attacks of others

Constant belittling

Excessive criticism

Routinely humiliating child

Openly telling child that he or she is worthless and no good

Excessive name calling

Scapegoating child

Calling child derogatory or demeaning names

Cursing child

Continually yelling at child

Attributing to child behaviors or characteristics that are totally unacceptable to child

Table 9-10. Parental Overpressuring Behaviors
Excessively advanced expectations of child
Excessively critical of age-appropriate behaviors, calling them inadequate
Punishes child for acting in age-appropriate manner, calls it "immature"
Ostracizes child for not achieving far above normal abilities
Does not provide assistance with remedial work, refusing to acknowledge that child would need assistance with such "simple" materials
Refuses to provide age-appropriate experiences, insisting on providing experiences that are advanced
Begins toilet training very early and insists that child control body functions
Makes comparisons of child to those who are very advanced, consistently leaving child "poor by comparison"
Routinely buys toys that are far too advanced for child, with clear expectations that the toy will be used inappropriately, setting the child up for almost certain failure

not really trying rather than having done a "good job." The overpressured child is praised and valued for what is accomplished but not for just being himself or herself.

Case Example

Sara's parents expected her to be "Harvard material." She was expected to do well in everything, playing the piano, sports, and academics. But she was average. Her parents regularly expressed their expectations and disappointment with her level of achievement, her appearance, and her choice of friends. At 15, she was convinced that she was a failure and attempted suicide "to save her parents the embarrassment," the note said.

RESULTING CHARACTERISTICS

Parents can set high standards for their children and still demonstrate acceptance and love. Nurturing parents demonstrate positive feelings to their children, recognize their achievements, and convey pride. Overpressuring parents, however, fail to demonstrate that they feel acceptance, love, and pride toward their children. As a result, the overpressured child feels worthless, discouraged, lazy, unreliable, unacceptable, and inferior. The child feels inadequate or unacceptable as she is since her parents are always trying to change her. The child's identity is in terms of accomplishments rather than based on an appreciation of self. Stress-related illnesses are common in these children. Because they lack parental support and good self-esteem, they are more vulnerable to negative experiences. These children commonly suffer from depression and are at high risk for eating disorders, suicide, and poor peer relationships throughout their lives.

◆TOILET TRAINING

Beginning to toilet train too early says to the child, "you are not acceptable as you are and need to change." Often parents combine the age-inappropriate toilet training with terrorizing and threats of what will happen to the child if he does not gain control of his bowels and bladder. These children may later be seen in the physician's office with extreme constipation and/or urinary tract infections as the child continues to try to gain control of his or her "environment" by control of body functions. When children repeatedly hear parents or grandparents say, "Your dad or mother was potty trained at 9 months," they feel the pressure to be toilet trained but lack the muscle control. The children feel inferior because they are unable to perform as wanted by these significant adults. To the child this is a subtle but consistent putdown for not performing at the same level as the parent. When this putdown is combined with other forms of overpressuring, the results are frequently stress-related illnesses and excessive anxiety.

◆CAUSES OF PSYCHOLOGICAL ABUSE

Many theories exist regarding the causes and correlates of child abuse. The four theories discussed here are (1) the psychiatric approach, (2) the social approach, (3) the developmental approach, and (4) the ecological approach.

PSYCHIATRIC APPROACH

The psychiatric approach to psychological abuse of children assumes that the perpetrating parent suffers from some mental illness. Perhaps 10% of all maltreating parents are psychopathic or sociopathic. Studies of mentally ill patients show they are at high risk for failing to meet a child's psychological needs because of the amount of effort they must expend to meet their own emotional needs. As compared to a control group, psychologically abusive parents have shown significantly more psychosocial problems, more difficulty coping with stress, more difficulty building relationships, and more social isolation. According to one study, psychologically abusive parents described themselves as having poor child management techniques and being victims of maltreatment in their childhoods. The mother who is overwhelmed with her own depression and psychologically stressed after childbirth lacks the physical or emotional energy to give the child what is needed. The parent preoccupied with the death of a parent, sibling, or spouse may also be unable to meet a child's needs. Although postpartum depression and grief tend to be short term and reversible, they negatively impact the parent-child relationship and can adversely affect the developing child. Mothers who are psychologically unavailable to their children appear to impair both socioemotional and cognitive development of the children. Psychological abuse stemming from the mental illness of parents is one possible explanation but explains only a small number of psychological abuse cases.

SOCIAL APPROACH

Social approach theory places emphasis on the role of stress as a force impacting the family dynamics and causing psychological abuse. Nearly 60% of all abuse cases are associated with stress. Social stress interacting with other variables leads to aggression in the form of psychological abuse. The stressors for all families include limited resources, problems at work, death of the significant other, unemployment, health problems, overcrowding, isolation, substance abuse, high levels of mobility, poverty, and marital problems.

Individuals respond differently to stress. Women as a group demonstrate a tendency toward depression rather than violence as a response. Men as a group respond to stress with violence. Stressed women usually are psychologically unavailable to their children, thus ignoring, rejecting, or isolating them. Men, on the other hand, tend to physically or verbally assault their children. The family's socialization to violence determines if the father is physically or verbally assaultive.

Since all parents experience stress, the following mediating variables can assist in identifying which parents will abuse their children and which will not:

1. Presence or lack of appropriate coping mechanisms

2. Degree of family integration or isolation

3. Presence or absence of positive social networks

These mediating variables and the underlying causes of the stress determine the length and degree of the psychological abuse and, consequently, the amount of damage to the child's development.

DEVELOPMENTAL APPROACH

The developmental approach to psychological abuse is based on a theory that parenting attitudes and behaviors parallel Piaget's stages of cognitive development and Kolberg's stages of moral development. The stages require increasing cognitive sophistication and moral reasoning. At the lower developmental level, behavior is marked by immediate, direct, and unmodulated responses to external stimuli and internal need states. At higher levels of maturation, behavior is characterized by the appearance of indirect, ideational, conceptual, and symbolic or verbal behavior. Parents at the higher levels are more apt to use words and reasoning as part of parenting. Parents at the higher levels look at each child as an individual and at what is best for that individual. Parents at the lower levels are more impulsive, directive, and physical in their parenting. Parents at the lower levels parent from their own point of view and to make themselves feel good. Abusive parents, therefore, are parenting at their developmental level.

The orientations toward the parent-child relationship are egoistic, conventional, individualistic, and analytic orientations. **Table 9-11** describes the characteristics of parental reasoning at each of these cognitive-developmental stages.

Table 9-11. Cognitive-Developmental Stages of Parental Reasoning

Egoistic (Self) Orientation

The basis for parental activity and for understanding of the child is the child's actions in relation to the parent's needs. Child care tasks and parenting are seen as being carried out in response to external cues which affect the parent's emotional and physical comfort or which offer approval to the parent. Intentions of the child are recognized, but as a projection of parental feelings, and are not separate from actions. The organizing principle is achieving what the parent wants, and the object of socialization of the child is to maximize parental comfort.

Table 9-11. Cognitive-Developmental Stages of Parental Reasoning (*continued*)

Examples:

What do you feel children need most from their parents?

Love and attention.

When you say love, what do you mean?

Holding them, telling them you love them, making them behave so they won't get on that dope and stuff when they get older. I want my kids to feel proud of me. I know eventually when they get older maybe I'll fail, but I'm gonna try my darndest when they're younger and just hope they don't turn out that way.

Conventional (Norms) Orientation

The basis for parental activity and for understanding of the child is the child's actions and inferred intentions in relation to preconceived, externally derived expectations. The child is conceived as having internal states and needs which must be acknowledged, but the parent conceives of the child's subjective reality in a stereotypical way. The child is not seen as unique, but as a member of the class of "children," and the parent draws upon tradition, "authority," or conventional wisdom, rather than solely upon the self, to form expectations and practices. The parent and child are understood to have well-defined roles which are their responsibility to fulfill. The parent-child relationship is conceived as mutual fulfillment of role obligations.

Examples:

What do you feel children need most from their parents?

Love.

Explain.

Just letting them know you love them. Letting them know you care, that you are concerned about what they do, and just trying to be the best parent you can.

Why do you think that is most important, conveying that love?

Because if children know they have love, then they are secure.

Individualistic (Child) Orientation

Each child is recognized to have unique as well as universally shared qualities and is understood in terms of his or her own subjective reality. The parent tries to understand the child's world from the child's particular point of view and conceptualizes the parent-child relationship as an exchange of feelings and sharing of perspectives, rather than only fulfillment of role obligations.

Examples:

What do you feel children need most from their parents?

Love and time. They need to have their needs considered, that they aren't always happy with things that we do and with the things that we want to make them do and with the things we want to make them happy. You have to look at them and if they don't tell, you have to ask them. You have to really try to find out what each child wants and what is going on in his head.

Analytic (Systems) Orientation

The parent can view the relationship between parent and child as a mutual and reciprocal system and understand that the child has a complex psychological self-system. The parent can understand

Table 9-11. Cognitive-Developmental Stages of Parental Reasoning (*continued*)

that the motives underlying a child's actions may reflect simultaneous and conflicted feelings. The parent can also recognize that there may be ambivalence in his or her own feelings and actions as a parent, yet still love and care for the child. Individuals and relationships are understood not only in terms of their stable elements, but also as a continual process of growth and change. The parent-child relationship is built not only on shared feelings, but also on shared acceptance of each other's faults and frailties as well as virtues, and on each other's separateness as well as closeness.

Examples:

What do you feel children need most from their parents? I will say love and you will say to me, "What do you mean by love?" and I will say, "I think it is an acceptance, unqualified, for what that person is in time...." It has nothing to do with grades or cleanliness. I would like her to be clean and tidy, but it has nothing to do with love and feeling that someplace in this world you are loved for what you are by the people who know you best and nevertheless love you. I think that it is something that will help the children begin to love themselves.

What do you mean to begin to love themselves? Well, I think that people can be so cruel to themselves, "Oh, I'm dumb, I'm stupid." Words which tear down instead of build up. And I think one way to serenity about the way you are and the way you see the world, even if life is difficult, is if you can be gentle with your errors and failures and see them as part of a process. Then I think you will have a kind of stability and mental health that is a legacy from parents who love you unqualified.

(From Newberger & Cook, 1983).

ECOLOGICAL APPROACH

The ecological approach to psychological abuse of children involves all of the various aspects of the family's life, including what the parents bring to the relationship, the child, the social context of the family and its support system, and the total societal influences and values. The parents bring to the parent-child relationship various influences, such as how they were parented, their parental developmental level, their feelings toward the child, their knowledge of child development, their marital relationship, and their individual mental health. The child himself influences how he will be parented through such factors as health, temperament, ordinal position in the family, and other family relationships. Additionally, the support systems of the family and the total societal expectations are influencing factors. The interaction of all the influencing factors determines the type of parenting.

◆IDENTIFYING PSYCHOLOGICAL ABUSE

Psychological abuse, although the core of all types of maltreatment, is very difficult to specifically identify and diagnose. With careful multidisciplinary documentation, each professional can provide a valuable part of the total picture. Many young psychological abuse victims, especially ritualistically abused victims, may initially have few overt indicators. The complete picture becomes evident as the child feels safe with more professionals. The assessment of the child's situation begins with a professional seeing some minor abnormalities and then becoming more concerned as he or she obtains additional information. **Table 9-12** summarizes indicators of psychological abuse in children. Psychological abuse generally results in reduced cognitive and emotional function. Identifying reduced cognitive function is more easily accomplished than determining reduced emotional development and function.

Although both impairments are usually present, it should not be assumed that cognitive ability is always reduced.

Table 9-12. Indicators of Psychological Abuse	
Socioemotional Indicators	**Cognitive Indicators**
Impaired capacity to enjoy life	School learning problems
Refuses to defend self	Short attention span
Pseudo-mature behavior	Hypervigilance
Sexually precocious behavior	Hyperactivity, attention deficit
Lies notably when it is not to protect self but often in circumstances when there is nothing to lose by telling the truth	Language delayed
	Motor delayed
Cheats, steals	Lack of exploration and curiosity
Refuses to accept responsibility for actions; blames others	**Physical Indicators**
	Nonorganic failure to thrive
Psychiatric Symptoms	Slowed growth in trunk and distinctly short limbs, dwarfism
Tantrums	
Bizarre behavior	Circulatory problems
Low self-esteem	Accident prone
Withdrawal	Awkwardness
Opposition	Small abrasions that heal slowly on limbs
Compulsivity	Coarse, dry, brittle hair and dry scalp
Aggressive, defiant, domineering	Self-destructive both physically and socially
Controlling but lacks self-control	Eating disorders, anorexia nervosa, bulimia, obesity
Extreme behaviors	
Seeking love, acceptance, and affection outside of home	Gastrointestinal and bowel problems, including chronically loose stools, refusal to void
Pregnant adolescent wanting her baby to love her	Poor posture
	Reduced energy level, lethargy
Apathy	Catatonia
	Sleep disorders

◆ BEHAVIORAL INDICATORS

The psychologically abused child's behavior is characterized by a wide range of behaviors, including apathy, crying and irritability, refusal to be calmed, and avoidance of eye contact with adults, especially parents.

NEGATIVE AFFECT

Emotionally maltreated infants commonly show a negative affect to anyone in the environment. They also fail to grimace or show pain when appropriate, such as not crying after a fall or a shot. They don't respond as other children would when things such as toys or food are taken away from them. In situations where a normal child would cry or seek comfort, these children have no affect, appearing indifferent.

FAILURE TO THRIVE

In extreme cases of psychological abuse, the infant can undergo the process of nonorganic failure to thrive characterized by insufficient weight gain, impaired health, slow physical growth, retarded language development, distorted social responses, irritability, an anxious attachment, apathetic solitariness, and catatonia.

PASSIVITY

Abused children appear numb to either negative or positive environmental stimuli. If left alone with familiar objects, they do not have normal age-appropriate play skills and do not demonstrate normal pleasure and satisfaction from either solitary play or play with adults. They are excessively passive and obedient.

NEGATIVE SELF-IMAGE

Young children who have experienced psychological abuse demonstrate a negative view of their world and themselves. They see themselves as unworthy and view the world as a hostile place. They are fearful, angry, anxious, aggressive, and sometimes violent. They may engage in both physically and socially self-destructive behavior. They are often depressed, withdrawn, passive, and shy, exhibiting poor interpersonal communication skills. These children are often suicidal. They may frequently complain of headaches and sleep disturbances.

Children who externalize their feelings tend to be disobedient, impulsive, and overactive. They lack self-control and often are violent toward other people and their environment. Maltreated children who are aggressive exhibit a continuous and generalized aggression. The aggression is a state of being rather than a response to a specific action or individual. They behave according to impulses rather than social norms. Children who internalize their feelings are withdrawn, indifferent, submissive, and hostile.

ABNORMAL RESPONSES

Some psychologically maltreated children have low levels of social responsiveness or hesitant response patterns. They approach unfamiliar adults indiscriminately, seeking attention while avoiding physical contact with them. Other psychologically maltreated children cling to adults other than their parents and remain distant from peers. In both instances, the child's social behavior can be situationally inappropriate. In most instances the child is unable to respond to environmental rewards such as children asking them to join in group activities, smiles, and verbal praise. The child is often indifferent to positive feedback about his or her own success and responds negatively with social challenges or peer rejection.

Maltreated children respond negatively to parents and/or merely attempt to avoid the parent to avoid more maltreatment. The child may also try to take care of the parent's needs to reduce the instance and degree of maltreatment in the future. In the home, as in other social environments, the child may rebel and aggressively act out or may withdraw and attempt to escape physically or emotionally.

BEHAVIOR EXTREMES
Child abuse victims characteristically exhibit behavior at the extremes of the normal spectrum (**Table 9-13**).

Table 9-13. Extreme Behaviors of Victims of Child Abuse
Compulsively neat and meticulously clean, or destructive and extremely messy
Very polite, compliant, or very noncompliant and belligerent
Overly obedient, willing to do anything to please, or overly controlling, resistant
Socially very polite, kind, overly generous, or egocentric, revengeful, self-centered, antisocial behavior
Passive, or openly hostile and angry
Indiscriminately friendly, "shows affection" to or hugs anyone, or cold, indifferent, avoids peers, family, strangers
Overly obedient, helpful, "loving," or extremely disagreeable, angry, "purposefully hurts others"

These children have no moderation in their behavior. One child can be at both extremes on the spectrum in different areas of behavior but is more likely to be consistently on one end of the spectrum in all areas of development.

◆ CHILD AND FAMILY ASSESSMENT
The early indicators of psychological maltreatment should alert child care professionals to possible problems, prompting early intervention and treatment. Assessment tools combined with observational data from all professionals who work with a child and his or her family can give an accurate evaluation of family functioning. Most cases of psychological abuse are mild and will not enter the protective services system; instead the family in trouble will seek assistance with their own problems. If protective services and the courts become involved, the case should include professional summaries from a variety of professionals and an assessment by a psychologist with at least three of the assessment tools listed in **Table 9-14**.

Although many different professionals can observe behavioral indicators of psychological abuse, assessment for state involvement either by the protective services agency or the courts commonly requires that the case records include assessment by a licensed psychologist. The multidisciplinary assessment of child maltreatment involves a psychologist who has specialized training in administering developmental tests to evaluate (1) the child's cognitive developmental level, (2) the child's personality characteristics, and (3) the quality of the parent-child interaction. Most commonly used instruments for personality assessment include Minnesota Multiphasic Personality Inventory (MMPI), Rorschach Test, Thematic Apperception Test, and Draw-a-Person Test. A variety of instruments can be used for assessing infant, child, and adolescent psychological maltreatment and parent-child interaction.

Table 9-14. Instruments Used to Assess Psychological Maltreatment and Child-Parent Interaction

Bayley Scales of Infant Development (Bayley, 1969)

Tennessee Self-Concept Scale (Fitts, 1965)

State-Trait Anxiety Inventory (Spielberger, 1971; Spielberger et al., 1970; Rohner et al., 1978)

Child Behavior Checklist (Achenbach, 1978; Achenbach & Edelbrock, 1979)

Child Assessment Schedule (Hodges, 1982)

Table 9-15. Characteristics Common to Psychologically Abusive Parents

Psychologically abused as children

Stressed

Lack of appropriate coping skills

Mental illness, e.g., schizophrenia, character disorder, depression

Angry

Hostile

Ambivalence toward parenthood

Few resources (financial, social, etc.)

Inappropriate expectations of children

Lack of knowledge of normal child development

Marital problems

Lack of impulse control

Chemically abusive

◆ PARENTAL AND ENVIRONMENTAL INDICATORS

Most researchers and practitioners caution against overemphasis on identifying potential child abusers. Professionals, however, should be aware of parental behaviors and family dynamics that foster the child's behaviors that indicate that psychological abuse could be occurring. Emotionally abusive parents as a group share some common characteristics (**Table 9-15**), although nonabusing parents can also have some of these same characteristics. Because parents have some of the identified characteristics does not mean that they are or will become abusing parents, but it denotes the potential for abuse.

◆ PARENTS MALTREATED AS CHILDREN

Not all maltreated children grow up to maltreat their children. Parents who were maltreated as children, however, lack the role model of appropriate parenting and can suffer from lowered self-esteem, higher anxiety levels, and a more negative view of the world—all conditions that may have a negative impact on their child-rearing practices.

MENTAL ILLNESS AND CRIMINAL BEHAVIOR

Parents with a history of mental illness or criminal behavior, especially violent criminal behavior, are enough to alert protective service workers and other professionals to the possibility of child maltreatment. Many individuals involved in criminal activity corrupt and/or terrorize their own children.

PARENT-CHILD INTERACTION PATTERNS

A recent study identified the following pattern of parent-child interaction that consistently appeared in psychological abuse cases:

1. Verbal communication between mother and child was virtually one-way, with the mother using words as commands rather than initiating or allowing dialogue.

2. The mother repeatedly gave confused messages to the child about what was wanted; contradictions sometimes occurred within seconds.

3. The mother carried out activities for the child (for example, putting clothes on a doll) at the child's instigation. This was done without involving the child in the task and consequently did not lead to play or the teaching of skills.

4. The child was not involved in "doing things together with baby." The situation provided numerous (missed) opportunities for activities likely to provide environmental benefit for the child and also facilitate interaction between the child and her younger brother (Furnell, 1986).

Psychologically abusive parents, like all maltreating parents, have a negative view of their children and their children's behavior. This negative view of their children will be obvious to professionals working with the family. Some of the characteristic responses of abusive parents to their infants are listed in **Table 9-16**. The negative attitudes toward infants will persist as the child grows and develops if conditions remain the same. Professionals can observe similar parent-child interaction with children of any age. As compared to control groups of parents, the abusive parent sees the infant as purposefully acting in ways to "get even with" or "annoy" the parent. This may be due to the parent's lack of knowledge about child growth and development, as well as the parent's alexithymia and lack of trust of others. **Table 9-17** summarizes parental behaviors that may indicate emotional abuse.

Table 9-16. Characteristic Responses of Abusive Parent to Infant
Considered abortion or giving child up for adoption
Excessively irritated by baby's crying
Repulsed and irritated at having to change diapers
Describes the child in negative terms—ugly, deformed, makes repulsive sounds
Passive, unconcerned about child's needs
Disciplines—spanks, slaps, yells at—infant under 6 months for bad behaviors
Does not talk to the child
Tells others of disappointments with appearance, sex of infant
States that the infant does "things on purpose to irritate or to get even with parent(s)"
Not involved with child
Plays very little with child
Very concerned about how soon infant will have control of bowels and bladder
Calls the child derogatory names, e.g., little bastard, fart-head, freak

Table 9-17. Summary of Parental Behaviors that Indicate Potential for Psychological Abuse

Seldom shows emotions; when present, emotions tend to be negative

Routinely ignores or denies child's basic needs

Belittles child or calls child derogatory names in public

Consistently yells at child rather than talking in normal tone

Isolates child from normal contact with peers and community

Routinely ignores child behaving inappropriately

Fails to define appropriate behavior for child; instead punishes

Routinely verbally assaultive in public

Consistently demonstrates inappropriate expectations from child

Demonstrates a lack of basic knowledge of normal child development

Demonstrates sadistic behavior toward child

Threatens child with guns, knives, bondage, abandonment

Routinely humiliates child in public or in front of peers

Scapegoats child

Consistently demonstrates impulsive behavior

Routinely places own needs before child's to child's detriment

Consistently uses bizarre or frightening form of punishment

Teaches child antisocial or criminal activity

Knowingly allows child to engage in antisocial or criminal activity

Sexualizes activities with child

Consistently criticizes or calls child a "baby" when child behaves in age-appropriate manner

Begins toilet training very early and harshly disciplines child for "accidents"

Demonstrates jealous behavior toward child

Has diminished capacity due to mental retardation, psychopathology, substance abuse

Feels that his or her life is out of control

Has history of violent behavior

Lives in poverty

Describes self as "no good"

Lacks parental warmth toward child

◆CONSEQUENCES OF PSYCHOLOGICAL ABUSE

Consequences of psychological abuse vary with the child's age, relationship to the abuser, and level of development of the self at the time the abuse occurs. Table 9-18 lists some of the common consequences of psychological abuse. The consequences of maltreatment will become evident by differing behaviors as the child progresses through different developmental stages. When psychological abuse is combined with sexual maltreatment, the psychopathology appears to be most evident before puberty. Disturbances in body functions as a result of maltreatment are most evident in children under the age of 4 years, whereas psychoneurotic conflicts mostly manifest during paradolescence. Behavior disorders and psychomotor delays appear at all ages. Longitudinal research has prospectively related psychologically unavailable caregivers and verbally hostile caregivers to the development of child deviance and delay.

Ignoring and rejecting a child's basic needs appear to result in children who are destructive, impulsive, low in ego control, passive, low in impulse control, less flexible, less creative, and less persistent and who avoid their mothers. Young children lack the self-esteem and trust necessary to explore the environment or attend to cognitively oriented tasks. Since individuals view themselves as they believe "significant others" view them, and parents are the most "significant others" of young children, rejected children view themselves as unworthy of love and inadequate as individuals. Negative self-esteem and negative self-adequacy lead children to be less tolerant of stress, less emotionally stable, emotionally insulated, more dependent (clingy, intensely possessive), more defensive, more emotionally detached, and angrier. Rejected children in all cultures view God, the gods, or whatever form the supernatural takes as being malevolent. They believe that God is hostile and punitive and inflicts death, sickness, and misfortune.

Table 9-18. Consequences of Psychological Abuse
Psychiatric disorders—depression, character disorder, borderline personality disorder, multiple personality disorder, attention deficit
Self-destructive behaviors
Antisocial and delinquent behaviors, often violent
Increased vulnerability
Language delayed
Cognitive delayed
Fine and gross motor delayed
Decreased exploratory activity
Relationship problems
Low self-esteem
Negative view of self and others
Sleep disorders
Eating disorders
Maternal deprivation syndrome
Deprivation dwarfism
Nonorganic failure to thrive
Circulatory problems
Munchausen Syndrome by Proxy
Learned helplessness

INCREASED VULNERABILITY

Threats, trauma, or deprivation in a child's life increases vulnerability to other maltreatment. For instance, the emotionally deprived child is more vulnerable to negative experiences in day care than are children from enriched home environments. Children can overcome the experiences of physical assault or sexual abuse, provided they have been nurtured and valued by psychologically supportive parents.

EATING DISORDERS

Anorexia nervosa, bulimia, obesity, and other eating disorders in individuals at all ages are a common consequence of emotional abuse. The food behaviors of an abuse victim can range from refusing to eat or holding food in the mouth but refusing to swallow, to gulping food down, scavenging, stealing, and hoarding. These children are enuretic and encopretic; loose stools are common. Victims of psychological abuse commonly attach more emotional than physical significance to food.

MUNCHAUSEN SYNDROME BY PROXY

Munchausen Syndrome by Proxy victims manifest psychologically impaired development. These infants fail to develop a basic sense of trust in infancy and therefore are developmentally impaired throughout life. The children develop eating disorders, become withdrawn or hyperactive, and develop oppositional behaviors. They are passive and tolerate medical procedures. Older children and adolescents grow to cooperate with their parent's deceptions and begin to fabricate their own history of symptoms. The child victims of Munchausen Syndrome by Proxy become Munchausen Syndrome patients. It is very difficult to stop this cycle of learned behavior because of the extreme denial and manipulation that occur in both generations.

LANGUAGE DELAY

Most maltreated children demonstrate some degree of language delay. The more securely attached infants with better infant-mother attachment, however, consistently demonstrate better linguistic output and general language development.

DELAYED COGNITIVE FUNCTIONING

Maltreated children are delayed in their cognitive functioning. Children who have been verbally assaulted are less persistent in exploring their environment and have increased difficulty with problem solving and task completion. These skills are necessary for learning to occur. The abusive environment appears to encourage the development of aggressive behavior as an adaptive coping strategy. Cognitive-affective imbalance in maltreated children can cause them to interpret ambiguous stimuli as being threatening and aggressive. Maltreated children are more likely than normal children to interpret behavior as aggressive and respond in a like manner. This results in difficulty when interacting with their peers. Perhaps this can explain why maltreated children have more negative expectations of interpersonal relations.

ATTACHMENT DISORDERS

Parental threats to abandon the child and commit suicide can be seen as forms of psychological abuse, specifically as rejection, and can have pathogenic effects on the child's attachment mechanism. These pathological conditions can emerge as early as the preschool years and are manifested as childhood borderline disorders, attention deficit disorders, dissociative disorders, and childhood depression. Children of psychologically unavailable mothers tend to be more aggressive, less involved with peers, unpopular with peers, nervous, overactive, and lower overall in academic performance.

Psychological abuse of children as a result of mothers being psychologically unavailable appears to impair both socioemotional and cognitive development of the children. Interaction with their mothers is frequently characterized by negativity, noncompliance, lack of affection, and a high degree of avoidance.

♦ SUMMARY

Following psychological abuse, children experience impairment in all areas of development. The impairment can be minimized when the child is securely attached, when the abuse is not combined with other forms of maltreatment, and when the abuse is mild or takes place over a short period of time. However, in all cases some impairment occurs in all areas of development. The child's self-esteem is lowered. The child enjoys life less and either becomes withdrawn and passive or aggressive and hostile. Cognitive and language ability are also delayed. Physically the child's growth and motor abilities may be delayed. Ritualistic or multiple-victim multiple-perpetrator abuse leaves the most profound impairment because it is systematically planned, is continuous, and involves multiple types of maltreatment, including "brain-washing" of the child.

♦ SUGGESTED READINGS

Achenbach, TM: The child behavior profiles. I: Boys aged 6-11, *J Consult Clin Psychol* 46:478-488, 1978.

Achenbach, TM, and Edelbrock, CS: The child behavior profiles. II: Boys aged 12-16 and girls aged 6-11 and 12-16, *J Consult Clin Psychol* 47:223-233, 1979.

Bayley, N: *Manual for the Bayley Scales of Infant Development*, Psychological Corporation, New York, 1969.

Brassard, MR, Stuart, NH, and Hardy, DB: The psychological maltreatment rating scales, *Child Abuse and Neglect* 17:715-729, 1993.

Edmundson, SE, and Collier, P: Child protection and emotional abuse: Definition, identification and usefulness within an educational setting, *Educational Psychology in Practice* 8:4, 1993.

Elkind, D: *The Hurried Child: Growing Up Too Fast Too Soon*, Addison-Wesley Publishing Co, Reading, MA, 1982.

Finkelhor, D: *Child Sexual Abuse*, Free Press, New York, 1984.

Fitts, WH: *Manual: Tennessee Self-Concept Scale*, Counselor Recording and Tests, Nashville, 1965.

Furnell, JRG: Emotional abuse of children: A psychologist's contribution to legal establishment, *Med Sci Law* 26(2):179-184, 1986.

Gardner, LI: Deprivation dwarfism, *Sci Am* 227(1):76-82, 1972.

Hodges, KK: The Child Assessment Schedule (CAS) diagnostic interview: A report on reliability and validity, *J Am Acad Child Psychiatry* 21:468-473, 1982.

Newberger, CM, and Cook, S: Parental awareness and child abuse: A cognitive-developmental analysis of urban and rural samples, *Am J Orthopsychiatry* 53:512-524, 1983.

Ney, PG, Fung, T, and Wickett, AR: Child neglect: The precursor to child abuse, *Pre- and Perinatal Psychology J* 8:95-112, 1993.

O'Hagan, KP: Emotional and psychological abuse: Problems of definition, *Child Abuse and Neglect* 19:449-461, 1995.

Rand, DC: Munchausen Syndrome by Proxy: A complex type of emotional abuse responsible for some false allegations of child abuse in divorce, *Issues in Child Abuse Accusations* 5:135-155, 1993.

Rohner, RH, Saavedra, JM, and Granum, EO: *Development and Validation of the Personality Assessment Questionnaire: Test Manual*, ERIC Clearinghouse on Counseling and Personnel Services, Ann Arbor, MI, 1978.

Spielberger, CD: Trait-state anxiety and motor behavior, *J Motor Beh* 3:265-279, 1971.

Spielberger, CD, Gorsuch, RL, and Wishene, RE: *The Trait Anxiety Inventory*, Consulting Psychologists Press, Palo Alto, CA, 1970.

Wright, SA: Physical and emotional abuse and neglect of preschool children: A literature review, *Australian Occupational Ther J* 41:55-63, 1994.

THE CYCLE OF ABUSE

JAMES J. WILLIAMS, M.D.

Relatively scant societal attention and resources have been directed to the study of human violence. While societal awareness of interpersonal violence has been raised by various groups who have come forward and identified it in their own lives, children are largely a silent group. To this list of sufferers must be added children who are themselves abusers. Our ideas about human violence are flawed when they ignore child maltreatment and its links to human violence. Abusive children have probably always existed, and they are a manifestation of a number of tragic circumstances. Family violence and neglect should be among the most preventable of situations. This chapter will deal with that particular cause, describing the cycle of abuse.

◆ FAMILY VIOLENCE

Family violence is not entirely mysterious. To a large degree, it is predictable and understandable. When unchecked, its costs reach far beyond the tragedy of individual families. To the immediate costs of therapy are added the social costs of school failure, substance abuse, impaired parenting, psychiatric hospitalization, and criminal violence. These costs are more substantial for the victims but ultimately affect us all. Child protection has always varied with the value society has placed on the lives of its children. Successful intervention first requires recognition that abusive children exist and then a social commitment to respond to their suffering.

Though victims of family violence now receive increased public attention, the medical, legal, and social professions are still largely unaware of children who abuse other children. Revelations that children are battered or denied the necessities of life evoke contradictory and complex mixtures of denial and horror, disgust and fascination from the professions, media, and the public. It is even more incredible and unpleasant to contemplate that small children are the aggressors in situations of physical and sexual abuse. The response of the protective services system to young child perpetrators has been nearly nonexistent. The children remain essentially invisible, and society has great difficulty acknowledging them.

Historically, the widespread recognition of violence between family intimates is a modern phenomenon. Certain family functions, such as how children are disciplined and how spouses react to anger and frustration, have been addressed in western societies, exposing problems that have probably always existed. Paradoxically, the increased recognition has come in the same social context that minimizes spouse abuse. Child abuse exploded into public awareness in the 1960s and was championed by the child protection movement. In the 1970s, society became more aware of spouse abuse. Apart from the obvious physical differences between the sexes, social inequality explains why women and children remain the most vulnerable targets for men in family violence. Women and children continue to be viewed as being *owned* by the male head of the household.

Sexual abuse was brought into the open as incest survivors told their stories of unacknowledged pain. With the additional recognition of elder abuse, violence is now seen to span the generations, making the family itself the center of concern. Despite the progress in recognizing these problems, major concerns remain. We need to consider the violence instigated by children as a marker for assessing family violence. Ignoring the violence impedes efforts to protect children and to understand family functioning.

The home retains its aura of privacy for citizens in our society, making well-designed studies of family violence difficult to pursue. Yet the home is where aggressive interactions begin.

Reliable information on the levels of violence by children is particularly difficult to find. Several factors may allow this violence to be overlooked. Parents tend to ignore their children's violence. When society accepts sibling rivalry and abuse as normal, parents view sibling conflicts as a routine part of family relations, not as particularly violent. Many parents expect their children to engage in minor acts of violence as an inevitable part of growing up, and only intervene to discourage more serious conflicts. Parents may believe that rivalry and aggression prepare the child for the competitive world outside the home and enhance self-image and social competence.

Corporal punishment is another overlooked factor in children's violence. Parents who strongly believe in using physical punishment often do not recognize their children's violence or dismiss it as normal and routine. In homes characterized by spouse abuse and high levels of corporal punishment, young males may receive a double message: that their bodies are not safe from stronger males' violence and that it is part of their identity to be aggressive toward more vulnerable family members.

♦PHYSICALLY ABUSIVE CHILDREN

Despite the limited literature on abusive children, research has shown that they have a common background of family violence and/or neglect. Many have experienced coercive parenting, witnessed spouse abuse, suffered severe abuse or neglect, or seen other family members being abused or neglected.

At the core of child maltreatment is a breakdown in the parent-child interaction. Parents may promote childhood antisocial behavior through poor monitoring of the child's activities, little or no parental empathy with the child, and harsh and inconsistent discipline. No variable alone can be traced to the development of abusive behavior, but each factor influences the course of the parent-child relationship which the child considers as normal and applies to interactions with other people.

Brutalized by experiences with family members, the severely abused child incorporates these personal interactions into a deranged schema of the self and the world. An adult who learned as a child to blame herself for abusive treatment said, "Even after years of therapy, there's a part of me that still blames myself for what happened." This forgetfulness or blocking of the events, denial of one's true feelings, and acceptance of the intrusion of others' judgments is called "victimization."

Victimization is a leading pathway to human violence. The child's experiences may develop into a persistent and dynamic state of post-traumatic pain, which is central to the pursuit of aggressive behaviors. The rules of violence learned by the victim become crucial to the perpetuation of violence from one generation to the next (**Table 10-1**). At the time of the abuse, confusion, fear, anger, and sometimes arousal are too intense for the child to feel safely. To survive the repeated episodes of abuse, the child gives up any expression of distress and learns how not to feel. The child learns to accept the judgment of care providers concerning the experience of abuse. "My mother told me that nothing was really happening," one incest victim said, "so I remembered that my older brother teased me but I forgot the terrible things he did to me." Other survivors minimize the abuse they experienced. "My father hit me a few times, but I deserved it," a physical abuse victim said, "and I'm grateful that I was never allowed to get away with being bad." The thought patterns of the child survivor remain stable and firmly embedded in the personality long after the abuse has ceased.

Table 10-1. Social and Family Factors Involved with an Increased Likelihood of Child Abuse
History of abusive experience
Corporal punishment in the home
Being a witness to family violence
Lower educational status
Poor quality primary attachment with the parent
Poor parental supervision
Single parenthood and unwanted pregnancy
Other sources of family disruption:
Spouse abuse
Drug/alcohol addiction
Child neglect

With increasing repetition and severity of abuse, the child's emotional numbness develops into habitual cognitive and behavioral patterns that some have described as "soul murder." Harmful care providers are then reinterpreted, delusionally, as good. The delusions protect the child and allow him or her to survive the abuse and the loss of self-image. The delusion can persist and lead to destructive behaviors directed at self and others later. The family system perpetuates and reinforces the child's negative self-image, leading to possibly higher levels of violence.

◆ DEFINITIONS

Like abuse by adults, which has been studied for more than a generation, there is no adequate definition of what constitutes abuse by children. Despite the lack of precision, child abuse has been addressed from various directions—medicine, law, education, social work, sociology, and research—which greatly contributes to its recognition and treatment.

◆ PREVALENCE AND EARLY STUDIES

The biblical story of Cain slaying his brother Abel (Genesis, Chapter 4) has been cited as the earliest recorded instance of sibling abuse. Throughout the ages, many children have died as the result of adult brutality or neglect.

However, little attention has yet been paid to sibling abuse. Many jurisdictions in the United States do not even recognize sibling abuse as grounds for an investigation.

Children have many opportunities to learn and practice aggressive behaviors within the privacy of the home. Conflict between children is perhaps the most prevalent single form of family violence. Developmentally, all but the most severe violence decreases as children age, but aggression by older children may be more purposeful and severe than that seen among younger children. Conflicts occur most frequently when the only children in the home are male and they are less than 4 years apart in age. The high rate of sibling conflicts leads to the conclusion that childhood aggression is learned within the family and may be a characteristic of *normal* children, not just those referred for conduct disorders.

◆ CHILD MALTREATMENT AND AGGRESSION

Various concepts in child development and psychology provide a background from which to review childhood aggression. Fundamental to most formulations is the conviction that a person's early experiences are foundational and become internalized to influence later life experiences.

ATTACHMENT

Failure to recognize behavioral cues and personal boundaries is commonly found in physically and sexually abusive persons. Humans depend strongly on social supports for continued growth and development, which begins with the initiation of an affective bond with a parent. By the end of the first year of life, the child uses the parent as a base from which to explore the environment and to return during need; later, the parent is the child's base for developing social skills. Children who receive consistent and positive nurturing from the parent internalize these dimensions and will act similarly in future caregiving roles. During periods of stress and frustration, secure children can then remember empathetic attachment figures to regulate and label their emotional states. Conversely, insecurely attached children have an impaired sense of self and are vulnerable to recurrent failure in relationships. Such a child may become an insecure adult parent who believes that the physical protection of his or her children is impossible. To protect this insecurity, the parent may prefer to withdraw from perceived threats rather than face them.

SOCIAL LEARNING

Learning by modeling the self on others is crucial in human development. An abuser's modeling, reinforcement, punishment, and threats determine a great deal of what the child learns from maltreatment or neglect. Accordingly, children resort to violence after they have witnessed or experienced abuse or neglect and internalized its negative messages. A framework of retaliatory norms and strategies develops before they are able to reject what they have learned.

The basis for children's relationships is through attachment and interaction with the parent and later with persons they associate with who model and reinforce behaviors. In a sense, sibling aggression reflects what children see parents doing or neglecting to do for them and what they see parents doing to each other. Children at a pre-operational level of cognition perceive aggression and punishment to be the same. Parents, who may seek to curtail misbehaviors by severe corporal punishment one time and by ignoring them at another time, only add to the child's confusion about when aggressive behavior may be proper. The aggressive child evokes punitive behavior from the parent who, in turn, elicits a negative and frustrated emotional state in the child, further contributing to his high level of assertiveness. The pathology in the parent-child relationship must be discovered long before the child begins to abuse other children.

Neglectful parents can be unaware of what is happening between siblings. Children have felt murderous rage at younger siblings who displace them in the mother's affections. Unable to grasp the permanence of death, children have even killed younger siblings. Neglectful parents tend to disbelieve their child when he or she complains of being hurt or dismiss it as sibling rivalry, saying in effect, "you must have deserved it." Parental interventions, even in severe situations, are often ineffectual or nonexistent if their attention is diverted, for example, by an unwanted pregnancy, mental illness, substance abuse, or spouse abuse. Parents can be immature, disinterested in raising children, or feel trapped in their current situation.

Modern family life presents a less protective environment for children than has been previously assumed. The changing composition of the American family, with increasing numbers of nonrelated children living in the same household, gives new meaning to sibling rivalry and child protection. The vulnerability of children is increased when the parents expect the child to take over some or all of the care of younger children in the home during the parent's absence. Tragic instances have occurred when children, acting as caregivers, are too immature to understand how to parent. The older children may refer to their own experiences of violence and engage in destructive behavior.

Children's attachments and modeling progress during school age into peer group relationships. These contribute to the child's learning about empathy and social cooperation. Children in the third year of life typically begin to describe their negative feeling states through increasingly complex language. They are more and more able to discern another's inner psychological state along with their maturing ability to read social cues. However, abusive children have an inadequate basis on which to develop empathy, since they have learned not to label and share their distress. Instead, their distressing experiences have been kept out of conscious awareness. The victimization remains alive, however, possibly to erupt inexplicably in future situations of stress. Eventually, aggressive children's behaviors increase the likelihood of rejection by less aggressive peers, association with antisocial peers, and academic failure in school.

Aggressiveness is a stable personality trait over time. Critical contributions to the development of empathy and interpersonal cooperation are not made where there is parental and peer rejection. Aggression becomes a more likely outcome. Rejected male children tend to try to lessen their painful feelings by identifying with the aggressor. As victims who have become victimizers, the children are even less able to express feeling for the victim's distress.

The commonsense belief that "violence breeds violence" has been used by professionals to explain the origins of child abuse. Child abuse and adult violence are said to form an intergenerational continuum. Child victims carry their inner- or outer-directed distress into relationships with other children and, as adults, into the lives of their own children. Adults who resolve disputes by verbal or physical methods tend to use these methods in disciplining their children. Their children then tend to use similar behaviors in relationships with siblings and peers.

◆EFFECTS OF PHYSICAL ABUSE

The age and developmental level of the child at the time of the abuse have an important bearing on its lasting effects. The child's response is determined by how the experience is perceived. Equally important is how the abuse affects family functioning and the parent-child interaction. Violent intrusions challenge the child's most basic assumptions about personal safety and the world as a predictable place. Emotional exploitation, the background of all child maltreatment and neglect, attacks the child's basic sense of self as lovable and worthy of care. Abuse at an early level of cognitive development is more likely to be internalized to mean that the child is *bad*, a feeling that is carried into future relationships. Severe maltreatment leads to impaired emotional development, poor social competence, and deviations in cognitive development and character formation. Among the personal troubles experienced by children from violent homes are having few friends, receiving failing grades in school, and engaging in aggressive fights with family members and persons outside the home. As they grow older, aggressive male children tend to report that their negative behaviors are often directed toward restoring a low self-image. As adolescents, severely abused children may be institutionalized for psychiatric illnesses or have antisocial, delinquent, or self-destructive behaviors. As adults, abuse victims are at risk for abusing their own children, being abused by others, or having emotional disorders, criminal records, and substance abuse problems.

As violent behavior becomes accepted as "normal" by the victimized child, it is more available to him to employ against siblings and peers. When he gains greater physical strength, such violence is more readily available in confrontations with parents and other adults. The level of violence between children seems directly related to the amount of violence between their care providers. Child abuse may also lead to withdrawal and self-destructive behaviors.

Controlled empirical studies have shown the following:

—Abused infants, 14 months old, were more likely to turn away from their parent's attentions than controls.

—Abused toddlers, 1 to 3 years of age, avoided peers four times more often than controls. They hit peers, verbally or physically assaulted care providers, and were less likely to approach care providers in response to friendly gestures than nonabused children.

—Abused children, 4 years old, were more likely than controls to engage in aggressive behaviors with peers.

—Abused children, 6 to 7 years old, were more aggressive than controls in fantasy, free play, and the school environment.

—Abused children, 5 to 12 years old, were more likely to depict themselves as sad, unpopular, poorly behaved, and outwardly aggressive toward others than nonabused controls.

THE CENTRALITY OF VIOLENCE

Aggression develops at a cognitive-emotional as well as a behavioral level. Young aggressive children, compared to their peers, have biased and deficient patterns of processing social cues. They over-attribute hostile intent to their playmates, even when it is unwarranted, and they become less accurate in their attributions when they are under stress. They display far more aggression than they receive. Their bias leads peers to expect greater hostility from them. Given the series of inevitable negative interactions, their perceptions perpetuate a cycle of hostile attributions, aggressive behavior, school failure, and peer rejection.

Nevertheless, cognitive biases only partially explain the origin of aggressive behavior. It has been suggested that abused and aggressive children's deficits are conceptually similar to the inhibition deficit found in impulsive children, who fail to inhibit inappropriate behaviors that are more readily available. Abused and aggressive children can not only be cognitively delayed, but also develop along a deranged path resulting from early relationships and socialization.

◆ SEXUALLY ABUSIVE CHILDREN

Sexually abusive prepubertal children have been greatly understudied and are poorly recognized in the constellation of family violence. Yet the increasing numbers of reports of severe outcomes of sexual assault have forced clinicians to reconsider the nature of sexual activity between children. The position taken here is that children's abusive behaviors arise from severe prior sexual or physical victimization. Sexual abuse by children is the sexual expression of aggression, not the aggressive expression of sexuality. When these problem behaviors are present, they are among the few specific indicators that sexual abuse has occurred. Younger children who manifest extreme sexual aggression are likely to have been victimized in a preexisting abusive family context.

Why has sexual abuse by children remained unnoticed? In western culture, sexuality is not usually ascribed to children. There is little empirical knowledge of what is typical sexual behavior between children despite clinical impressions by many that it is common. Society has assumed that sexually abusive behaviors are perpetrated by adults so that what occurs between children is often dismissed as "just a phase." When adolescent perpetrators were identified in high numbers in the 1980s, clinicians came to realize that children may also be sexual abusers. Sexually abused children have similar adverse outcomes despite the age level of the perpetrator. Also, "sex play" has been misused as a cover for behaviors as diverse as "you show me yours and I'll show you mine" to forced oral, genital, or rectal penetration. Next, it has been assumed that sexual activity between children in the home is less serious than with contacts outside the home. Increasing numbers of sexual abuse have been reported in which biologically and nonbiologically related children living in the same home have been the identified perpetrators. The former distinction between inside and outside the home cannot be made a discriminator for abuse.

◆ EXPERIMENTATION OR ABUSE?

Doctors are often called upon to distinguish between consensual sexual play of nonabused children and reenactment behavior of sexually abused children. Children's typical sexual behaviors are age, activity, and culturally dependent.

Sexual behaviors may appear shortly after birth. Genital self-stimulation occurs in the first year of life as infants develop motor coordination and awareness of the penis or clitoris. By 3 years of age, most children have identified themselves as either boys or girls. Between 3 and 6 years of age, children become increasingly aware of anatomical genital differences, and genital play is common during this time. Usually, the play involves age-mates in some degree of undressing and touching in games, such as "doctor" or "house." This has sometimes been misinterpreted as a sign of earlier sexual abuse. The current understanding, however, is that typical childhood behavior is mutual and noncoercive in nature and in keeping with the child's developmental level (**Table 10-2**). Simulated intercourse will sometimes occur after viewing overt sexuality in motion pictures or in the home. More invasive acts, such as penetration of the genitalia or rectum, with or without coercion, are not typical and require investigation. During latency, sexual exploration continues to increase, although more covertly, within the peer group. With the onset of puberty, peer and family-related exploration diminishes and interest in sexual roles and sexual identity is added to curiosity and pleasure in motivating sexual contacts. In doubtful cases, an interview with the child may be most helpful in distinguishing the motivation.

Table 10-2. Consequences of Sexual Abuse
Age-inappropriate sexual behavior
Adult sexual adjustment problems
Being at increased risk for sexual victimization
Sexually victimizing others
Physical aggressiveness
Acting out
Conduct disorders
Self-destructive behaviors
Marked anxiety, fear, withdrawal, depression
Guilt, low self-esteem
Overly compliant, anxious to please
Dissociative disorders, split personality

◆ PREVALENCE

While the data on the prevalence of child sexual abuse by adults are unreliable, there are no data on the extent of child sexual offenders. However, it is clear that sexual abuse occurs in the lives of many children. Abusive sexual activity between siblings, cousins, and nonrelated children who are age-mates is considered to be common by many but is infrequently documented. While most of the perpetrators seem to be adolescents, we have no idea of the frequency of incestuous sexual abuse by children under 12 years of age.

◆ THE IMPACT OF SEXUAL ABUSE

To understand children with sexual behavior problems, we must first try to conceptualize the negative impact of sexual abuse itself. Sexual victimization can be understood as a combination of post-traumatic stress responses and socially learned cognitive and behavioral adaptations.

TRAUMATIZING FAMILY PRECURSORS

Sexual abuse often results from complex, pathological family interactions. Children become involved in sexual activity for a variety of reasons. Many children acquiesce to the abuser's sexual advances because the love, care, and approval they need are otherwise lacking in their lives. Their care providers may be physically or emotionally absent, neglectful, distracted by other needs and/or substance abuse, or sexually punitive; they offer little protection to the child and may have a history of being victimized themselves.

TRAUMATIZING ABUSE

The impact of abuse varies with the child's perceptions of it. Traumatic powerlessness occurs when the child perceives that his or her personal boundaries have been invaded and damaged. This can lead to severe post-traumatic pain and to later significant impairment of the ability to control aggressive behavior. Feeling in control of oneself is a foundational element of social development that is missing from the abused child's self-image. Male victims of abuse are more likely to turn outward in anger with antisocial and aggressive behaviors. They may define themselves as the abuser. "I wanted it," one male child victim said, "and I seduced him, not the other way around." Stigmatization is experienced when the child feels internally disfigured and shamed by the abuse. Betrayal is experienced when an emotionally significant person on whom the child depended for his or her identity, care, and safety is perceived to have caused harm. Traumatic sexualization occurs when the child's emotional growth is thwarted by the introduction of developmentally inappropriate behaviors. These factors result in an acceleration of sexual knowledge but at the cost of distorting the child's sense of intimate friendship. The victim can feel that the abuser owns his or her body. Male victims may become confused over sexual identity or attempt to master their pain by repeating the victimization on younger children. The *traumagenesis model* explains the multiplicity of symptoms found in sexual abuse. It points out that more severe symptoms occur in situations (1) where the perpetrator is closely related or emotionally significant to the child, (2) where the abuse is repetitive or of long duration, (3) when physical force is used, (4) when the victim is older and can understand what happened, and (5) when the experience involves oral, genital, or rectal penetration.

TRAUMATIZING FAMILY RESPONSES
The coping abilities of the child and the family have a great influence on recovery. Greater damage occurs to the child who lives in a family environment that is itself abusive. Such families are characterized by exploitation, coerciveness, invasiveness of physical and emotional boundaries, and betrayal of trust. Care providers can engage in coercive sexual or physical behavior toward each other, the child, or others, and they often lack empathy and functional interpersonal skills. Maintaining family secrecy is central to this family's value system. It is not surprising, therefore, that if the child discloses abuse, his or her revelations are likely to be delayed, unconvincing, and often followed by their retraction and denial.

◆ THE EFFECTS OF SEXUAL ABUSE
Children who sexually abuse other children are likely to have suffered prior sexual or physical victimization. Empirical studies find sexual abuse to be associated with a wide range of psychological and behavioral effects (**Table 10-3**). Some abused children are described as "wild" and "out of control," with their distress channeled outward into aggressiveness and inappropriate sexual activity. As with physical abuse, child sexual abuse victims are at risk for compulsive repetition of the abuse and loss of conscious memory of the trauma. Symptoms may also be directed inwardly and include somatic complaints, sleep problems, academic failure, running away, substance abuse, self-hatred, disturbed relationships with others, and inability to trust others and protect oneself. With severe victimization, self-destructive behaviors, particularly starving and cutting oneself, can occur.

SEXUAL BEHAVIOR PROBLEMS
Researchers have attempted to distinguish sexually abused from nonsexually abused children based on problematic sexualized behaviors. It is not clear

whether these behaviors represent reenactment of the victimization or premature and distorted activation of sexual capacities. Still, there are no reliably predictive profiles of who will become a sexual abuser. Not all sexually abused children will develop problem behaviors. However, it should be assumed that the abusive experience is so potentially toxic to developing sexuality that therapeutic measures should be taken accordingly.

SEXUALLY REACTIVE CHILDREN

Children with sexual behavior problems have been tentatively described as either sexually reactive or sexually aggressive. The sexually reactive child exhibits physically or sexually inappropriate behaviors reflecting the acute issues of recent abuse. The symptoms may result from confusion about self-boundaries. He may be a toddler, for example, who engages in increased masturbation, sexual exploration, exposure of genitals, sexualized play, or inviting others to become inappropriately sexually involved. These behaviors may have elements of aggressiveness, but they are noncoercive in nature. Generally, they reflect a sexualization of activities only, and do not imply an underlying psychopathology. The frequency of these behaviors is not known because care providers may minimize them as transitory or "sex play."

Table 10-3. Criteria for Defining Sexual Abuse Between Children

Sexual contact between children may be considered inappropriate or abusive in the presence of any of these conditions:

1. Sexual activity between children who are not of a similar age (within 5 years) or developmental level.

2. Sexual activity that is not consistent with the developmental level of the child.

3. Sexual activity in which force or threats are used.

4. Sexual activity between children in which there is outside influence from another, older individual.

5. Sexual activity that results in documented injury or predominantly negative feelings in the victim.

SEXUALLY ABUSIVE CHILDREN

Other children are referred to therapy because of behaviors that far exceed those typical of sex play. These behaviors involve overt and often coercive sexual activity. The child's aggressiveness has been firmly entrenched for some time. It has been maintained by ongoing abuse, by caregivers who treat the child like a scapegoat, and by a neglectful family environment. Children whose sexual behavior is driven by anger, depression, and anxiety are often male and their history of sexual abuse is severe and prolonged. Typically, they have been victimized repeatedly, often by multiple perpetrators. They also frequently have a preexisting physical abuse history. Less severe behavior problems, rejection by peers, and failure in school may occur before the sexually coercive behaviors toward other children become obvious.

The proportion of male to female sexually abusive children parallels that of adult sex abusers. Most of the reported offenders are boys. Girls, however, seem to suffer more abuse or neglect before becoming sexually abusive themselves. However, girls are less likely to follow the path toward abusing other children.

A high degree of personal and parental psychopathology, predating their abuse of other children, has also been associated with sexually abusive children. Even nonabusive parents of these children show a high rate of depression and substance abuse and often covertly reinforce the children's aggressive behavior by labeling them as *bad*, categorizing them as being the same as offending adults. Family issues center on inconsistent and neglectful parenting and lack of empathy.

♦ ABUSED-TO-ABUSER CYCLE

Research is leading clinicians to speculate on the possibility that there exists a cycle of violence for victims of physical and sexual abuse. Sexual abuse in childhood appears to increase the risk for later sexual aggression, probably for the more severely traumatized children. The greater the trauma of the abuse, the more likely the experience will be deflected from awareness, perhaps to reappear as abusive activity in the future. Studies of sex offenders have revealed that many began their activities in mid-childhood after being sexually molested. Sexual abuse as a child and the later development of juvenile delinquency and/or adult criminality have also been associated. Boys who are physically and sexually abused, unsupported in disclosing the abuse, and socially rejected are more likely to become delinquent or criminal than boys from supportive families. Many adult sex offenders may have been sexually abused in adolescence even before puberty.

Although the limited research cannot reliably predict who will become abusive, there is ample evidence of the damaging influence of abuse. While little direct evidence exists for an intergenerational transmission of sexual abuse, the complex traumatic components of child maltreatment are clearly associated with the behavioral symptoms, especially the physical and sexual aggressiveness of abused children.

♦ FACTORS IN ALTERING THE CYCLE OF ABUSE

Maltreated or neglected children are not necessarily predestined to develop into sexually or physically offending adults. The actual transmission rate of physical abuse is estimated as 30% to 50%. Although 30% is six times the rate of abuse in the general population, the implication is that most abused children escape at least the severe outcomes of the cycle and do not come to official attention.

Clinical research is not so naive as to attempt to prove direct causality in the cycle of violence. The child copes not only with the effects of victimization or witnessing family violence, but violence also results from the multiple family changes it sets in motion. These effects include (1) reduced maternal parenting effectiveness, (2) increased family dysfunction, and (3) increased (male) child aggressiveness as a result of modeling an abusive parent's behavior. As the child's efforts to cope with the violence place greater strain on the parents' relationship, a vicious cycle is set in motion. Similarly, mental health professionals' efforts at therapeutic interventions to correct a child's deviant aggressive behavior have often been undermined by continuing spouse abuse.

The relationship between trauma and an aggressive outcome is not straight-forward. Clinical experience has shown that variables within individuals, the family, and the social environment modify and buffer its impact. They include good cognitive abilities, absence of major psychopathology, and available nonabusing adults and peers.

A negative self-image, derived from early abusive relationships, is carried forward unless it is interrupted. Children who are given a chance to make sense of their abuse with a nonabusing adult are less likely to repeat the patterns of victimization in their later lives. The same is true in abuse prevention for adults who have a high risk of abusing their children. Parents who became abusive have had neither a supportive adult available during their childhood nor extensive psychological counseling at any time during their lives. Therefore, the availability of alternate relationships is important in interrupting the cycle of abuse.

◆ TREATMENT PERSPECTIVES

The family's response to the physically or sexually aggressive child is critical for the success of treatment. Parent training in how to respond to the child's sexual behaviors and a peer support group may be all that is needed for the child who is reactive to abuse. Parents who deal in a consistent and caring manner with the recently molested child, who is acting with increased masturbation, for example, will go far in eliminating the behavior by helping him to understand the proper boundaries regarding touching. On the other hand, parents who view the child as a scapegoat or as *damaged goods* add to his or her trauma.

Sexually or physically abusive children present far greater challenges. Their behaviors are more firmly established than those who have been abused but do not act aggressively. Typically, their families possess few, if any, mitigating resources. While therapy may start with small and easily achievable goals, there are larger patterns of failure requiring attention, including parent training, social competence and peer relations, and academic performance. Both parents and child need intense behavioral, cognitive, and affective therapy. Therapy must be based on such factors as the child's developmental age at the onset of the abuse, the age at which the child's aggressions began, the duration of the behaviors, and prior efforts at intervention. It is also necessary to evaluate all siblings for collateral abuse and their need for treatment.

Foster home placement, while sometimes necessary, is insufficient to treat the emotional damage of abusive children. Abused children in foster placement can display as much physical aggression as abused children in their natural homes. Foster care may be inadequate to reduce the level of aggression and problems at school.

Family system failure must also be addressed. The families of sexually aggressive children often have a long history of coercive interactions and inconsistent parenting. Their response to the child's aggressive behaviors has often been inappropriate or even encouraging. Greater assistance from local protective service agencies is needed to involve the parents in the treatment of their abusive children. Many are wary of or indifferent to professional involvement. Without an official agency's firm support, the parents often do not follow through and bring the child to treatment. Therapy will take a long period of time. Parents do not realize the length of the commitment nor do they have the energy or interest to invest in it.

Therapeutic intervention involves alternate adult and peer models of social interaction for the children and their parents. Integrating abused children into programs with normal peers and parents into support groups aids with more appropriate behavior models. Research is greatly needed in this area.

◆ SUGGESTED READINGS

Bandura, A: *Aggression: A Social Learning Analysis*, Prentice-Hall, Englewood Cliffs, NJ, 1973.

Bank, SP, and Kahn, MD: *The Sibling Bond*, Basic Books, New York, 1982.

Ben-Aron, MH, Hucker, SJ, and Webster, CD, eds: *Clinical Criminology: Current Concepts*, M&M Graphics, Toronto, 1985.

Bender, L, ed: *Aggression, Hostility, and Anxiety in Children*, Charles C Thomas, Publisher, Springfield, IL, 1953.

Burr, WR, Hill, R, Nye, FI, and Reiss, IL, eds: *Contemporary Theories About the Family*, Volume 1, Free Press, New York, 1979.

DeMause, L: *The History of Childhood*, Harper & Row, Publishers, New York, 1974.

Elmer, E: *Children in Jeopardy*, University of Pittsburgh Press, Pittsburgh, PA, 1967.

Finkelhor, D: *Sexually Victimized Children*, Free Press, New York, 1979.

Fontana, V.: *Somewhere A Child Is Crying*, Macmillan Publishing Co, Inc, New York, 1973.

Freud, S: *Beyond the Pleasure Principle*, Volume 18 (Strachey, J, ed and trans), Hogarth, London, 1920/1955.

Gerber, G, Ross, C, and Zeigler, E, eds: *Child Abuse: An Agenda for Action*, Oxford University Press, New York, 1980.

Wyatt, GE, and Powell, GJ, eds: *The Lasting Effects of Child Sexual Abuse*, Sage Publications, Newbury Park, CA, 1988.

Chapter 11

THE ROLE OF LAW ENFORCEMENT IN THE INVESTIGATION OF CHILD MALTREATMENT

Gus H. Kolilis, B.S., Education

Technically, the role of law enforcement in the investigation of child maltreatment is clear. The abuse, neglect, and exploitation of children is a crime. Police officers report and investigate crime; however, the investigation of crimes involving children and families is only a sliver of law enforcement's overall responsibilities. Other than in the largest departments, there are very few police officers dedicated to the investigation of children's events. The lack of specialized training and experience in very difficult and complicated cases contributes to the ongoing dilemma of how to prove or disprove allegations or suspicions of child maltreatment. Formal multi-disciplinary teams of police officers, medical personnel, and social workers provide an efficient and effective approach to these very complex and emotional cases.

All investigations begin with a suspicion or allegation. Most reports of crime to police departments are by victims eager to provide details and information. Adult reporters generally hope that the investigation of the event reported will be successful. The police officers taking these reports usually can initiate effective and appropriate actions with a reasonable expectation of solving the crime. However, crimes against children are considerably different from crimes involving adult victims. The report or disclosure of the event is seldom deliberate. As a rule, children do not report being abused. Depending on the child's age and developmental level, he may not understand what has happened or even the fact that he was abused. Many child victims are confused, afraid, and intimidated. Infants and very young children may lack the ability to comprehend or communicate what has occurred. In addition, in many cases, the systems in place to protect children and investigate and prosecute offenders are complicated and ineffective. Child abuse investigations are among the most difficult cases handled by law enforcement agencies. In fact, children can be perfect victims, for the following reasons:

1. Because of their physical, mental, and emotional development, children are usually unable to "protect" themselves from abuse, neglect, and exploitation.

2. The crimes are usually conducted in a private place, in a one-on-one setting, meaning there are no witnesses and no accomplices.

3. Defendants in such cases usually do not brag about their crimes, so, unlike with other criminal activity, they are unlikely to be informed on by others.

4. Children are often viewed as less credible or competent than the suspected adult offender.

5. Communities are in denial of the problem. People do not want to get involved, or they don't want the negative publicity to reflect on their community.

6. Interviews of children require special training, understanding, and patience.

7. For many reasons, children do not tell about abuse or the disclosure is delayed and/or delivered piecemeal over an extended period of time.

8. Children often do not want the offender punished; they may only want the abuse to stop. They may not even understand that they are being abused.

9. Crimes against children are not isolated incidents. They take place over a period of time and may involve multiple victims.

10. Crimes of abuse often have no physical or medical evidence. If such evidence does exist, it does not necessarily prove who the suspect is.

11. Child maltreatment cases often involve concurrent civil, criminal, and sometimes administrative investigations that result in investigative conflicts and obstructions.

12. Cases often cross jurisdictional and political boundaries, making determination of venue difficult.

13. The criminal justice system was not designed with the special needs of children considered. Children may be frightened and intimidated by the court room/trial process.

14. Child abuse and neglect crimes are often investigated by personnel with little specialized training or experience in dealing with children's events.

Initiating an investigation of suspected child maltreatment begins with a clear allegation. The abuse may be physical, sexual, emotional, or involve some form of neglect. It is the responsibility of the investigator(s) to use every legal means to validate the allegation by collecting verifiable evidence and information to prove or disprove that the crime has occurred. The majority of information is collected by interviewing the victim(s), witness(es), expert(s), and suspect(s). How these interviews and interrogations are conducted will, in large part, determine the ultimate outcome of the investigation, which will, in turn, determine what interventions are needed to protect the interests of the child victim. It may also identify other children at risk, as well as crimes not directly associated with the allegation.

♦ INTERVIEW GUIDELINES

GENERAL INTERVIEW PREPARATION

An interview is simply the process of one person obtaining information from another by a question-and-answer method. It is important to gather all available case and background information pertinent to the nature of the interview. If necessary, revisit the scene and review photographs. Make sure you know the offense and what happened to the victim. Never assume guilt or innocence. Every event should be evaluated and investigated on its own merit.

All persons interviewed must be properly identified in your notes and reports. Ensure that the following are documented:

- Correct spelling of person's name

- Date of birth and Social Security number

- Home address—apartment number, floor, and location (front or rear)

- Telephone number—both home and work

- Secondary contact person—name, address, telephone numbers—both home and work

Attempt to conduct the interview(s) away from other victims, witnesses, or suspected perpetrator(s). Suggested sites include:

- A place convenient and familiar to the subject.

- A neutral setting—the two most undesirable places for a victim or witness interview are where the alleged abuse took place (especially for the victim) and at the police station. However, the police station is an appropriate place to interview the suspected perpetrator(s).

- With a child interview, any place that is child friendly—where privacy is assured—is appropriate.

Interviews should take place as soon as possible after the event has occurred so that witness' statements are not affected by memory loss, by talking to others, etc. One person should conduct all interviews, if possible. Remember to communicate thoughts clearly and accurately. Do not display bias in nonverbal communications, and, above all, be professional.

Determine what information is to be obtained from the person being interviewed. Stay focused on the injury/event being investigated. Keep in mind the alleged offense when directing questions. When formulating questions, follow these guidelines:

- Keep questions short, clear, and easily understood.

- Confine questions to one topic at a time.

- Avoid "yes," "no," and leading questions that begin with "did" or "does."

- Use comparison-type questions to pinpoint details.

Even though each interview is unique, there are seven general steps to conducting any interview:

1. Develop interview objectives (what needs to be known).

2. Use an introduction and warm-up.

3. Use the opening statement to set the tone of the interview.

4. Ask what happened and then **listen.**

5. Start over and get specific details (including what occurred before, during, and after the injury/event).

6. Obtain any other information required for the investigation.

7. Bring the interview to a conclusion.

◆ THE VICTIM INTERVIEW

When interviewing a child, remember both the developmental level and communicative abilities of the child and the circumstances surrounding the interview. Be aware of young children's eating and sleep schedules. Do not interview them if they are hungry, sleepy, or otherwise physically uncomfortable. Minimize the size differential between you and the child by getting on the same physical level. Interviewing tools (such as dolls, drawings, paper, crayons, doll house, etc.) may be used, but should not detract from the interview. Only use such tools if you have received proper training. Allow for sufficient time to conduct the interview. Assure the child that she is not in any trouble.

Information gained before the interview should help you relate to the child on his developmental level. Keep questions and sentences simple, using words that are familiar to the child. Use the child's words for body parts. Do not assume that your meaning of a word is the same as the child's. Be careful using pronouns (like he or she) and words like "there" and "that." The child may be unable to follow your meaning. Tell the child it is okay to answer "I don't know" or "I don't understand" rather than guess.

Ask questions that encourage the child to give more than a "yes" or "no" answer. Avoid leading questions that start with "did" or "does." Most of all, avoid "why" questions; they imply blame or identify a specific person. Reassure the child that she is believed and that she is not at fault for what happened.

Be aware of the child's nonverbal communication and allow him plenty of time to respond to any question asked. Be careful of your own nonverbal communication (i.e., touching, facial expressions, eye contact, body posturing, hand gesturing, body distance) because it can affect the child's responsiveness during the interview. Don't use the child's or your body parts to evaluate the child's knowledge of anatomy.

CONDUCTING THE INTERVIEW

At the beginning of the interview, make introductions and give a simple explanation of the job of an interviewer. Take time to establish rapport with the child. Some sample questions that can assist in establishing rapport are as follows:

- What is your name? How old are you?

- Where do you live? Who lives with you? Who visits you?

- What are your mother's and father's names?

- What school do you go to? What grade are you in?

- What is your favorite subject? Your least favorite?

- What is your teacher's name? Who was your teacher last year?

- What makes you happy? Sad? Mad? Scared?

- What do you like best about the people you live with? Least?

- What kind of things do you like to do alone?

- Why are you here today?

Ask as few direct questions as possible, but attempt to obtain the what, who, how, where, and when of the allegation (**Table 11-1**).

CONCLUDING THE INTERVIEW

On completing the interview, ask the child if he has any questions and answer them honestly. Comfort the child, but do not make promises that may not be kept.

Ask the child what she expects will happen, then explain what is likely to happen. State whether there will be further contacts or interviews. If additional interviews are needed, remember it is less traumatic for the child to deal with the same interviewer

---

Table 11-1. Questions That Can Be Asked of the Child Victim

What happened to you?
This question allows the child to describe the event in his own words. Help the child expand on the information by asking the following:

What were you wearing? What was the suspected perpetrator wearing?

What happened to your clothes? Suspected perpetrator's clothes?

What did he or she say? What did you say to him or her?

Who did you tell this to?

Are you hurt or sick now?
Never delay emergency medical care. If the child indicates that she is hurt, ask "where?"

What happened next?
This question encourages more detail. When a child begins to disclose, you may prompt him with questions such as the following:

What else do you remember? What else do I need to know?

Could you tell me what you mean by _____? I need to understand a little more here.

Were pictures taken? Of what? By whom? Where are the pictures?

Were you asked not to tell anyone? Who asked you? What were you asked not to tell? Who were you not supposed to tell? This helps to determine the use of threats or bribes.

Who did this to you?
If information is not volunteered, it is important to ask the name and/or relationship of the abuser.

Were you touched by anyone? Who? Where?

How do you know him or her?

Has anyone else done this to you? Who? Where?

How did this happen?
Asking this question will encourage an explanation of the event.

What were you touched with (an object may have been used)?

Table 11-1. Questions That Can Be Asked of the Child Victim *(continued)*

When did this happen?
Determining when the event happened may require association with other dates, such as holidays, visits, day or night, etc.

Time of day? Month? Year? With a younger child, you may need to link this with the clothes he was wearing, before or after a meal, during a television show, describing the weather, birthdays, anniversaries, holidays, etc.

Has this happened before? When? Where? (If sexual abuse is alleged, look for grooming and events leading up to the act.)

Who saw this happen?
Asking this question corroborates witness information and addresses the possibility of multiple victims or suspected perpetrators.

Was anyone else in the room when this happened? Who was there?

Were you seen by anyone else? Who?

Was there anyone else this happened to?

Was anyone else touched? By whom? Where?

Was anyone else at home? Where were they?

Has anyone else done this to you?

If the child has not disclosed abuse but there are indicators that abuse did take place, it may be necessary to refer him to a qualified counselor. However, if prosecution is a possibility, counseling, therapy, or other abuse-related treatment (including hypnosis) could compromise the criminal case. Discuss such treatment with the prosecutor before arranging for these types of services.

♦ THE WITNESS INTERVIEW

BASIC REQUIREMENTS OF WITNESSES

Some of the more important factors to be considered when conducting an interview are discussed here. However, before attempting to weigh their effect on the witness' story, you must first determine that the witness meets three essential requirements:

1. The witness was present during the event or a portion of it.

2. The witness was conscious (aware) of what was happening.

3. The witness was attentive to what was happening. (This final element is the most difficult to establish.)

CONDUCTING THE INTERVIEW

When interviewing a witness, first allow the person to tell what happened or what he or she observed in a narrative style. Specific questions can be asked later to gather more detail and to jog the witness' memory.

Be sure that you (1) ask the witness for the correct spelling of names and for the addresses and phone numbers of other persons talked about; (2) ask if the victim disclosed the incident to the witness; (3) ask if there is anything that you have failed to ask; (4) ask if there is anything else the witness wants to discuss; and (5) obtain a written statement, if possible.

At the end of the interview, tell the witness that there are no further questions at this time, but as the investigation continues, he or she may be needed later to talk about new information or clarify what has just been revealed. Encourage the witness to contact you with any additional information. Never tell the witness that by talking now he or she will not have to appear in court.

♦ INTERROGATING THE SUSPECTED PERPETRATOR

Always follow local dictates. Procedures or practices should be guided by the investigative ageny's rules/procedures and applicable local, state, and federal laws.

A background check on those involved can be invaluable. It is important to gather as much background information as possible before interviewing the suspected perpetrator(s), including:

- Criminal history

- Social history

- Medical history

- Driving record

- Credit history

- Family, friends, hobbies, likes, dislikes, and personal history

- Evidence or previous report of domestic violence in residence

In addition, read original reports (e.g., police) and check with other professionals (e.g., social worker).

If two interviewers are present, one should conduct the interview while the other one takes notes and shows support by displaying positive gestures.

CONDUCTING THE INTERVIEW

Make introductions and identify why the interview is being conducted. This will set the stage for the interview, so be candid, honest, and polite. Shake the person's hand. First impressions are lasting impressions. Communicate on the same level as the person being interviewed. Don't use big, difficult words to impress or embarrass the other person. Be attentive at all times. Maintain eye contact and use reflective listening techniques—mirroring back to the person what is said indicates that you are really interested in what he or she has to say. Be patient, make sure sufficient time is scheduled for the interview, and be empathetic.

If dealing with a person in custody, begin the interview by reading the Miranda rights and have him or her sign and date a waiver. If a person not in custody starts making incriminating statements, advise him or her of the Miranda rights and have a waiver signed and dated by the person before the interview continues. These steps should be guided by the investigative agency's policy and procedures.

During the interview process it should be your goal to build rapport. Encourage openness by sharing noncritical information. Don't be judgmental—exhibiting personal feelings and emotions, such as anger or disgust, can influence the interview. Demonstrate interest in the suspected perpetrator as a person through control of your actions and reactions. Let the suspected perpetrator talk about himself or herself. Pay attention to his or her interests and fantasies, and appeal to the person's emotions. You may even want to show photographs of the victim. Do not, however, allow the suspected perpetrator to show disrespect for the victim.

To reduce any feelings of threat, emphasize positive characteristics to bolster the suspected perpetrator's ego. Be open-minded and empathize with the weaknesses and defects of the suspected perpetrator. Help the suspected perpetrator look at the problem with a lowered level of personal threat, perhaps stating, "I understand how these things can happen; sometimes we just lose control." You may want to suggest that "There are always two sides to every story. This may be your last chance to tell exactly what happened and why. It's never as bad as you think."

Keep in mind certain information that must be obtained: who, what, when, where, why, and how, if possible. Don't ask the direct question, "Did you do it?" If applicable, ask if drugs or alcohol were used and whether they could be responsible for what happened. Also ask if photographs were taken and/or videotapes made.

Look for and recognize the importance of verbal and nonverbal cues. Remember, most of the time the person being interviewed is looking for help or a release from guilt. He or she may be remorseful if the correct emotional response can be triggered. Distinguish between denials and objections. Guilty people often object; innocent people use denial or profess guilt. Don't take objections personally. Provide a face-saving situation for the suspected perpetrator, if applicable. When appropriate, close the interview on a cooperative note, remembering that the suspect may have to be interviewed again.

The use of videotaped or audiotaped recordings during interviews and interrogations is becoming increasingly popular. They may be used as monitoring devices or to document interviews/interrogations. Follow investigative agency procedures and check with the prosecutor. Use the best equipment available, and be proficient in its use.

◆ PRELIMINARY INVESTIGATIVE CHECKLIST

To facilitate a more timely and comprehensive assessment of the case, checklists are an excellent investigative aid. They act as reminders to obtain specific information and provide a means to organize and measure the status of the investigation. Checklists can be adapted to meet most agency requirements. The checklist in **Table 11-2** outlines information essential to the investigation of suspected child maltreatment. Encourage field investigators to evaluate the list and make modifications appropriate to specific case needs and objectives. Remember that this checklist is only a reminder and guide. Every effort should be made to verify and expand on information as it becomes known. It is essential to a credible investigation to differentiate between investigative leads and verified facts.

Table 11-2. Preliminary Investigative Checklist
How was the allegation received?
Nature of allegation(s)?
Victim(s)—full pedigree?
Parent(s)—full pedigree?
Medical treatment—Was it needed?
If sexual abuse is alleged, has a sexual assault forensic examination been completed on the victim?
Has the victim been interviewed?
Suspected perpetrator(s)—full pedigree?
Records checks completed?
Is there physical evidence?
Are there witnesses?
Have documented statements been taken from witnesses and others?
Child protective services/juvenile court actions taken to date?
Criminal justice action taken to date?
What agencies and investigators are involved in the investigation?

◆ SERIOUS CRIME/EVENT SCENE PROCEDURES

Child maltreatment often comes to the attention of police officers as they respond to a call for service. While the call may concern a report of child abuse, it may originate as a domestic disturbance or the report of an accidental injury. Based on what is seen and heard, the responding officer(s) may suspect abuse. In some cases, it may be necessary to immediately protect the child by removing him from the home. Regardless of how the call is received or what actions are taken by police officers, assignments involving the possibility of child maltreatment are potentially very dangerous.

◆ PREPARING A REPORT

Assemble all obtained information into a logical sequence of events, accurately reflecting the results of the entire investigation. Observations, statements, evidence, sketches, photographs, and medical and technical findings should clearly portray all the known facts of the case. If new or additional information becomes available, prepare a **supplemental** report and distribute it to all participating agencies.

Record all investigative results (interviewing, disposition of evidence, names of responders and what they did, etc.) according to the policy and procedures of the investigative agency. You may need to take hand-written notes, record electronically, videotape, or use a combination of all these methods. Whatever the means, **record and document** every step of the investigation.

While the primary role of law enforcement in the investigation of child maltreatment is to investigate alleged crimes, the ultimate responsibility is to identify and protect children at risk. Beyond the case being investigated, law enforcement officers should be alert to any situation that puts a child in harm's way. The assessment and immediate actions taken by law enforcement may save a child's life and improve the opportunity to preserve the family.

◆ SUGGESTED READING

Walsh, B.: *Defining the Role of Law Enforcement in the Intervention Process,* presented January 17-21, 1994, Huntsville, Alabama.

Chapter 12

LEGAL ISSUES

JESSE A. GOLDNER, M.A., J.D.
CASSANDRA K. DOLGIN, B.A., J.D.
SANDRA H. MANSKE, R.N., M.A., J.D.

The identification and investigation of alleged child abuse and neglect for purposes of medical treatment, social service intervention, or criminal prosecution are likely to involve some aspect of the legal system. First, various state statutory provisions provide definitions of "child abuse" and "child neglect," although they may differ both from state to state and within a given state, depending on the objective in making the identification: for purposes of reporting to child protection agencies, for establishing a standard for juvenile court intervention, and for defining behavior deemed unlawful and meriting punishment through the criminal justice system. Second, state laws and regulations, as well as other legal rules, prescribe the manner in which child abuse and neglect cases are handled. They address both the method of reporting the incident to the appropriate state agency and how that agency is to respond to the report. Third, the legal system not only controls what may transpire in a juvenile, criminal, or divorce court setting but also dictates some of what should occur in medical facilities.

♦AN HISTORICAL PERSPECTIVE

The United States initially adopted the legal view that children were a form of property of their parents from English common law. Although the law did recognize the parental obligation to maintain, educate, and protect one's own child, the widely accepted maxims, "a man's home is his castle" and "spare the rod and spoil the child," reflected the reality that parental duties were relatively free from legal restrictions. Consequently, only cases of severe child abuse, involving cruel and merciless punishment or permanent physical injury, resulted in intervention and criminal prosecution.

During the Industrial Revolution there was a greater willingness to recognize the need for child protection. Legislation limited child labor and provided for other forms of child protection. In the early nineteenth century, state statutes were adopted that authorized the removal of children from neglectful environments. Not until 1874, however, with the founding of the Society for the Prevention of Cruelty to Children, an outgrowth of the Society for the Prevention of Cruelty to Animals, was there a significant push for legislative reform in child maltreatment.

State juvenile court systems, modeled after the Illinois Juvenile Court Act of 1899, emerged in the early 1900s. The development of these courts represented a direct exercise of the state's *parens patriae* authority, which justifies state intervention, over parental objection, in order to protect children. *The exercise of such state power over a child is generally controlled by three principles:*

1. It is presumed that children lack the mental competence and maturity possessed by adults.

2. Before intervening, the state must show that the child's parents or guardians are unfit, unable, or unwilling to care for the child.

3. The state may exercise the *parents patriae* power solely to further the best interests of the child.

The development of juvenile courts corresponded with the movement toward professionalism in social work and increased social services directed at child protection. Today, the juvenile court exercises jurisdiction over minors brought within the system due to alleged abuse, neglect, abandonment, incorrigibility, and delinquency.

These courts, as opposed to those which are part of the criminal justice system, afford the judge broad discretion in addressing the problems encountered by invoking state coercion to achieve the social welfare system's goal of rehabilitation and treatment of abusive parents and other caretakers. The court's determination that a child needs supervision or assistance may result in court-ordered family services, placement of the child in foster care or a state youth facility, or, in extraordinary circumstances, termination of parental rights.

Differentiating between physical abuse and symptoms or injuries resulting from disease processes or accidents often proved to be a difficult task. The work of two physicians provided guidance. Radiologist Dr. John Caffey, in the early and mid-twentieth century, related previously unexplained X-ray findings to trauma which may have resulted from parental action. In the 1950s and early 1960s, Dr. C. Henry Kempe and his colleagues at the University of Colorado Medical School defined the "battered child syndrome" as an observable clinical condition capable of medical diagnosis. Together, these discoveries had legal as well as medical significance.

Medical identification of certain nonaccidental physical injuries contributed to increased criminal prosecutions and to legislative efforts to require reporting of suspected cases of child abuse. In 1963 the U.S. Department of Health, Education and Welfare's (now Health and Human Services) Children's Bureau developed a model child abuse reporting statute. By 1967 each state had enacted such a law. The aim of these first reporting statutes was simply to identify suspected child abuse, and only physicians were designated as mandatory reporters. As knowledge regarding child abuse increased, however, states refined these laws, expanding their purpose beyond mere identification to investigation and intervention, and broadening the group of mandated reporters.

Recently, the rehabilitative approach to dealing with child abuse and neglect cases, which has been favored in the treatment of physical and sexual abuse, has been subject to extensive attack. Some critics have cited frustrations with the courts' ability to effectively intervene in many cases where such intervention seems necessary. Other critics point to the inability of professionals working in the area of mental health and child protection to change deviant behavior, particularly in a cost-effective way.

Consequently, attention is shifting in two other directions. On the one hand, over the last decade, in an effort to increase the success of reliance on the judicial system to aid in the handling of these cases, many jurisdictions have passed statutes or issued judicial rulings designed to make testimony by a child easier and less traumatic in some or all of the proceedings involving child abuse. These generally involve efforts to minimize the need for the child to be in the presence of the alleged abuser, while at the same time protecting the rights of defendants and others involved in these cases. Options include the use of closed circuit cameras, videotaped testimony and courtroom screens, and the increased admissibility of hearsay evidence. Some limitations on the use of such techniques are reviewed later. In addition, increased efforts are being made to focus on prevention as perhaps the most cost-effective way of dealing with child abuse and neglect in the long run.

Generally, it is the state that responds to child maltreatment, but during the past quarter century federal legislation has greatly influenced the states' legal response to child maltreatment. Beginning in 1974, the National Center on Child Abuse and Neglect was established by Congressional mandate (Child Abuse Prevention and Treatment Act, 1974). The law imposed various requirements on the states as a condition for receiving federal funds for "developing, strengthening, and carrying out child abuse and neglect prevention and treatment programs." Presently, eligibility for funding under the legislation requires the establishment of the following: state reporting laws, statutory immunity provisions for those who report suspected cases of abuse and neglect under state law, a state agency responsible for carrying out investigatory and treatment procedures, a state-wide central child abuse registry, provisions for confidentiality of registry records, and the appointment of a *guardian ad litem* for the child in cases involving judicial proceedings.

In 1980 additional federal legislation was passed (Adoption Assistance and Child Welfare Act, 1980) that requires states to make reasonable efforts to avoid removing maltreated children from parental custody and mandates court or administrative review of state-supervised foster care placement at least every 6 months. This review determines the continuing necessity for and appropriateness of the placement, the compliance with an established case plan, and the extent of progress made toward alleviating or mitigating the cause of the placement. The review must also include a projected date for the child's return home or, when return to the biological parent's home is unlikely, recommend placement for adoption or legal guardianship. The enactment of federal statutes concerning Native Americans (Indian Child Welfare Act, 1978) requires state agencies to make "active efforts" to provide services "designed to prevent the breakup of the Indian family."

Finally, federal legislation has enhanced intervention in child sexual abuse cases. Recent statutory measures impose criminal sanctions upon any person who uses, or assists another in using, a minor to engage in sexually explicit behavior for the purpose of producing physical depictions of this behavior with the intent to distribute the material in interstate commerce (Federal Protection of Children Against Sexual Exploitation Act, 1986).

◆REPORTING STATUTES AND CHILD PROTECTIVE SERVICES

The identification of abuse and neglect, the assessment of family social service needs, and the implementation of treatment programs and other intervention strategies for abused children and their families are carried out predominantly by state and county child protective service (CPS) agencies. Authorization for such action typically is found in state laws that establish and provide funding for these agencies and define the criteria for and mode of intervention. The primary purposes of CPS agencies are "(1) to protect and insure the safety of children who have been or are at risk of maltreatment, and (2) to provide services to alter the conditions which create risk of maltreatment in the future."

A report to the state's child abuse and neglect hotline, made either by a professional involved with the child or by a neighbor or other nonmandated reporter, generally results in a referral to a CPS agency. Often such a referral results from a report to the local police. Occasionally the report is initiated by one parent with respect to the other in the context of a child custody dispute.

Child abuse and neglect reporting laws dictate the manner in which referrals are made to the CPS agency and also how the agency is to respond. Additionally, the statutes mandate other duties and rights of health care personnel and other reporters. These laws govern the central registries that maintain information regarding cases which have previously been investigated by the CPS agency. Finally, the laws often define the relationship between the CPS agency, the juvenile court, and various law enforcement agencies.

REPORTING STATUTES

Each state, as well as the District of Columbia, Puerto Rico, and the Virgin Islands, has enacted its own child abuse and neglect reporting legislation. As a result, there is a lack of uniformity in statutory language and in the effect of the various laws. In particular, the statutes vary as to the precise definition of child abuse and the standards and procedures used for reporting suspected cases. All of the statutes, however, share a common purpose and tend to follow a similar format based on the federally mandated requirements.

The purpose of every child abuse and neglect reporting statute is to protect the child from additional injury. Accordingly, statutes are written to encourage and facilitate reporting of suspected abuse or neglect. They are designed to promote early identification of the child in peril so that adequate investigation and treatment of the child, as well as of the family, when appropriate, can begin.

Every state reporting statute contains essentially the same elements, including the following:

1. What must be reported (reportable conditions/definition of child abuse)

2. Who must or may report

3. When a report must be made (including the degree of certainty a reporter must have)

4. Reporting procedures

5. The existence and operation of a central registry

6. Rules regarding protective custody

7. Immunity for good faith reporters

8. The abrogation of certain privileged communication rights which might otherwise apply

9. Sanctions for failure to report

In addition, many child abuse reporting statutes provide for the taking of photographs or X-rays of the child when physical abuse is suspected, even in the absence of parental consent.

WHAT MUST BE REPORTED

Every state reporting statute requires that mandated reporters report suspected child abuse and neglect. Each state, however, defines child abuse and neglect differently; therefore, reportable conditions vary among the states. In general, reportable conditions include nonaccidental physical injury, neglect, sexual abuse, and emotional abuse.

WHO MUST REPORT

Each state reporting statute designates who is required to report suspected child abuse and neglect. Typically, these individuals include physicians, health care professionals, educators, and law enforcement personnel. Many states, however, have an even broader base of mandated reporters, including such professionals as coroners, dentists, probation officers, social workers, or other persons responsible for the care of children. Over 20 states require "any person" to report. In addition, the majority of state reporting statutes also provide for permissive reporting by nonmandated reporters.

WHEN MUST A REPORT BE MADE

Child abuse reporting statutes dictate when a report must be made. Most statutes require reporters to make an immediate oral report by telephone, followed shortly thereafter by a written report to the appropriate state agency. This procedure facilitates an immediate investigatory response by the CPS agency, ensuring that the child is protected. It also establishes a permanent record of the alleged incident.

The degree of suspicion a reporter must reach before making a report is set out in the reporting statute and likewise varies from state to state. The original child abuse reporting statutes provided for a report to be made when there was "reason to believe" that a child had been abused. Many states have expanded the requirement and now use language such as "cause to believe" or "reasonable cause to suspect" that a "child has been or may be subjected to abuse or neglect or observes a child being subjected to conditions or circumstances which would reasonably result in abuse or neglect." Practically, "cause to believe" and "reasonable cause to suspect" mean essentially the same thing for reporting purposes. As noted later, however, there may be a distinction in cases where civil liability for failure to report is at issue.

REPORTING PROCEDURES

Each state statute specifies at least one agency to receive reports of suspected child abuse and neglect. Traditionally, four different agencies have served as potential recipients for child abuse reports: social service agencies, police departments, health departments, and juvenile courts.

Most states have designated the department of social services, or a division within that department, as the appropriate agency to ultimately receive these reports. Some states designate only the department of social services, while other states designate two or more agencies, such as the police and the department of social services, to receive reports. These states generally require that all reports ultimately flow into the department of social services. A few states, however, permit the reporting to two or more agencies without requiring the coordination of information by any agency.

In many states the reporting statute specifies what information is to be included in the report. In other states the receiving agency determines, on a case-by-case basis, what information is required. Required information typically includes name, age, address, present location of the child, type and extent of the injuries, name and address of the parent(s) and/or caretaker(s) if known, and any other information that the reporter believes might be relevant. Most states require a mandated reporter to divulge his or her name and position but permit a permissive reporter to remain anonymous.

Reporting statutes generally prescribe the time within which the CPS agency must initiate its investigation. In most instances this is within 24 hours of the receipt of a report.

CENTRAL REGISTRIES

Reports received by a state's child abuse hotline are recorded in a central registry. Central registry records usually contain additional case information such as prior reports of child abuse and neglect and CPS case outcomes, treatment plans, and final dispositions at the CPS level. Nearly every state has established a central registry of child protection cases. Current exceptions include Minnesota, New Mexico, and Utah.

State law generally deems central registry records confidential and regulates their disclosure because they contain highly private data about individuals and families. Three general statutory approaches govern record accessibility: (1) Only individuals within a CPS agency may have access; (2) the CPS agency may issue regulations authorizing access by certain persons outside of the agency; or (3) state law may enumerate precisely which persons may have access. This third approach is most prevalent today. Those typically having access are law enforcement personnel investigating a report of child maltreatment, the treating physician, the CPS agency, the court, and persons conducting bona fide research. In addition, the child's attorney or *guardian ad litem* generally is permitted to review registry records in instances when the CPS agency or law enforcement personnel refer the case to juvenile court and court involvement ensues. Registry information often is available for purposes of screening applicants for licenses to establish child care facilities, agencies, or services or applicants for employment or volunteer work with such operations or with schools. Almost all states provide that prohibited disclosure is punishable as a misdemeanor.

PROTECTIVE CUSTODY

Nearly every state authorizes certain categories of individuals to take a child into protective custody if the individual concludes that the child would be seriously endangered if he or she remained with or was released to the parent or other caretaker. The child abuse reporting statutes designate who may take the child into custody, when, and under what circumstances. Depending on the particular statute, such individuals may include one or more of the following: police officers, physicians, juvenile or probation officers, and CPS professionals.

Some states require a court order, at least over the telephone if not in writing, before taking the child into custody against the parent's wishes. Other states directly authorize protective custody, provided that written notice or another document is filed with the juvenile court within 24 to 48 hours after the action is taken. In either case, a custody hearing will typically be held at the juvenile court within a short period of time thereafter to review the initial decision to hold the child. Some states provide for protective custody when an authorized individual deems that there "is an imminent danger to the child's life or health." Other states allow protective custody when returning the child to his parent "would endanger his health or welfare."

IMMUNITY FOR GOOD FAITH REPORTERS

Individuals may be reluctant to report suspected child abuse. Potential reporters may fear that the suspected perpetrator will bring a lawsuit against them if the abuse is unconfirmed. To encourage reporting and alleviate this fear, every state's reporting statute extends some type of immunity from civil and criminal liability to persons making reports. Although such immunity provisions may not completely insulate the reporter from a lawsuit, that is, they cannot prevent the filing of an action against a reporter, they can make the successful litigation of such suits nearly impossible.

Some jurisdictions grant absolute immunity to mandated reporters. This means that the mandated reporter is protected even if the report was false and the reporter knew it to be false. Most jurisdictions, however, provide immunity only to an individual making a good faith report. In these states, a reporter is liable only when the plaintiff can prove that the reporter made a false report and that the reporter knew that the report was false, or otherwise acted in bad faith or with a malicious purpose.

ABROGATION OF PRIVILEGED COMMUNICATIONS

Certain professionals owe their patients or clients a duty of confidentiality. This duty is incurred by virtue of the ethical obligations which the individual undertakes on becoming a professional and adopting the standards of that profession. Any breach of this obligation would ordinarily lead to a malpractice suit against the professional in which money might be awarded to the patient or client as compensation for damages sustained as a result of the breach of confidentiality. If the disclosure is mandated by a state statute, as in the instance of child abuse, however, no liability will result. Moreover, as discussed later, in such instances, the failure to make the disclosure, even in the face of an otherwise existing obligation of confidentiality, may, in fact, result in liability.

In addition to this obligation of confidentiality, certain professional communications are protected by a judicially or legislatively created testimonial privilege. Generally, a privilege operates to exclude information obtained in the course of a particular relationship from being presented as evidence at judicial proceedings.

The most common types of privileged communications are those between doctor-patient, husband-wife, attorney-client, social worker-client, and priest-penitent. States differ, however, as to which communications are protected by testimonial privilege. Most states abrogate all types of privileged communications in a child abuse case, except attorney-client. Many states also refuse to intrude on the priest-penitent relationship.

Mandatory reporters must report suspected abuse or neglect, regardless of whether the abuse or neglect became apparent as a result of a confidential communication with the patient or client. Also, the professional must testify in juvenile court child protection cases when subpoenaed. In many jurisdictions, this requirement to testify may also exist in criminal cases and in child custody cases in which allegations of child abuse are involved. Failure to testify when a judge orders that the testimony be given is likely to result in holding the witness in contempt and jailing the witness. In some states, however, if a claim of privilege is appropriately made, the testimony may be limited to information required to be reported under the reporting statute rather than to more extensive information about which the witness may have become aware.

CRIMINAL SANCTIONS FOR FAILURE TO REPORT

Most states have provisions in their reporting statutes that make it a crime for a mandated reporter to knowingly fail to report suspected child abuse. Almost all of these statutes classify the offense as a misdemeanor and specify a maximum fine and/or jail sentence. Although criminal prosecutions for failure to report are rare, courts have ruled that physicians, including psychiatrists, may be subject to criminal penalty under the child abuse statute for failure to report suspected child abuse. The inclusion of a penalty provision serves a useful function for some reluctant professionals. They may find it more palatable to report suspected child abuse if they can explain to the child's family or caretaker that it is a crime for them not to make the report.

SOCIAL SERVICE AND LAW ENFORCEMENT RESPONSE

A report of suspected child abuse or neglect to a state-wide maintained telephone "hotline" or to a local office in accordance with the state's child abuse reporting statute usually initiates the CPS process. At this early stage of the process, child abuse and neglect are often broadly defined. Individual local CPS offices and workers exercise wide discretion in how the agency will respond to individual reports of child maltreatment.

VALIDATION OF REPORTS

As noted in the preceding discussion of reporting procedures, each state has enacted legislation prescribing criteria for case follow-up, which generally requires an investigation within a limited period of time. The primary aim of the investigation is to determine the validity of the report. If the case is "substantiated," "founded," or "indicated," a decision must be made regarding how to proceed.

If the child is not in the protective custody of a physician, the police, or the juvenile court at the time of the investigation, the CPS investigator must determine if there is imminent risk of harm to the child that would warrant the child's immediate removal from the home. If such action is needed, the police or the juvenile court may be contacted to facilitate this removal.

If the available evidence is insufficient to merit a finding of abuse or neglect, or if the investigation could not be completed, the case may be deemed "unsubstantiated" or "unfounded." The case may then be closed and all references to the report and case deleted from the central registry within a designated period of time, if no additional reports are made.

Central registries involve state collection of potentially inflammatory personal information. This gives rise to constitutional concerns regarding the rights to privacy and due process. Accordingly, many states have enacted procedures, by statute or state regulation, for the expungement of registry records. Expungement of records is based either on the child's attainment of a certain age, passage of a designated period of time since services were terminated, or a finding by the CPS agency that the report was unsubstantiated. In some states individuals may formally challenge information contained in the registry through administrative or court procedures for the expungement or modification of records.

INVESTIGATIVE PURPOSES AND PROCEDURES

Reporting statutes often detail the purpose of the investigation. Generally the goal is to evaluate the nature, extent, and cause of the abuse or neglect and to identify the person responsible. Efforts are also made to ascertain the names and conditions of other children in the home, the nature of the home environment, and the relationship of the subject child to the parents or other caretakers.

The investigative caseworker typically begins the process by contacting the individual who made the hotline report to confirm the information originally provided and to obtain additional information. The investigation consists of a series of interviews. Often the child is the next person interviewed. Preferably, this takes place in a neutral setting. The parents are also interviewed, often during a home visit. Thereafter, other persons named in the report who may have relevant information are questioned. These persons typically include teachers, physicians, neighbors, and other relatives.

The CPS purpose when responding to a report of child maltreatment is distinct from the objectives of the criminal justice system. Yet, as noted, law enforcement personnel may be contacted by the CPS worker during the investigatory stage or they may already be otherwise involved. This is true in cases involving serious abuse, where there is a reason to believe that the parents are or may likely be resistant to CPS intervention, or if the CPS caseworker is concerned for his or her own safety.

State law provides the authority for CPS home visits, either expressly or implicitly, although if individuals refuse to cooperate, a warrant or court order may be needed to gain access to a home. In addition, many states' statutes, regulations, or case law authorizes CPS or law enforcement investigators to conduct examinations of the child or to refer the child for evaluation by medical personnel.

CONSTITUTIONAL CONCERNS

Constitutional considerations are raised in the CPS investigative stage because the Constitution protects individuals against state action. CPS caseworkers act under "color of state law," that is, they carry out their investigative tasks pursuant to legislative authority. Protection under both federal and state constitutions may be implied in such areas as home visits, child and parent interviews, and examinations of the child.

Search warrants are generally not required to conduct such visits or examinations. The burden of obtaining a warrant would seriously impair, if not frustrate, the state's effort to protect the child, particularly in emergency situations. There may, however, be constitutional limits on the nature and circumstances under which investigatory visits take place. Usually the parent or guardian consents to the caseworker's or police officer's entry into the residence. Absent consent, or if the search exceeds the scope of the consent, any evidence that is found may be deemed inadmissible in any subsequent criminal proceeding. Similarly, statements made to investigators by a parent or other perpetrator may be inadmissible if a court finds that at the time of the questioning the individual was in custody or otherwise deprived of his freedom in some significant way.

TREATMENT AND REFERRAL OPTIONS

Following a determination of the validity of the allegation of abuse or neglect, a report is made to the agency's central registry. If the hotline referral is substantiated, a CPS caseworker, who may or may not have been involved in the initial investigation of the report, is usually assigned to the case. The caseworker develops a treatment plan and presents it to the family. CPS agencies offer various mental health and social services and seek voluntary acceptance of these recommended services. If the parent or guardian does not cooperate with the CPS agency, or if such voluntary treatment will not adequately protect the child, the investigative or treatment caseworker will request that a juvenile or probation officer file an abuse or neglect petition with the juvenile or family court or file such an action himself. Such an action will seek court intervention with the child and his or her family. Intervention may include temporary removal of the child from the home, court-ordered treatment, or, in some circumstances, termination of parental rights.

When the police have not been involved in the investigation, referral to a local law enforcement agency upon completion of the CPS investigation may be mandated under state law, when the abuse is "substantiated" or meets the statutory requirements for criminal child or sexual abuse. In the absence of legislative direction, CPS regulations may require referral to prosecuting authorities or the police.

CIVIL LIABILITY AND CHILD MALTREATMENT

Health care professionals and others engaged in protective services may be exposed to civil liability during the identification and investigation of alleged child abuse.

FAILURE TO REPORT BY MANDATORY REPORTER

Violation of a statutory duty, such as the duty imposed on a mandated reporter to report suspected child abuse or neglect, is negligence *per se* (negligence in itself). Under this theory, an injured child and his family could successfully sue a doctor or another mandated reporter for willingly or negligently failing to detect and report known or suspected child abuse. The suit could result in a judgment awarding monetary damages to compensate the patient for all injuries that occurred as a result of abuse or neglect after the time when a report should have been made.

OTHER BASES OF LIABILITY OF REPORTERS AND POTENTIAL DEFENSES

In rare instances, civil actions may also be brought against health care professionals or others based on their conduct in connection with a child abuse or neglect case. Typically these lawsuits allege that the physician, social worker, or police officer and their respective agencies negligently acted under the reporting statute, thereby causing harm to the parent or the child. A parent or child may bring an action seeking monetary damages for a wrongful report of child abuse, defamation and slander, negligent diagnosis or treatment, breach of confidentiality, overintrusive investigation, wrongful removal of a child from his or her home, wrongful institution or prosecution of an alleged offender, and wrongful examination of the child for signs of abuse. Willful conduct may also be alleged, including battery, false imprisonment, and/or malicious prosecution.

These claims are usually based on state tort (private or civil wrong or injury) law which, through statute or common law (judicial precedent), recognizes that individuals in certain situations owe duties to one another. Violation of these duties can form the basis of an action for monetary damages. Similarly, an alleged violation of constitutional rights, either federal or state, may form the basis of a claim for damages.

As previously noted, all jurisdictions provide absolute or limited immunity for the reporting of suspected child abuse. The same immunity provisions typically apply to other authorized actions taken by any individual in connection with the making of the report. Such actions include, for example, the taking of photographs and X-rays, the removal or retaining of the child, the disclosure of otherwise confidential or privileged information to CPS investigators, and the participation in any judicial proceedings that results from the reporting. Immunity provisions may preclude liability, but they cannot prevent the initiation of a civil action.

Initially the court assumes that the plaintiff's allegations in the petition or complaint regarding the defendant's actions are true, without hearing any testimony. The court then determines if the immunity granted by the child abuse reporting statute was applicable. In jurisdictions that have adopted a rule of "absolute" immunity for statutorily prescribed activities of the defendants, the judge will dismiss the proceeding. If, however, the jurisdiction has adopted a rule of "qualified" immunity, that is, immunity only for actions undertaken in "good faith," the court will allow the case to go to trial. The jury, or the judge acting as the finder of fact, will then hear testimony on behalf of each party from various witnesses regarding the allegations of the petition. If the alleged actions are proved to be true, but the trier of fact concludes that they were taken in good faith, the proceeding will be dismissed. Liability attaches only if the facts adduced at the trial prove both that the defendants engaged in the alleged behavior and that the defendants did not act in good faith.

ADDITIONAL CAUSES OF ACTION BASED ON FAILURES TO PROTECT THE CHILD AND RELATED DEFENSES

In situations involving state-employed child protection workers resulting in the death or additional serious injury to the child, the child and an innocent parent or guardian may bring an action alleging that the public employees should have taken various steps to protect the child. The lawsuits may allege a failure to accept reports for investigation, a failure to adequately investigate reports, a failure to remove the child from the home, a failure to protect the child following return to the home or to foster care or a child care facility, or a failure to provide services leading to the return of the child. These actions are also typically brought under state tort law.

Similar suits for damages have been brought charging violations of the federal Constitution. The typical allegation is that the officials' failure to act deprived them of their liberty in violation of the Due Process Clause of the Fourteenth Amendment to the United States Constitution. Specifically, the plaintiffs assert that substantive due process requires state agents to protect children referred as abused to child protection agencies. Nevertheless, in 1989 (*DeShaney v. Winnebago County Dept. of Social Servs., 1989*) the United States Supreme Court limited the type of suit that could be brought in some of these cases. The Court concluded that a state's failure to protect a child, not in the actual custody of the state, against violence generally will not constitute a violation of the Due Process Clause, because the Clause imposes no duty on the states to provide members of the general public with adequate protective services. While the Clause forbids the state from depriving individuals of life, liberty, and property without due process of law, it only limits the state's power to act and does not impose an affirmative obligation to ensure any minimal level of safety and security. Thus, the constitutional issue is not whether the CPS agency, or another public actor, was aware of the danger to the child, but rather whether it limited or prevented the child from acting on his or her own behalf. Liability still could be found, however, under state rather than federal law, based on negligent conduct, or in instances where a child is within the custody of a state agency.

In addition to any immunity provided under the reporting statute, civil liability may also be precluded by the "public duty" doctrine or rule. This rule generally applies only to health care professionals or other child care workers who are state employees. The rule provides that a public official is generally not liable to individuals for his or her negligence in discharging public duties. The rationale behind the rule is that the duty is owed to the public at large, rather than to any one individual.

Liability will attach, however, where the duty is specifically owed an individual under state tort law. A special relationship between an individual and a public official or agency may be sufficient to give rise to liability for negligence in carrying out that duty. State reporting laws may be viewed as creating such a duty. Consequently, the public duty doctrine generally will not protect a physician or other health care professional employed by a public agency who undertakes to treat a child but then fails to report child abuse or otherwise fails to comply with the specific requirements of the reporting statute.

Finally, in addition to legislating a statutory immunity for actions taken by reporters under the child abuse reporting laws, a number of states have enacted general immunity statutes that protect public employees from liability for injuries caused while acting within the scope of their employment. The underlying rationale is that the fear of being sued will infringe on the individual's discharge of his or her duty. In addition, even in the absence of a statutory provision, as a matter of common law, immunity may be affirmatively pled and judicially invoked by public employees.

As with the immunity provisions under the reporting statutes, "absolute immunity" applies to "public officials whose special functions or constitutional status requires complete protection from suit," and extends to judges, legislators, and prosecutors acting within their official capacity. Only "qualified" or "good faith immunity," on the other hand, is available to officials performing discretionary functions. But even such limited immunity may be sufficient to terminate a lawsuit based on insubstantial claims involving bare allegations of malice by government employees.

◆ THE LITIGATION OF CHILD ABUSE AND NEGLECT CASES

Court involvement in child abuse or neglect cases may occur in the form of a civil proceeding under specific child abuse or neglect statutes in a juvenile or family court or in a criminal proceeding for homicide, assault or battery, or criminal child abuse or neglect. The issue may also be litigated in a child custody case related to a dissolution of marriage proceeding. A recent study examined over 800 substantiated cases of intrafamilial child abuse and neglect reported in three counties across the country in the mid 1980s. Statistical analysis indicated that juvenile court proceedings were brought in just 21% of the cases and criminal prosecutions in only 4%, although treatment plans developed in some 75% of the cases and out-of-home placement occurred in 50% of the sample. Thus, it is apparent that criminal prosecutions of the perpetrator remain relatively infrequent. Usually, the state's goal of protecting the child in peril is met in a civil proceeding that takes place in a juvenile court or a family court.

This section reviews how child abuse cases generally proceed in juvenile, criminal, and divorce courts. It concludes with a discussion of the evidentiary rules which may arise in any trial dealing with child abuse.

THE ROLE OF THE JUVENILE COURT AND ITS PROCEDURES

The role of the juvenile court or family court in child abuse cases is to (1) protect the child from further injury; (2) provide a fair and impartial hearing on the allegations in the petition; (3) consider recommendations of the child protection agency and other social service agencies; (4) implement a treatment plan for the child and/or the parent(s) when appropriate; and (5) protect the constitutional rights of both the child and the parents. The function of the court is not to punish but, rather, to work closely with the social service agencies to effect a treatment plan designed to protect the child. Generally, the court attempts to improve the family situation so that the family is preserved, unless the child has suffered serious harm and would continue to be endangered if allowed to remain within that family.

Statutory provisions give these courts their specific powers. Typically, juvenile courts are authorized to adjudicate proceedings involving claims of abuse and neglect, dependency, and delinquency, as well as requests for the termination of parental rights. There has been a long-standing debate, however, on whether the focus of juvenile court jurisdictional statutes, from a policy perspective, should be directed to intervention where there has been a showing of potentially harmful behavior of the parents or caretaker or only where there is a showing of harmful effects of such behavior on the child.

Some states have structured their juvenile justice system around family courts. Family courts generally have a broader jurisdiction than juvenile courts, including divorce and child custody, intrafamily assaults, and juvenile traffic offenses. Juvenile courts and family courts are courts of limited jurisdiction, and thus are involved only in those types of cases which the state's statutes specifically authorize the court to hear. Moreover, these courts can issue orders only as specifically authorized by statute. Separate sets of state and local court rules may also govern the conduct of juvenile and family court procedures.

Child abuse and neglect proceedings usually involve bifurcated hearings. For the court to take any action with respect to the child, it first must determine that the child has, in fact, been abused or neglected and thus qualifies to be a "ward" of the court or "dependent" of the court for care and protection. This is often referred to as the "adjudicatory" stage or phase of the proceeding. If the court concludes that abuse or neglect has taken place, the child is considered to be under the jurisdiction of the juvenile court and the second phase, or dispositional hearing, is held. The dispositional hearing is designed to determine the appropriate intervention and to initiate a treatment plan.

The court may then order one or more of a variety of dispositions for the child. Additionally, the court may order dispositions for one or both of the parents. Generally, if the parent fails to comply with the juvenile court's order, the court cannot punish the parent by fines or imprisonment but is restricted to conditioning the child's return to the home on the parent's obeying the court's order. In very limited instances, in which the remedy of changing custody is not available or appropriate, the court may be authorized to hold the parent in contempt and jail the parent until the parent complies with the court's order.

Juvenile court proceedings generally are confidential and closed to the public and the press. In most instances, only those individuals directly involved are allowed access.

PARTICIPANTS IN THE JUVENILE COURT PROCESS

Participants in a juvenile court child abuse proceeding may include the judge, the petitioner, the child, the parent or parents, an attorney for the petitioner, an attorney for the parent(s), a *guardian ad litem*, and sometimes an attorney for the child.

Judge

Child abuse cases in juvenile court are heard by a judge assigned to the juvenile court on a permanent or a rotating basis or by an attorney who is appointed to hear cases in juvenile court. These attorneys are called commissioners, masters, or referees.

The judge's initial responsibility in juvenile court child abuse cases is to protect the child's well-being, and in seeking to attain that goal, to see to it that proper procedures are observed. In addition, the judge is the trier of fact. Generally, there are no juries. The judge rules on the admissibility of evidence and then decides, based on the evidence which has been admitted, whether the child should be adjudicated and placed under the jurisdiction of the juvenile court. In the dispositional hearing, the judge reviews the various recommendations and determines the appropriate disposition for the child.

Petitioner

State statutes often restrict who may bring actions in juvenile court. Generally, a suit may be filed by probation officers, juvenile officers, officials of the state or local social service agency, or local county or prosecuting attorneys. In some states "any interested person" can initiate a proceeding. The decision to initiate juvenile court proceedings is based on a variety of factors, including (1) the nature of injury involved; (2) the attitude of the family toward voluntary cooperation with social service agencies; and (3) prior history of abuse or neglect within the family.

Child

The child is the subject of the juvenile court proceeding. The case is often named or "styled" "In the Interest of John Doe, a Child." The child may be called as a witness at the hearing by any of the parties and may be subject to cross-examination by other parties.

Parents

Each parent of the child is entitled to notice of the hearing and in most jurisdictions is considered a party in the case. The parent, too, can be called as a witness and would then be subject to cross-examination. A parent can claim his or her constitutional right under the Fifth Amendment to refuse to respond to any question which might tend to be incriminating. Such a right may be limited if the state grants immunity to the parent, whereby testimony given by the parent cannot then be used against him or her. In addition, the U.S. Supreme Court has held that, even without such a grant of immunity, a parent can be required to produce a child, in his or her custody, for a court hearing, at least in those instances where a parent has custody of a child pursuant to a court order resulting from child protection proceedings. Such action can be mandated even though it might tend to incriminate the parent and aid the state in criminally prosecuting the parent.

Attorney for the Petitioner

In most juvenile courts there will be a county, city, or corporation attorney who is employed full time to represent the party instituting the court action. In some jurisdictions, CPS agencies have their own attorneys whose functions include bringing such juvenile court actions. In some localities the government contracts with private attorneys for representation. The petitioner's attorney drafts and files the petition and other necessary pleadings or motions. At the adjudicatory hearing the attorney for the petitioner attempts to establish, through the presentation of evidence, that the allegations in the petition are true. Then, at the dispositional hearing, the attorney attempts to convince the court to follow the recommendations of the petitioner regarding the child's future.

Attorney for the Parent(s)

Because it is often the parent who is suspected of inflicting the harm or neglecting the child, the parent will typically want to be represented by an attorney in the juvenile court proceeding. In every state the parent has a right to be represented. In most jurisdictions the state will appoint an attorney if the parent is indigent, although this is not required by the United States Constitution. The right of a parent to appointed counsel may be granted by state statute. The United States Supreme Court (*Lassiter v. Department of*

Social Servs., 1981) has held that the Constitution does not require the appointment of counsel for parents in every parental termination proceeding. The Court ruled that in the absence of an applicable state statute or rule regarding the appointment of an attorney for indigent parents, the decision to do so must be made by the trial judge on a case-by-case basis.

The attorney for the parent, of course, is required to protect the interests of the parent. In the adjudicatory hearing, the parent's attorney usually tries to persuade the court that no abuse or neglect occurred, that any injury sustained was accidental, or alternatively that the perpetrator was someone other than the parent and the parent cannot be faulted for the perpetrator's conduct.

If the child is adjudicated to be within the jurisdiction of the juvenile court, the parent's attorney in a dispositional hearing will typically seek to have the child remain in the custody of his or her client or otherwise minimize the extent of official intervention in the family. The attorney must also protect the other interests of his client. The attorney must caution the client not to make statements which could be used against that parent in a later criminal prosecution. If there is a conflict of interest between the parents, it may be necessary for each parent to have his or her own attorney.

Representation for the Child

Many states have enacted statutes providing representation for the child in child protection proceedings. State laws vary, however, as to whether the child is to be represented by a *guardian ad litem* (guardian for this particular law suit), an attorney, or both. Frequently, one individual is appointed to both positions, although the responsibilities of the two differ. Both the *guardian ad item* and the attorney may present evidence and question witnesses at the adjudicatory hearing, and both may offer recommendations regarding the child's placement and treatment at the dispositional hearing.

The *guardian ad item* represents the child's best interest in the child abuse or neglect proceeding. He or she must use independent judgment to determine the best interest of the child. The *guardian ad item* is not the child's legal guardian and has no duties after the proceeding. An attorney must be an advocate for his client, in this case the child, and when the child is mature enough to express an opinion, counsel must generally advocate what the child determines to be in his or her own best interest.

JUVENILE COURT PROCEDURES
Petition

A juvenile court case involving abuse or neglect usually begins with the filing of a petition or complaint that alleges one or more specific instances of child abuse, neglect, or dependency. The petitioner is usually a juvenile probation officer or a representative of the state's department of social services charged with the investigation of allegations brought to the court by social service personnel, police, or other individuals. With the assistance of the attorney, the petitioner decides whether or not to file the action.

Custody Hearing

The juvenile court will typically conduct a custody or detention hearing within a short time after a petition is filed. This allows the judge to review the initial decision to hold the child and to authorize continued placement outside the home. The hearing occurs only if the child has not been returned to his or her home pending further proceedings but, rather, remains in a hospital, other temporary shelter, or with relatives without the parents' consent. The temporary placement may have been authorized or arranged by the juvenile court, a probation officer, or a CPS worker. Before ordering the continuation of the protective custody, the judge generally must ascertain, pending a full hearing, that there is a substantial risk of immediate harm to the child and that there is no viable alternative for reducing that risk.

Adjudicatory Hearing

In an adjudicatory hearing the state presents the evidence of abuse or neglect to the court. The only issue to be resolved is whether the child has been abused, neglected, abandoned, or otherwise comes within the jurisdiction of the court. In many instances the parent will admit the allegations or at least a sufficient part of them for the court to conclude that it is authorized to take jurisdiction or to adjudicate the child to be a ward of the court. In other situations, however, it is necessary for the attorney representing the petitioner to call witnesses to substantiate the facts alleged in the petition. Typical witnesses are doctors, police, teachers, child protection workers, relatives, parents, or other individuals who possess relevant information. Often, a subpoena is issued to compel the witnesses' attendance at the proceedings.

The burden of proving child abuse or neglect in a juvenile court is on the party asserting the abuse or neglect, typically the state. The petitioner does not have to prove that a specific individual committed a certain abusive act, but only that the child's environment is injurious to his or her welfare or that those legally responsible for the child's care did not carry out their legal responsibility.

The standard of proof refers to the level of certainty by which the trier of fact must be convinced that the allegations in the petition are true. In a juvenile court child abuse case the standard is not that of "beyond a reasonable doubt," as in a criminal matter. State laws differ, however, as to whether the petitioner must prove child abuse or neglect by the standard of a "preponderance of the evidence" or by "clear and convincing evidence." "Clear and convincing" is higher than preponderance but lower than "beyond a reasonable doubt." Proof by a "preponderance of the evidence" means that the petitioner must convince the judge that it is more likely than not that certain facts are true, that is, by a 51% degree of certainty. A "clear and convincing evidence" standard requires proving that it is highly probable that the existence of those facts is true. The United States Supreme Court has concluded, however, that a burden of proof of at least "clear and convincing evidence" is constitutionally necessary when the petitioner seeks to terminate parental rights. Some states, however, do require the higher standard of proof of "beyond a reasonable doubt" for termination of parental rights.

In most jurisdictions the judge has the authority to exclude individuals from the courtroom upon a finding that it is in the best interests of the child to do so. A judge may, for example, exclude a parent when the child is testifying to acts of abuse or neglect. Similarly, the judge may exclude a child, who might otherwise be entitled to be present, during medical or other testimony.

Rules of evidence do apply in juvenile court proceedings, but their application may be less strict and court procedures less formal than in criminal cases. Direct evidence, that is, evidence by an eyewitness to the incident, is not necessary to prove child abuse or neglect; circumstantial evidence can be sufficient. The inference of abuse or neglect can be drawn from a combination of evidence such as the nature and extent of the injuries, the lack of explanation for the injuries consistent with medical knowledge, the age of the child, and the fact that the parent was the custodian of the child at the time of the alleged abuse.

If the state fails to establish child abuse or neglect by the requisite standard of proof, the case is dismissed and no further action is taken. If, however, the child is adjudicated and the court takes jurisdiction over the child, the case proceeds to disposition.

Dispositional Hearing

The appropriate placement for the child and the appropriate treatment, if any, for the child and the parent are determined at the dispositional hearing. The hearing may take place immediately after the adjudication or may be scheduled for a later date, pending the collection of additional information that might aid the judge in deciding the terms for the court order. Evidence submitted at the hearing usually focuses on the recommendations made to the judge by a court social worker, and in some situations by the *guardian ad litem*, regarding placement and treatment. Generally, state statutes give juvenile courts the authority to order a broad range of dispositions, but the specific powers granted to the court differ from state to state. Additionally, some states add a phrase such as "and such other orders as the court deems necessary." *Common dispositional powers include the following:*

1. Returning the child to the home with or without supervision

2. Giving physical custody to a relative

3. Placing the child in foster care

4. In severe cases, terminating the rights of the parent to the child

Once a child has been adjudicated a ward of the juvenile court, the court retains "jurisdiction" or control over the child until the child either reaches the age of majority (as defined by state law, usually 18) or until the jurisdictional status is otherwise terminated by the court. Most juvenile courts hold periodic reviews to measure the progress of the case and to determine the need to modify previous orders. Review hearings are usually scheduled every 6 months to a year.

The most drastic measure a state may take to protect an abused or neglected child is the termination of parental rights. In essence the court orders that the parent(s) no longer has any rights or duties with respect to the child. Termination of parental rights may be either voluntary or involuntary. State statutes define the grounds and the specific circumstances under which parental rights may be terminated. Usually involuntary termination is a disposition of last resort.

The most common grounds for termination of parental rights are abandonment, child abuse, or neglect. Statutes specify what conditions constitute abandonment for termination purposes. In some states termination of parental rights is not an authorized disposition in the initial child abuse or neglect proceeding. Rather, it can only be ordered in situations where there is chronic failure to support the child or a consistent pattern of specific unacceptable parental behavior with respect to the child. Ordinarily, the parent must be given sufficient time and opportunity to become a more adequate parent before termination. In some states a parent's severe chronic mental illness rendering him or her unable to adequately care for the child may also be grounds for termination of parental rights.

CHILD ABUSE AND NEGLECT IN CRIMINAL COURT

The prosecution of individuals accused of crimes perpetrated against children, while not necessarily commonplace, has increased in recent decades, particularly in the area of child sexual abuse. This increase is, in part, due to advances made in identifying battered and sexually abused children and to the relaxation of evidentiary rules relating to victim competency, in-court testimony, and certain out-of-court statements.

Although the juvenile court's involvement in these cases is based on the state's role as *parents patriae,* the criminal justice system's (CJS) involvement is exercised under the state's police power, which authorizes official action to prevent identified harms to society. The use of this power serves to dissuade private retribution on the part of victims by placing responsibility for prosecuting alleged violations of the criminal law solely within the government's ambit. CJS activities include law enforcement investigations, criminal prosecutions, and sentencing proceedings. The substantive criminal law defines what conduct is criminal and provides the punishment to be imposed on an adjudication or finding of guilt.

SUBSTANTIVE CRIMINAL LAW

State legislatures are responsible for declaring what conduct within their own jurisdictions is deemed criminal and subject to punishment. Similarly, the United States Congress provides for the punishment of activity determined to be harmful to society that occurs within certain territories under federal supervision.

In most jurisdictions, "child abuse" or "child neglect" is viewed as violating the prohibition of one or more of the following statutory crimes: murder, homicide, manslaughter, felonious restraint, false imprisonment, assault, battery, rape, statutory rape, deviant sexual assault, sexual assault, indecent exposure, child endangerment, reckless endangerment, and corruption of minors. A majority of jurisdictions do, however, have specific crimes of child abuse and child neglect. Depending on the alleged conduct and resulting harm to the victim, a criminal prosecution may be sought for one or more of these offenses. Conviction of more than one substantive crime arising from the same series of actions may be authorized, if the proof of each particular crime differs or overlaps.

Crimes are further differentiated as felonies and misdemeanors. The boundary between which offenses constitute felonies and misdemeanors varies from state to state. In some jurisdictions, the distinction between the two is based on whether ordered incarceration will take place in a local jail or in a state penitentiary, but more frequently the difference is in the prescribed minimum penalty in the event of a conviction. In general, a felony offense typically is punishable by 1 year or more of imprisonment. Sanctions imposed for a misdemeanor conviction usually involve incarceration for less than a year and/or a fine of $500 or less. The distinction between misdemeanors and felonies is not only relevant to the potential punishment, but also to the resulting procedural consequences. Greater constitutional protection is offered to defendants in felony prosecutions, such as the right to a trial by jury. Defendants are entitled to appointed counsel for all felonies and in misdemeanors where the convicted defendant's punishment involves confinement.

PROCEDURE IN CRIMINAL CASES

The precise procedure in criminal cases varies somewhat from state to state, but the sequence is basically the same. Most frequently, the initial stage in the CJS process is the police investigation. In cases of alleged child abuse, police involvement may (1) precede reporting to the CPS agency; (2) coincide with or accompany the CPS investigation; or (3) follow the CPS agency's substantiation of a reported allegation of maltreatment and referral to juvenile court and/or the law enforcement agency. Regardless of the time and manner in which law enforcement officers are notified of a suspected case, the police investigation is directed at goals separate from those of child protection investigations. The law enforcement agency's primary function is to determine whether a crime has occurred, and if so, whether there is sufficient evidence indicating the guilt of a particular person to justify arresting and charging the individual. CPS agencies are concerned with the identification of abuse for prevention and intervention purposes in the furtherance of child protection.

Investigation

Police officers use a variety of investigative techniques, including pre-arrest questioning of possible suspects, interviewing witnesses or others with pertinent information, and collecting physical evidence (See Chapter 11) . Care must be taken, however, to ensure that a health care professional does not breach the obligation of confidentiality in an effort to cooperate with law enforcement personnel. Access to an individual's medical records or information should not be given to law enforcement personnel without a valid release of information, specific statutory authority, or a court order.

Health care professionals may wish to obtain a release of information authorizing the disclosure of information to police and prosecutors. Only half of the state statutes explicitly authorize and require the reporting of child abuse cases to the police. Such statutes may permit disclosure to certain law enforcement agencies or personnel of either specific facts or general medical or other reliable information known to health care personnel. In the absence of such specific authority, on occasion, police sometimes attempt to gain access to this information by threatening the health care professional with criminal charges based on other statutes. Such threats ought to be resisted.

A few states still have misprision of felony statutes, which create an affirmative obligation to report a felony on the part of anyone with knowledge of its occurrence. Although some jurisdictions have statutes prohibiting the obstruction of justice or the hindering of prosecution, these, as well as misprision of felony laws, generally require an affirmative interference with an officer's lawful discharge of duties in order for the statute to apply. Thus, it would be permissible for the health care professional to refuse to disclose to the police otherwise confidential or privileged information.

On occasion health care personnel may be presented with a *subpoena duces tecum* commanding the production of medical records. Subpoenas are generally issued in the name of a court clerk at the request of an attorney, but at this stage there has been no judicial determination that the record should, in fact, be disclosed without consent. In the absence of a release of information from an authorized individual such as a parent, a judge should be asked to rule on the question of whether the medical record should be released to avoid the possibility of liability for breach of confidentiality.

As the police proceed with their investigation, possible suspects may be questioned. If an individual has been taken into custody or otherwise deprived of his freedom of action in any significant way, prior to questioning by law enforcement officials, the suspect must be given his "Miranda warnings." These warnings contain specific cautionary language informing the individual that he has a right to remain silent, that anything he says may be used against him in a court of law, that he has a right to an attorney, and that if he cannot afford an attorney one will be appointed for him. If the warnings are not given, or if any statement or confession made was not voluntary, then the information may be excluded from evidence in any subsequent related criminal trial.

Arrest and Booking

Prior to making an arrest, that is, formally taking an individual into custody, law enforcement officers must have probable cause to believe that the arrestee is committing or has committed a felony, or that the arrestee committed a misdemeanor in the officer's presence. If, however, the crime is a misdemeanor not committed in the officer's presence, the policeman must obtain an arrest warrant from a magistrate or other judicial officer.

Once the police have probable cause to justify an arrest, they usually take the suspect into custody and process or "book" him or her. Fingerprints are made and "mug shots" or booking photos are taken. How long the suspect can be held without judicial review is determined by state law. If an arrest warrant is not issued by a court before the termination of the prescribed time period, the police must release the suspect. In many jurisdictions, an individual arrested has the right to have a bond commissioner or judge decide if he or she is to be released on personal recognizance or if a bail amount is to be set, pending prosecutorial review of the case and the possible issuance of formal charges.

Prosecutorial Discretion

The investigating police officer presents the case to the prosecutor's office. The prosecutor possesses broad discretion regarding whether or not to file formal charges. This latitude finds support historically in American law. A number of factors generally influence the decision to file charges, including the strength of the available evidence, the harm caused by the offense, the victim's attitude toward pressing the case, the arrestee's prior criminal record, and the adequacy of alternative remedies apart from prosecution.

Prosecutors sometimes are particularly reluctant to prosecute child abuse cases. Sometimes there is the belief that a criminal prosecution of a parent may impede treatment and reunification of the family. More importantly, quite frequently a young child is the victim or otherwise is the primary or sole witness and concerns arise regarding both the child's credibility and the absence of other admissible evidence. Extensive cross-examination of a child witness may lead to confusion. Fears also exist that the child may be highly suggestible to influence by the perpetrator or other family members, causing an alteration of the content of the child's testimony at trial from the description of events provided earlier to the police and prosecutors. Sex abuse cases generate concerns that the jury will view the child as being prone to fantasy or being curious about sexuality and therefore apt to be confused. The extent to which these notions are valid is debatable. Many prosecutors, however, believe that the jury's possible concerns make it difficult to establish the elements of a criminal offense to the satisfaction of a jury "beyond a reasonable doubt." Those relatively few cases in which prosecutions are brought generally involve sexual abuse, severe maltreatment, a nonparent perpetrator, an ethnic minority perpetrator, a female victim, or a victim who is 7 to 12 years of age.

Over the past decade, however, many prosecution offices have organized special units or assigned a limited number of prosecutors to pursue these cases. In such instances expertise with these cases is developed and successful prosecutions may be more likely to occur.

If the prosecutor elects to bring criminal charges, a complaint is filed and if an arrest warrant has not previously been obtained, the court generally will issue one upon the filing of the complaint. Further screening out of cases may occur as a result of a preliminary hearing of grand jury action, as described later in this chapter.

Initial Appearance

The arrestee, now referred to as the defendant, is presented before the court and advised of the formal charges contained within the complaint. This proceeding must occur within a specified period of time after arrest, as prescribed by law. At this hearing bail and other possible conditions of release will be set or reviewed if initial determinations on these issues were made earlier. In felony cases a date will be set for a preliminary hearing on the charges, as described later in this chapter, unless such a hearing is waived by the defendant or a grand jury issues an indictment in the interim. Defendants charged with misdemeanors are generally not entitled to preliminary hearings or grand jury indictments and the case will be brought based solely upon the prosecutor's charge.

Right to Counsel

At the initial appearance, the court will generally inquire whether the defendant has retained counsel or wishes to do so. If, however, the defendant is indigent, the court will appoint an attorney to represent the defendant. The attorney will either be a public defender or an attorney in private practice who has agreed to represent indigents. In either instance, the attorney will be paid by the state.

Bail

Bail is usually viewed as a means of securing the defendant's presence at subsequent proceedings, and it also has come to be viewed as a way of helping to ensure the safety of the community. State and federal statutes may specify factors for the court to consider in determining whether bail should be set and in what amount. Typically, these factors include the seriousness of the offense, the strength of the case, the defendant's prior criminal record, and the defendant's background. The court may impose additional conditions of release. Appropriate conditions in child abuse cases may include a prohibition on contact with the victim, other members of the victim's family, or other witnesses.

Sometimes, particularly in homicide cases, the court will refuse to set bail or other conditions of release and instead will order that the defendant be held in jail pending the trial. Such preventive detention may be warranted upon a finding of future dangerousness or when there is a serious likelihood that the defendant will flee or otherwise attempt to obstruct justice. This measure may be appropriate in child abuse cases when there are concerns that the perpetrator will return to the child's home and either engage in further abuse or attempt to influence the child to recant accusatory statements.

Preliminary Hearing

The preliminary hearing or grand jury is the next stage in the process. In many jurisdictions, individuals accused of crimes have a right to an adversarial preliminary hearing before a magistrate or judge. There the court determines, based on the evidence presented, whether probable cause exists to believe that a crime was committed and that the defendant was the perpetrator. Both the prosecution and the defense have the right to present evidence by subpoenaing witnesses and questioning them, as well as by the submission of documentary evidence such as medical and other reports.

The government carries the burden of proof. The defendant rarely presents affirmative evidence on his own behalf at this stage, although prosecution witnesses may be rigorously cross-examined. Probable cause will be found in practically all cases because the magistrate or judge generally does not have to weigh the credibility of the various witnesses unless the testimony is implausible or incredible. The only question is whether or not a jury, if it believed even some of the evidence presented, could find that a crime was committed and the defendant did it. If the judge concludes that a jury could so find, then the case is "bound over" for trial. The prosecutor will then issue a charge, usually called an information, based on what took place at the preliminary hearing. If no probable cause is found, the case must be dismissed and the defendant released.

The preliminary hearing gives the defendant an opportunity to review the likely testimony to be presented against him. This may play a significant role in inducing him to enter a guilty plea. The defendant, of course, is entitled to attend the proceedings, although as described below, in some cases involving child abuse, limits may be placed on this right.

Grand Jury

In federal felony prosecutions, the Fifth Amendment to the United States Constitution requires that the case proceed only upon issuance of a grand jury indictment. A number of state constitutions contain comparable provisions. In some of those jurisdictions the preliminary hearing may be bypassed by the presentation of the case to a grand jury.

Grand jury review, whether or not subsequent to a preliminary hearing, also serves to provide a means of determining whether there is probable cause to proceed with prosecution against the defendant. But, unlike a preliminary hearing held before a judicial officer, the grand jury consists of a selected group of private citizens who review cases over a legislatively determined period of time.

The grand jury screening process differs fundamentally from the preliminary hearing in the manner in which it is conducted. The grand jury meets in closed session and only hears testimony from witnesses whom it or the prosecutor subpoenas. Members of the grand jury and the prosecutor may question the witnesses, but the defendant and his counsel are not permitted to attend the proceeding. The grand jury mechanism may be preferable in cases involving child maltreatment, because if the child is to be a witness, the grand jury procedure protects the child victim from the trauma of an additional confrontation with a perpetrator and an additional cross-examination by defense counsel. In some jurisdictions it may not even be necessary for the child victim to appear before the grand jury because a parent or law enforcement officer may be permitted to testify to what the child has stated or a videotape of the child's statement may be used in lieu of live testimony.

When a majority of the grand jurors find sufficient evidence to justify prosecution, an indictment is signed by the members of the grand jury and designated a "true bill." The indictment, which sets forth a description of the offense, is then filed with the trial court. Return of a "no true bill" requires dismissal of the charges against the defendant.

Arraignment
After the filing of either the prosecutor's information or the grand jury indictment with the court, the defendant is formally arraigned. The defendant appears before the court and is informed of the charges now pending against him or her. The defendant then enters a plea of not guilty or guilty. The question of the propriety of bail and other release procedures may again be explored.

Pre-trial Motions
Between entering a plea and the commencement of trial, the criminal defendant typically makes one or more pre-trial motions, challenging such technical matters as the institution of the prosecution; the sufficiency of the indictment; the admissibility of expected physical evidence, statements, or confessions; the court's jurisdiction; and the physical location of the trial. In addition, the defendant will seek to "discover" certain materials from the prosecution and otherwise obtain information from witnesses who may testify against him. The extent to which this occurs depends on applicable law.

Plea Bargaining, Guilty Pleas, and Dismissals
Before the arraignment, plea bargaining between the prosecutor and defendant frequently occurs. Agreements derived from plea negotiations may take various forms. Such agreements can involve a plea of guilty to a less serious offense, a plea of guilty to the charged offense with a promise by the prosecutor to recommend a reduced sentence, or a plea of guilty to one or more charges in exchange for dismissal of other charges or a promise not to file additional charges. Justification for plea bargaining is found in the notion that it provides a quick disposition of cases necessitated by a system of justice that is already heavily overburdened. Plea bargaining is an

important tool for the prosecutor when the child witness is reluctant to testify or the physical evidence of the crime is less than compelling.

The vast majority of criminal cases are disposed of by a guilty plea or by the dismissal of charges. In one study which examined a set of criminal filings in three counties across the country during the mid 1980s, 68% of the defendants entered guilty pleas to some or all of the charges and another 20% were dismissed before trial. These figures are consistent with national trends for all felony cases, where only 10% to 15% of the cases that reach the trial court actually go to trial.

Diversion

Diversion programs have emerged as a possible alternative to adjudication within the CJS. Diversion involves halting or suspending formal criminal proceedings against a defendant without a formal conviction and requiring his or her participation in a therapeutic program. Diversion programs are a response to the difficulties in successfully prosecuting child maltreatment cases, particularly those involving sexual abuse.

Diversion generally is used only for misdemeanors or less serious or first felony complaints and typically when the victim and the accused are family members. It may begin before the arrest or at any other stage before trial. Individuals selected for diversion are generally viewed as likely to participate in treatment and likely to benefit from it. Typically they are offered counseling directed at the abusive behavior, as well as career development, education, and supportive treatment services. If the participant responds favorably for a specified period of time, the court or the prosecutor or both will dismiss the case. If the defendant fails to meet the program's obligations, prosecution is resumed on the original criminal charge.

Jurisdictions vary in their use, if any, of diversion programs. Some states, by statute, specifically authorize diversion for particular crimes if certain criteria are met, while other jurisdictions provide for some decree of prosecutorial discretion or specific court involvement. Similar schemes may be used as part of a condition of probation after a guilty plea or conviction at trial.

Constitutional and Related Issues at Trial

The trial of any criminal case raises a broad array of constitutional and related issues, practically all of which are designed to protect the defendant and ensure a fair and impartial trial.

Presumption of Innocence and Burden of Proof

The defendant is entitled to a presumption of innocence. This means that the prosecution has the burden of producing evidence of guilt and must persuade the trier of fact (the jury or the judge alone in a "bench trial") of the truth of each of the elements or legally significant facts of the offense with which the defendant is charged. Moreover, each of the elements must be proven by a high degree of evidence—"beyond a reasonable doubt." Although it is difficult to define this standard, it is usually said that there must be "an abiding conviction, to a moral certainty, of the truth of the charge."

Privileges

The Fifth Amendment to the United States Constitution protects the defendant against compelled self-incrimination. This protection includes the right of the defendant not to take the witness stand and be forced to testify against himself.

In addition, statements admitting responsibility for abuse which are made to spouses, physicians, and other health care professionals may be excluded as a result of a claim of privilege. The privilege may apply in criminal cases with respect to at least some of the information provided to health care professionals, even in the face of an abrogation of the privilege for civil child protection proceedings under a state's reporting statute.

Searches, Seizures, and Confessions

As briefly noted in the discussion of social service and police response to reports of child abuse and neglect, an investigation of alleged child maltreatment may implicate a variety of constitutional issues that affect the admissibility of evidence at trial. These concerns are commonly based on activities such as the examination of the child, a search of a perpetrator's home, and statements obtained from the child's parent(s), guardian(s), or other possible perpetrators. The constitutional issues come into play not only in the context of potential civil liability of health care and child protection professionals, but in criminal cases involving charges brought against perpetrators of child abuse and neglect.

Generally, constitutional provisions protect against intrusions by state authorities. Such authorities may include the police, child care workers, and even medical personnel employed by or acting on the direction of law enforcement or other state agencies. If such constitutional violations do occur, evidence obtained as a result of the violation may not be admitted in criminal prosecutions. Thus, physical evidence that implicates a defendant may be excluded if it was seized in violation of the defendant's rights to be free from unreasonable searches and seizures under the Fourth Amendment to the United States Constitution. Similarly, confessions made in the absence of required Miranda warnings or as a result of police coercion may not be admissible at a criminal trial.

Confrontation Clause

The Confrontation Clause of the Sixth Amendment to the United States Constitution is an area of constitutional law which has recently attracted attention from the United States Supreme Court. The Clause often impacts the trial of criminal cases involving allegations of child abuse. The Clause provides, in part, that "[i]n all criminal prosecutions, the accused shall enjoy the right. . .to be confronted with the witnesses against him." The Clause confers on a criminal defendant a right to confront witnesses at trial, both face-to-face and through cross-examination, and is designed to increase the defendant's ability to challenge the charges against him and to ensure an adversarial proceeding at trial. Confrontation Clause rights are also buttressed by rights under the Fourteenth Amendment's Due Process Clause, which prohibits a state from depriving an individual of liberty without due process of law.

The tension between the right to confrontation and attempts by both legislatures and individual judges to protect child victims from the potential trauma of confronting the abuser at trial or in pre-trial proceedings is evident. Unlike the situation that may occur in both juvenile court and divorce-related hearings, where the court may be authorized in some circumstances to allow a child to testify "on camera" or in-chambers and outside the presence of the alleged perpetrator, such testimony in a criminal case may violate the defendant's right to a public trial under the Sixth Amendment to the Constitution. It may also violate his right to confront witnesses and be present at trial under the Confrontation Clause. Finally, the First Amendment rights of the press and related rights of public access to trials may likewise be implicated.

A number of states have passed legislation providing for closed circuit and videotaped testimony in an effort to balance the competing interests of the child victims and the rights of criminal defendants. In addition, as discussed in the evidentiary section later, the Confrontation Clause may play a role in connection with the creation of various exceptions to the hearsay rule.

A violation of the Confrontation Clause may occur when the defendant is denied face-to-face confrontation with the witness. Although the defendant's right to be present extends to every stage of the trial, some exceptions do exist. The Supreme Court (*Kentucky v. Stincer, 1985*) failed to find a violation of the Confrontation Clause when the defendant (but not his lawyer) was denied access to a pre-trial hearing to determine the competency of two children who were victims of an alleged sex offense. The Court noted, however, that the questions asked did not relate to the crime itself and therefore the lack of the defendant's participation did not bear a substantial relationship to the defendant's opportunity to defend himself at trial. Moreover, the same questions were asked at trial where the defendant was present and there was full and complete cross-examination.

The problem surrounding face-to-face confrontation is more likely when a child victim gives live testimony at trial, out of the presence of a defendant. In another case (*Coy v. Iowa, 1988*), the United States Supreme Court reversed the conviction when a state law permitted a trial judge to order the placement of a large screen between the defendant and two 13-year-old girls who testified that he had sexually assaulted them. The Court noted that the screen improperly prevented the witnesses from seeing the defendant and only allowed him to dimly perceive them. Justice O'Connor, who agreed with the reversal but filed a separate opinion, pointed out that the statute presumed that trauma would occur any time a young victim testified. She suggested that had there been an individualized finding by the trial judge that the child witnesses needed special protection, a different result might have ensued.

Soon thereafter, the Supreme Court upheld a conviction under somewhat similar circumstances. In a 1990 case (*Maryland v. Craig, 1990*), a state statute provided for a one-way television procedure if the trial judge decided that face-to-face testimony "will result in the child suffering serious emotional distress such that the child cannot reasonably communicate." The statute provided that once this finding was made, the witness, prosecutor, and defense counsel would withdraw to a separate room, while the judge, jury, and defendant remained in the courtroom. The defendant could watch direct and cross-examination of the child over a video hookup and remain in electronic communication with his counsel.

The Court concluded that the central concerns regarding the Confrontation Clause were addressed under such a procedure. The Court acknowledged the "growing body of academic literature documenting the psychological trauma suffered by child abuse victims who must testify in court." It concluded that as long as the trial judge decided, on a case by case basis, that such trauma would result if the child was faced with the defendant, and procedures such as those provided were followed to ensure the defendant's rights were respected, there was no constitutional violation.

Trials

Defendants charged with felonies or misdemeanors punishable by more than 6 months in jail are entitled to jury trials. Juries generally comprise 12 persons, but in some jurisdictions, in certain cases, a jury of 6 is permissible. A defendant can waive his right to a jury trial and be tried by a judge alone. A jury verdict either of guilt or acquittal, at least in felony trials, must be unanimous. If the jury cannot come to a unanimous agreement, a mistrial results and the prosecution is terminated without a decision on the merits of the case. The state may not retry the defendant after an acquittal, but a subsequent prosecution may follow a mistrial.

Sentencing

Following a guilty verdict, a sentencing hearing is scheduled. Before the hearing, a pre-sentence report is completed, usually by the state's probation and parole department, to guide the judge in the sentencing decision. The report includes information about the defendant based on interviews with a variety of individuals who have had contact with the defendant. The report may include the results of psychological testing or interviewing.

Both state and federal law define the range of permissible sanctions that may be imposed for the offense committed, including whether probation is available. In some jurisdictions, in some circumstances, the jury will recommend a punishment, which the judge can follow or choose to ignore in favor of a less severe penalty.

In some situations, the defendant may receive a prison sentence, but the sentence may be suspended with the defendant being placed on probation (with or without some limited period of incarceration) under the supervision of the probation department. A typical condition of probation in child abuse cases is a requirement for treatment of the defendant. The defendant's failure to attend or to participate in the treatment program can be viewed as a violation of probation and the court might then reinstate the prison term originally decreed. Other conditions of probation may include an order to stay away from the victim and required payment to the victim of his or her treatment costs.

Appeals and Post-Conviction Action

Following a criminal conviction, direct appellate review is limited to a statutorily defined period of time and allows challenges to any alleged errors committed by the judge which occurred at trial. These include the judge's rulings on various motions which the defendant's attorney made before or at trial, on objections made to the admissibility of evidence, and on instructions the judge gave to the jury regarding the applicable law in the case. If the defendant's appeal is unsuccessful, he may make a "collateral attack" on the conviction. A collateral attack is usually based on constitutional challenges, such as a claim of ineffective assistance of counsel at trial or on appeal. The state, however, may not appeal from an acquittal.

CHILD CUSTODY DISPUTES AND ALLEGATIONS OF ABUSE
ARENAS OF LITIGATION

Sometimes allegations of child abuse arise in child custody disputes. Often they include claims of sexual abuse. The parents may have been residing together as a family unit at the time, or the alleged behavior may have occurred subsequent to the breakup but pending judicial resolution of custody and visitation rights. Alternatively, the alleged incident might have taken place after a temporary or final custody decree, while the child was in the custody of a custodial parent, or during the course of visitation by the child with the noncustodial parent.

If no dissolution of marriage action has been filed, but there is a dispute concerning child custody, its resolution is likely to take place in the context of a juvenile court child protection proceeding as described previously. In addition, most states have enacted legislation that provides for "civil orders of protection" for victims of domestic violence. Many of these statutes provide for judicial determination of custody rights with respect to the children of the parties involved in the context of such litigation.

Finally, the issue of child abuse may appear in any one of a number of stages of a court action related to the dissolution of a marriage of the child's parents. For example, together with or shortly after the filing of a petition for divorce, a motion may be filed requesting the court to issue an order providing for temporary custody and visitation pending the final hearing on the petition for a decree of divorce. At the final hearing, in which the court must determine provisions for joint or sole custody and visitation rights, the issue of child abuse may also be contested. Subsequent to the court issuing a final custody order, one or both of the parents may file motions to modify that order, alleging a change in the circumstances of the child or custodial parent. There, too, the question of child abuse may be litigated. State law or state or local court rules will determine whether it will be a juvenile or family court or a court of general civil jurisdiction that will rule on the custody issue in each of these contexts.

Litigation of child custody disputes in each of these situations differs from that in the juvenile court/child protection context or the criminal context. The court here is engaging in a private dispute settlement function where it must choose between two or more individuals, each of whom claims an associational interest with the child. In the other situations described previously, the court is enforcing standards of behavior believed necessary to protect the child or the greater society at large and, perhaps, to punish a wrongdoer.

PROCEDURAL AND EVIDENTIARY RULES

The state's power to adjudicate private custody disputes, like its power in child protection cases, derives from the common law concept of the state as *parents patriae*. Each state, through legislation and judicial precedent, has prescribed both procedural and evidentiary rules that regulate how the issue is to be litigated as well as substantive rules which guide the court in determining what its orders regarding custody should be.

Depending on the particular state, rules exist that permit or require the appointment of a *guardian ad item* in child custody disputes. Similarly, under more or less restrictive circumstances, the trial judge may order that an investigation and report regarding custodial arrangements for the child be made by employees of public or private social service agencies or by other competent individuals. The child may be referred to professionals for diagnosis by the court or by the individual conducting the custody investigation. The investigator may consult with and obtain information from medical, psychiatric, or other experts who have previously dealt with the child. The judge may conduct in-chambers interviews with the child to ascertain custodial preferences or seek the advice of professional personnel in an effort to elicit such information most effectively. Some jurisdictions require the consent of all parties, in some circumstances, for the application of one or more of these unique procedural devices in a given child custody case. The manner in which a given state approaches these issues affects the court's ability to ascertain whether or not abuse or neglect has taken place. This, in turn, will control the extent to which the abuse or neglect then plays a role in the court's ultimate determination of contested custody questions.

Evidentiary rules control the extent to which professional privileges such as that between physician and patient, psychologist and client, and husband and wife limit the amount of information available to a court in making a child custody determination. Although most state reporting statutes seem to abrogate these privileges in child custody situations involving known or suspected child abuse or neglect, the precise language of the statutory provision which abrogates the privilege in a given state and possible judicial interpretations of that language could still affect whether or not related evidence is deemed admissible.

SUBSTANTIVE STANDARDS

A majority of states currently provide that custody decisions turn on "the best interests of the child" or comparable language, as the substantive standard for making custody determinations. Likewise, visitation rights may be subject to a similar analysis. "The best interests of the child," however, can be an ambiguous standard. This standard essentially requires that a prediction be made in relation to the child's needs and each parent's ability to meet them.

The analysis of the phrase, when specified by the legislature, may provide guidelines that take into account a lengthy list of factors. *These include matters such as the following:*

1. The wishes of the child's parents as to custody

2. The wishes of the child

3. The interaction and interrelationship of the child with his parents, siblings, and any other person who may significantly affect the child's best interest

4. The child's adjustment to his home, school, and community

5. The mental and physical health of all individuals involved, including any history of abuse of any individuals involved

6. The needs of the child for a continuing relationship with both parents and the ability and willingness of parents to actively perform their functions as mother and father to meet the child's needs

7. The intention of either parent to relocate his residence outside the state

8. Which parent is more likely to allow the child frequent and meaningful contact with the other parent

9. Other considerations of environment, physical and emotional needs, intellectual stimulation, financial resources, moral development, and family makeup

When custody is contested, the judge must choose among various alternative arrangements, allocating between the two parents the rights and obligations relating to the child that were formerly shared by them. Although most jurisdictions now authorize awards of "joint custody" under which the parents continue to share rights and responsibilities with respect to the child after divorce, such an award is not required. In cases where child maltreatment is alleged, the court necessarily seeks to determine the truth of the accusations. When the allegations are substantiated, the judge should, of course, choose a custody arrangement that will maximize the child's safety.

REVIEW AND MODIFICATION

Custody decisions are generally viewed as matters best left to the sound discretion of the trial court because of the fact-sensitive nature of the determinations, combined with the general lack of firm guidelines controlling "the best interests of the child" analysis. The wide latitude traditionally afforded to a trial court allows for a necessarily individualized case-by-case decision. It does, however, limit the scope of review of an appellate court to that of reversal only for an "abuse of discretion." Thus, on appeal, a higher court generally will not re-evaluate the facts to determine whether, in its own view, a finding of child abuse perpetrated by the accused should have been made.

Legislation providing for modification of a child custody or visitation order commonly requires a showing of a "substantial or material change of circumstances" and that a modification will be in "the best interests of the child." Allegations of abuse, formerly raised when custody was initially decided, will generally not constitute a change of circumstances, without new evidence of abuse.

EVIDENTIARY ISSUES

The law of evidence is the system of rules and standards which regulates the admission of proof at the trial of any lawsuit. In response to efforts to introduce various types of evidence, in the nature of both testimony and physical exhibits (sometimes called "real" evidence), objections may be made by opposing counsel. The trial judge must then rule on these objections and determine what actual evidence the finder of fact (which may be the jury, as in criminal cases, or the judge himself or herself, in juvenile court child protection cases or divorce cases) will be allowed to consider. The judge will rely on established rules that are part of the law of evidence in making these determinations.

General rules of evidence may affect virtually any question that is asked of a witness during the trial. Particularly unique and difficult evidentiary issues do arise, however, in cases involving child abuse and neglect and these warrant specific attention here. These issues include the possible use of circumstantial evidence, the competency of child witnesses, the use of hearsay testimony, limits regarding the scope of admissible expert testimony, and the use of various types of demonstrative evidence such as photographs and anatomically correct dolls.

Generally, the applicable rules of evidence in criminal child abuse prosecutions, civil juvenile court child protection proceedings, and child custody cases are the same. The rules may be somewhat "relaxed" in noncriminal proceedings in juvenile court or in divorce cases, because a judge rather than a jury is the fact finder and, at least theoretically, has been trained to ignore inadmissible evidence in making his or her determination.

DIRECT AND CIRCUMSTANTIAL EVIDENCE

Child abuse often does not yield a great deal of evidence which, under American rules of evidence, would be admissible in any of the trials or hearings related to child abuse. Most cases of child abuse occur in the child's home, and often the only people present are the child and the perpetrator. Even when others are present at the time of the incident, in many instances it is a member of the immediate family, such as a spouse who may be unwilling to testify or to testify truthfully, or a young child who is too immature to take the witness stand. Frequently the victim is too young or too immature to testify. Even if the child is mature enough to testify, he or she may be reluctant to do so or will change or recant his or her story. The alleged adult perpetrator typically contends that the child's injuries were accidental. Therefore, direct evidence is usually sparse or nonexistent. Direct evidence is evidence which, if believed, resolves the matter in issue.

Most of the available evidence in child abuse cases is circumstantial. Circumstantial evidence is evidence not based on actual personal knowledge or observation of facts or events in controversy. Rather, it is based on facts from which deductions may be drawn, showing indirectly that certain events did take place or that certain other facts sought to be proved are true. Circumstantial evidence, even if believed, does not resolve the matter at issue. Additional reasoning must be applied to reach the proposition to which it is directed.

For example, a witness' testimony that he saw X beat a child with a belt is direct evidence of whether X did, indeed, beat the child. Testimony that the child had belt marks on his back and legs, that the child was in X's custody, and that no one else had access to the child during the time when the marks were acquired would be strong circumstantial evidence that X beat the child. A case of child abuse may be proven entirely by circumstantial evidence, but there still must be sufficient evidence to convince the trier of fact.

In juvenile court proceedings some courts have applied the doctrine of *res ipsa loquitur* to support an inference of child abuse. *Res ipsa loquitur* means "the thing speaks for itself." For example, child abuse may be inferred from the mere fact that the child sustained a particular injury, given the character of the injury and the surrounding circumstances.

COMPETENCY

An individual must be competent to testify as a witness at any trial or hearing. Competence to testify involves four factors: (1) a present understanding of the difference between truth and false testimony and an appreciation of the obligation to speak the truth; (2) the mental capacity, at the time of the occurrence in question, to observe or receive accurate impressions of the event; (3) memory sufficient to retain an independent recollection of the observations; and (4) the capacity to communicate into words that memory and to understand questions about the event.

Historically, courts and legislatures created presumptions, depending on age, regarding the competency of children to testify. More recently, however, the trend has been to presume that all witnesses are competent to testify and to resolve doubts as to the credibility of the witness in favor of allowing the testimony and having the trier of fact decide what weight to give that testimony. A party can still challenge a witness, however, and the trial judge may prohibit the testimony if the judge finds that the witness did not meet one of the criteria listed. Because judges would otherwise have the discretion to exclude testimony on the basis of competence, a number of jurisdictions have recently passed legislation that makes admissible *all* testimony by a child regarding evidence of child sexual abuse.

HEARSAY

In general, a witness can only testify to those facts about which he or she has personal knowledge. The witness may not testify to what others have said in an out-of-court or extrajudicial statement to prove the truth of the matter stated. Such second-hand information is called hearsay. Hearsay evidence is usually inadmissible in a judicial proceeding. Hearsay is excluded to prevent the introduction of statements made by out-of-court declarants whose statements were not made under oath and whose credibility cannot be evaluated by the jury.

There are, however, certain recognized exceptions to the hearsay rule. Each of these exceptions has been recognized in some or all jurisdictions. The exceptions typically have been created when the situation and the circumstances surrounding the declarant's statement increase the reliability of the out-of-court statement and thereby make the statement more trustworthy. For such statements to be admissible, however, they must meet the jurisdiction's requirements for that particular hearsay exception and, in criminal cases, not violate the Confrontation Clause of the Sixth Amendment to the United States Constitution. A number of the recognized exceptions to the hearsay rule are important in child abuse and neglect cases.

Excited Utterances and Statements of Physical and Mental Conditions

One recognized hearsay exception is that for excited utterances. This exception allows for the admission of nonreflective statements regarding a startling event made while the declarant is still in a state of excitement. For example, a statement made by a child to a neighbor or the police that her mother beat her with a belt may be admissible if the court finds that the statement was made while the child was still excited and that the statement was impulsive and spontaneous rather than a product of reflective thought.

A related exception, recognized in most jurisdictions, is that for statements made to anyone regarding then existing physical conditions, including pain or other physical sensations. These are admissible to prove the truth of the statement. That is, they are admissible to prove that the physical condition or pain existed at the time the statement was made. Thus, a statement made by a child to her mother, while pointing to a genital area, that "it hurts," could be admissible under this exception.

Similarly, most jurisdictions admit statements of the declarant's then existing state of mind or emotion. Thus, for example, in child custody litigation incident to a divorce, a child's statement to another individual regarding affection for or dislike of a parent will be admissible. Similarly, statements indicating fear of an abusive parent may also be admitted.

Statements for Medical Diagnosis

In most jurisdictions there is a separate recognized exception authorizing the admission of statements made for purposes of medical diagnosis and treatment. Statements admissible under this exception may pertain to present or to past conditions, if they are made to a physician or the physician's agent, such as a nurse, technician, or receptionist. Such statements are admissible on the assumption that one generally does not fabricate statements to health care providers because the success of the patient's treatment depends on the accuracy of the information provided. Thus, an affirmative response by a child to a question asked by a physician of whether anyone "touched you there" would be admissible as evidence to prove that the molestation had taken place.

Some courts also will admit statements that refer to the cause of the condition for which the declarant is seeking treatment if the statements are reasonably pertinent to the diagnosis and are made in connection with the treatment. In the child abuse situation, a number of courts have reasoned that because the treatment of child abuse includes removing the child from the abusive setting, the doctor should attempt to ascertain the identity of the abuser. Therefore a child's statement to a physician to the effect that "Daddy hurt me" would be admitted.

Present Sense Impressions

A few jurisdictions recognize an exception for "present sense impressions." These are statements describing or explaining an event or condition that were made while the declarant was perceiving the event or condition or immediately thereafter. For example, if a child was rescued while the abuse was taking place, and immediately began to describe to the rescuer what had occurred, his or her statement may be admitted.

Admissions by Parties

Another recognized exception to the hearsay rule is when the out-of-court statement is that of a party to the litigation and is relevant to the party's defense. For example, a parent-perpetrator may tell a neighbor, "I beat my child because he wet his pants." In a criminal case against the parent, the neighbor could testify to this statement. Its admission in a juvenile court proceeding may depend on whether the parent is considered a party under the state's juvenile court rules.

Business and Medical Records

Finally, an additional exception to the hearsay rule allows the introduction of business records. This generally includes medical records. When business records are used to prove the truth of their contents, this constitutes hearsay. Such records, however, often will be admitted under a recognized exception to the hearsay rule for records kept by a business in the regular course of its operation. The theory is that if the "business" itself will rely on the accuracy of such records in carrying out its operations, a court should do likewise. For the record to be admitted, there must be "foundational testimony" to the effect that the entry to the records was made accurately and promptly, it was made in the course of usual business activity, and the person recording the information had first-hand knowledge of the matter.

In most instances, medical records may be admissible as substantive evidence of the child's diagnosis, condition, medical history, and laboratory and X-ray findings under the business records exception to the hearsay rule. Medical records may also be used to refresh the physician's memory regarding the specific case when the physician is testifying at trial or when giving evidence in a deposition. This use is appropriate whether or not the record is otherwise admissible as a business record.

Many courts are reluctant, however, to admit prognostic statements or statements about the cause of a condition that are contained in the medical record unless the doctor who wrote the statement is available for cross-examination or the statement was based on objective data rather than on data requiring speculation. For example, it would probably not be necessary to have a radiologist testify in court that the child has a spiral fracture of the femur. In this situation the record would be admissible to show that the child had the spiral fracture. Conversely, a doctor's statement that the spiral fracture of the femur was caused by child abuse rather than by an accidental fall would probably not be admitted into evidence unless the doctor was available for cross-examination.

Residual Exception

Some jurisdictions have recognized a so-called "residual" exception to the hearsay rule. This permits the receipt of "reliable" hearsay evidence, which does not fit into an established exception, under limited situations, as long as the statement has "equivalent circumstantial guarantees of trustworthiness" to the recognized exceptions. Courts have sometimes relied on this exception in litigation involving children.

Sexual Abuse Hearsay Exception

A number of jurisdictions, legislatively or by judicial decision, have created a new hearsay exception that authorizes admission of out-of-court statements by children about sexual abuse. Often the sexual abuse hearsay exception's applicability is limited to criminal or juvenile court proceedings or both. This exception is similar to the residual exception, but only applies to children's statements about sexual abuse. The time, content, and circumstances of the statement must provide sufficient guarantees of trustworthiness. In addition, the child must either testify at the hearing or must be unavailable. When unavailable, there must be additional corroborative evidence of the act that is the subject of the child's statement. These statutes allow a parent, doctor, or other individual to whom a child has made a statement regarding sexual abuse to testify to the child's description of what occurred, irrespective of whether or not the statement otherwise meets the requirements of another hearsay exception.

Videotaping Statutes

Some state legislatures have passed statutes permitting a child's testimony to be preserved on videotape for presentation to a jury, thus enabling the child to avoid repeated appearances in court. The statutes exempt from the ban on hearsay an audiovisually recorded statement of a child victim or witness that describes an act of sexual abuse or physical violence, if certain requirements are met. The court must find that (1) the minor will suffer emotional or psychological stress if required to testify in open court; (2) the time, content, and circumstances of the statement provide sufficient guarantees of trustworthiness; and (3) certain other procedural requirements were met. Generally, the presence of the judge, the accused, or counsel is not required at the taping, and any person can conduct the interview. Before the statement is admitted, however, on the defendant's request, the court must provide for further questioning of the minor. The admission of the statement, however, does not preclude the court from allowing a party to call the minor as a witness, if justice requires.

In addition, these statutes authorize presenting the evidence of the statement of the child as the equivalent of testimony in the case, either by audiovisually recorded deposition or by closed circuit television. Such statutes specify who is to be present at the recording and authorize the exclusion of a party on a finding that his presence may cause severe emotional or psychological distress to the child. The use of such a recording is permitted, provided the defendant can observe and hear the testimony and can consult with his lawyer.

Confrontation Clause Issues

Although the rules regarding hearsay and its exceptions are generally applicable in juvenile, criminal, and divorce cases, particular note should be made of the interplay between these hearsay rules and a criminal defendant's rights under the Confrontation Clause of the Sixth Amendment to the United States Constitution. As noted in the discussion of criminal trials as well as in the discussion of hearsay, state legislatures and trial courts have endeavored to reduce the trauma a child might sustain from testifying in a criminal trial. Such protective measures may, however, violate the Confrontation Clause.

The Confrontation Clause and the hearsay rules are not one and the same. Nevertheless they do advance a number of similar values. As a matter of constitutional law, the right to confrontation (1) ensures that the witness will give his statements under oath, thus impressing him with the seriousness of the matter and guarding against a lie by the possibility of a penalty for perjury; (2) forces the witness to submit to cross-examination, which aids in the discovery of truth; and (3) permits the jury to observe the demeanor of the witness in making his statement, allowing it to assess his credibility.

When the state seeks to admit hearsay evidence in a criminal case, the proper inquiry under the Confrontation Clause is said to be twofold. First, where the declarant was available as a witness at trial, it must be asked whether the defendant was permitted an adequate opportunity for cross-examination. Second, and more important for present purposes, if the declarant was not present as a witness at trial, it must be asked whether the absence of the witness was necessary and whether there was sufficient "indicia of reliability" surrounding the out-of-court statement. When the declarant is a child victim, the prosecutor must produce evidence of a good faith effort to obtain the presence of the witness, or establish that the witness is "not capable of testifying" as defined by state law. This may involve a showing that the witness is incompetent, or that the child should be excused from testifying because the experience will cause additional trauma.

In a 1990 United States Supreme Court decision (*Idaho v. Wright, 1990*), a female defendant and her companion were convicted of lewd conduct against the companion's 2 1/2-year-old daughter. The conviction was successfully challenged by the female defendant on the grounds that the trial court should not have admitted the pediatrician's testimony that the victim suggested to him that her father had abused her. The critical statements were made in response to the doctor asking whether her daddy touched her with his "pee-pee." The girl responded that "daddy does this with me. . . ." The trial judge determined that the daughter was incompetent to testify and refused to allow her testimony, but he concluded that her statements to the pediatrician were reliable and admitted them under the state's "residual exception" to the hearsay rule.

On appeal, the Supreme Court held that incriminating statements such as these, although otherwise admissible under an exception to the hearsay rule, may be prohibited under the Confrontation Clause. To be admitted, the prosecution must produce the declarant for cross-examination or establish the declarant's unavailability, as well as demonstrate that the statement bears adequate indicia of reliability.

The Court assumed that given the incompetency finding, the child had in fact been "unavailable" for testimony. The question then became one of the reliability or trustworthiness of the statements. The Court refused to adopt any hard and fast rules for professional interviews, such as a requirement that the statements be videotaped or that leading questions could not be used. It ruled that in determining reliability, factors relating to whether the child was likely to be telling the truth when the statements were made were to be considered and that these included the declarant's mental state, spontaneity, and consistent repetition; motive or lack of motive to make up a story; and the use of terminology unexpected of a child of that age.

In this particular case, the Court pointed out that the doctor had conducted the interview in a suggestive manner. Given the presumptive unreliability of the statements, the Court concluded that there was no special reason for supposing that the statements were particularly trustworthy.

EXPERT TESTIMONY

Generally, a witness is only permitted to testify to factual matters and may not offer an opinion or conclusion regarding the meaning of those facts. An expert witness, however, is allowed to give opinions in areas related to his or her expertise when the judge determines that such testimony is beyond the common knowledge of the trier of fact and will aid the trier of fact in deciding the issues in the case. An expert witness is someone with specialized knowledge obtained through training and/or experience. To qualify as an expert, the witness will be required to state facts about his or her education and experience. The opposing attorney or the judge may ask additional questions regarding the witness' expertise. The trial judge is given great discretion in deciding whether the witness qualifies as an expert on the particular matter in issue.

Generally, physicians and perhaps other licensed or certified health care professionals have sufficient training and experience to express a medical opinion to help the judge or jury understand the medical aspects of the case. Therefore, in most situations, an individual with a medical degree will qualify as an expert witness. There is no requirement for subspecialization. The weight the fact finder, be it a judge or a jury, gives the physician's testimony, may, however, be affected by such factors as board certification in the particular area involved, experience, publications, and the clarity of the witness' presentation on the pertinent condition.

Battered Child and Failure-to-Thrive Syndromes

When physical abuse is alleged, expert medical testimony is often essential to establish that the injury was not accidental. In child abuse cases, a physician usually qualifies as an expert who can give his opinion as to the nature of the child's injuries. Medical testimony that the child's injuries are consistent with the "battered child syndrome" is often allowed on the grounds that it is an accepted medical diagnosis. For example, patterned abrasions (belt, cord, stick), and certain fractures in young children (posterior rib fractures in different stages of healing) are powerful evidence of nonaccidental injury and child abuse.

"Failure-to-thrive" syndrome is another diagnosis generally recognized by the medical community and the courts. The syndrome describes a condition in which a very young child's height and weight are consistently below the third percentile on the standard growth chart. Although similar growth patterns may be indicative of certain organic disease processes, they may also be due to parental neglect or deprivation, such as inadequate feeding and poor nutrition. Courts generally have accepted an expert's conclusion that the problem is due to neglect when, subsequent to the child's hospitalization and receipt of proper nutrition, the child has gained substantial weight in a relatively short period of time.

Other Abuse-Related Syndromes

Psychologists, social workers, and other mental health professionals may be called as expert witnesses in child abuse cases to testify to matters within their competence. Such areas include testimony regarding the emotional status of the child, conditions of the child's home, and parenting techniques. "Child abuse family profile," "child sexual abuse accommodation syndrome," and the "battering parent syndrome" are terms used to denote specific behavior patterns and characteristics common to children and families where child abuse has occurred. In a very few jurisdictions testimony regarding the presence of these characteristics and syndromes common in abused children or in families in which abuse occurs may be offered into evidence by an expert to indicate the probability that the child has been abused. Courts in many jurisdictions are reluctant, however, to admit expert testimony regarding these syndromes because such syndromes are based on psychological factors that are speculative as compared to physical factors that are either concrete or qualitative.

Demonstrative Evidence

Demonstrative evidence consists of things rather than assertions of witnesses about things. Demonstrative evidence, such as photographs, medical illustrations or diagrams of the child's injuries, and X-rays, is frequently helpful in assisting the trier of fact in child abuse cases to understand a particular issue.

Photographs, Drawings, and X-rays

Generally, demonstrative evidence will be admitted if a proper foundation is laid. That is, it must be shown that the demonstrative object is a fair and accurate representation of the thing it purports to represent or illustrate. For example, if a physician testifies about a child's bruises and cuts observed in the hospital and then is shown a picture of the child taken at approximately the same time the doctor examined the child, the doctor will be allowed to testify that the photo is a "true and accurate representation" of what he or she saw. Consequently, the photograph can then be admitted into evidence and shown to the trier of fact. Similarly, drawings that indicate the location of injuries may be admitted when the proper foundation is laid.

In a criminal prosecution for child abuse, admission of photographs of the child's injuries is left to the discretion of the judge because such photographs may inflame and prejudice a jury. The judge must balance the probative value of the pictures against their prejudicial effect in ruling on admissibility.

Generally, the child's X-rays will be admitted into evidence if accompanied by testimony explaining their relevance. X-rays may reveal certain types of fractures, which, when found in a young child, are indicative of child abuse rather than accidental injury. For example, posterior rib fractures in different stages of healing in a young child are highly suggestive of physical abuse. Conversely, an X-ray may indicate an accident rather than child abuse. A fractured clavicle accompanied by bruises on the arms is indicative of an accidental fall.

Anatomically Correct Dolls

The use of anatomically correct dolls is designed to reduce the trauma to child witnesses in sexual abuse cases. The dolls may ease the child's experience of testifying and assist the child who has difficulty relating events using appropriate sexual or physiological terms to the trier of fact. Some states have enacted legislation expressly permitting the use of such dolls during children's testimony. In addition, expert witnesses are sometimes permitted to describe or comment on a child victim's interactions with the dolls. Because the use of such dolls has sometimes been viewed as controversial, some jurisdictions bar their use in the courtroom.

◆ SUGGESTED READINGS

Coy v. Iowa, 487 U.S. 1012 (1988).

DeShaney v. Winnebago County Dept. of Social Servs., 489 U.S. 189 (1989).

Hechler, D: *The Battle and the Backlash: The Child Sexual Abuse War*, Lexington Books, Lexington, MA, 1988.

Helfer, R, and Kempe, R, eds: *The Battered Child*, University of Chicago Press, Chicago, 1987.

Horowitz, R, and Davidson, H: Protecting children from family maltreatment. In R Horowitz and H Davidson, eds: *Legal Rights of Children*, Shepard's/McGraw-Hill, Colorado Springs, CO, 1984.

Idaho v. Wright, U.S., 110 S.Ct. 3139 (1990).

Iverson, T, and Segal, M: *Child Abuse and Neglect: An Information and Reference Guide*, Garland Publishing, Inc, New York, 1990.

Kempe, C, et al: The battered-child syndrome, *JAMA* 181:17, 1962.

Kentucky v. Stincer, 474 U.S. 15 (1985).

Lassiter v. Department of Social Servs., 452 U.S. 18 (1981).

Levine, R: *Caveat parents*: A demystification of the child protection system, *U Pitt L Rev* 35:1, 1973.

Maryland v. Craig, U.S., 110 S.Ct. 3157 (1990).

Myers, J: *Child Witness Law and Practice*, Wiley Law Publications, New York, 1987.

Nicholson, E, ed: *Sexual Abuse Allegations in Custody and Visitation Cases*, American Bar Association, National Legal Resource Center for Child Advocacy and Protection, Washington, DC, 1988.

Radbill, S: Children in a world of violence: A history of child abuse. In R Helfer and R Kempe, eds: *The Battered Child*, The University of Chicago Press, Chicago, 1987.

Reppucci, N, et al, eds: *Children, Mental Health, and the Law*, Sage Publications, Beverly Hills, CA, 1984.

Chapter 13

ABUSE, SCHOOLS, AND THE LAW

PEGGY S. PEARL, ED.D.

Schools have legal and ethical reasons to be involved in cases of child maltreatment. Whether the primary reporter of the maltreatment, the alleged perpetrator, or a collateral in an investigation, school personnel should know the legal issues pertaining to child maltreatment. For various reasons, teachers seem reluctant to report their concerns to child protective service agencies. But no reasoning removes the legal requirement for involvement. Beyond this, schools have ethical obligations to participate in community efforts to improve the well-being of all children.

◆ REPORTING STATUTES

WHO REPORTS?

Currently teachers in all fifty states, U.S. territories, and the District of Columbia are mandated by law to report to the state protective services child abuse hotline any suspected child maltreatment. Beyond legal issues, school personnel should file these reports to assist families in crisis obtain help. Since child abuse is a symptom of a family needing help, schools can best assist parents in accessing assistance by alerting the child protective services of possible child maltreatment. Each state's statutes define child abuse, provide confidentiality to reporters, and specify who shall and who may report. For a list of the state protective services agencies see Appendix I at the end of this chapter.

The law requires teachers to report immediately to the state protective services agency if they "**suspect or have reason to believe**" children are being mistreated. No state requires that individuals who make reports to the state child abuse hotline prove that the abuse has occurred before making the report.

The information necessary for making the report commonly includes the following:

— Name of the alleged victim
— Age of the child
— Home address or where the child can be located
— Parent(s) name, phone number, and address, if known
— Type of abuse

— Alleged perpetrator (Some states will ask, but most of the time the reporter will not know the perpetrator, and should not make unfounded allegations. If the child told the reporter, then this information should be included as part of the report.)
— Specific indicators of the maltreatment (what exactly led the reporter to make the report)
— Whether this is an emergency or if the child is in imminent danger
— Name, phone number, and address of the reporter (Some states allow anonymous reports, but knowing the name and phone number allows the state agency to obtain additional information.)

The determination of whether abuse occurred rests with the state protective services agency.

LEVEL OF PROOF REQUIRED TO REPORT

Since no state requires that those individuals who make reports to the state child abuse hotline prove that the abuse occurred before the report was made, most child protective services agencies do some initial screening when they receive a report. Therefore the individual taking the child abuse report will ask for as many details as the reporter can give. It is recommended that reporters write down specific facts prior to making the report. This will ensure that all the known details are reported to the child protective services. If left to memory, some important details may be inadvertently omitted.

PENALTY FOR NOT REPORTING

Nearly every state has a penalty for mandated reporters not reporting child maltreatment ranging from a misdemeanor to a felony charge. In recent years states have begun to prosecute individuals for noncompliance with reporting statutes. In some states mandated reporters may be convicted whether or not they knew a report was required and regardless of whether the failure was deliberate or a case of negligence.

Individuals and/or school districts may also be sued in civil court for not reporting suspected abuse. The civil action will not result in imprisonment of the negligent staff member but will result in a financial award to the individual filing the case. Considering the litigious nature of contemporary society, individuals and school districts should follow both state statutes and their moral obligations.

IMMUNITY FROM CRIMINAL PROSECUTION AND CIVIL LIABILITY

Every state, territory, and the District of Columbia provided immunity from civil liability and criminal penalty for mandated reporters who report in good faith. Good faith means that the individual understood the indicators of child abuse, observed those indicators, and/or was told by a child of maltreatment and therefore had reason to believe that abuse had occurred and made the report without malice or specific intent to harm.

◆ SCHOOL POLICIES ON REPORTING

PURPOSE OF THE POLICY

All school districts should have a clear and specific written policy dealing with reporting child maltreatment. This should be distributed to all school district professional staff and parents. Having a specific written protocol ensures that every child is protected equally under state laws. Additionally, it gives school personnel, including teachers, nurses, counselors, social workers, and administrators, the guidance needed regarding specific steps to be taken and how to fulfill the state statute. The school district protocol supports teachers and reduces their feelings of vulnerability when they are reporting. The standardized policy prevents some children's needs from being ignored, some parents from being the victims of prejudice, and some personnel from becoming overzealous. Review of the policy must be part of regular in-service training for all staff. Topics for staff in-service training include identification of symptoms indicating child abuse and neglect, protocol for reporting of child abuse, and techniques for working with child abuse victims in the classroom.

CONTENTS OF THE POLICY

The statutes of each state will determine the specific requirements to be included in a child abuse reporting policy. The protocol should be written by an interdisciplinary task force including, among others, parents and teachers. A sample policy is in Appendix II at the end of this chapter. The policy should address all forms of child maltreatment, including alleged abuse by school district personnel. Also included are the written notations to be placed in the student's files documenting specifically what was observed, when, and by whom. Since most child abuse is a pattern of incidences rather than a single event, the student's file may have several entries. However, if the behavioral indicators are clear or the child tells an adult of the abuse, it should be reported immediately. Policies vary according to who actually makes the phone call. Some school buildings designate one person (counselor, nurse, principal, or teacher) to receive all the information and make all calls, usually with the individual who began the process present. Other school districts instruct the individual with the concern to make the hotline call, usually in the presence of the counselor or building principal, and then to write a summary of what was said for the student file. Some states send mandated reporters a form to complete and mail to the child abuse hotline following the phone report. The summary should include the date and time of the report, the name of the person accepting the call, the details given to the hotline personnel, and the name of any other school personnel consulted in making the decision to report the suspected abuse.

After a case is reported to the child protective services agency, there should be a follow-up procedure. Some states automatically provide follow-up information to mandated reporters. In others, the reporter will need to inquire about the disposition of the case. State confidentiality requirements may prevent the sharing of this information.

The Federal Family Educational Rights and Privacy Act of 1974 (FERPA), which governs the release of information from school records, does not bar the reporting of suspected child abuse and neglect by educators. In most cases educators rely on their own knowledge and observations when reporting suspected child abuse and neglect, not school records. Therefore FERPA does not apply, since no school records are involved. In a small number of cases it may be necessary to consult school records to determine whether a suspected child abuse and neglect report should be made. Ordinarily parental consent is required before information contained in school records can be released. However, exceptions can be applied in cases of suspected abuse and neglect. Prior parental consent is not required when disclosing information from school records if a "health or safety emergency" exists. It is the position of the National Center on Child Abuse and Neglect (NCCAN) and the Fair Information Practice Staff (the federal unit that administers FERPA) that child abuse and neglect generally are considered a "health or safety emergency" if the state definition of child abuse and neglect is limited to situations in which a child's health or safety is endangered. NCCAN and the Fair Information Practice Staff agree that the responsibility for determining whether a "health or safety emergency" exists must be accepted by the school official involved on a case-by-case basis. Thus if a school official determines that an emergency exists, information in records can be disclosed without parental consent and without violating the provisions of FERPA.

Another exception to the prior consent rule exists if the release of information in school records is made to: "State and local officials or authorities to whom such information is specifically required to be disclosed pursuant to State statute adopted prior to November 19, 1974." The National Education Association 1984 Study of legal regulations affecting teachers compiled all state child abuse and neglect reporting statutes requiring reporting by educators to state or local authorities. Most were enacted before November 19, 1974, so in most states the release of information from school records to state or local child protective services agencies is permitted under FERPA. Educators and school districts should check with legal counsel to be certain whether a particular state enacted a reporting law before November 19, 1974, and to determine whether this exception to the FERPA provision applies in their jurisdiction.

INSTITUTIONAL ABUSE REPORTING POLICY (WHEN THE ABUSE IS AT SCHOOL)

School districts should include in the child abuse reporting policy the protocol to be followed when a school employee is the alleged perpetrator. If the individual has direct supervision of children, the school district must determine if the school employee can continue with this assignment. Several options must be considered while the investigation is being conducted. Will the employee be moved to another position without contact with children? Placed on unpaid leave? Placed on paid leave? Will there be a change in the supervision of the employee? Will the employee retain access to children? Most investigations take about 30 days, often longer. When the individual's position does not require direct supervision of children, such as school district office personnel, financial officers, or maintenance staff, removal from the position during the investigation is usually not warranted.

When a report is made, the principal or other school administrator should attempt to gather facts rather than defend the staff member or school system. It is inappropriate for the school official to become defensive. All findings must be documented. School officials must determine if or when legal counsel for the school and/or staff member should be involved in the process. As with any case of suspected child abuse and neglect, the interview of the child should be conducted by protective services and/or law enforcement investigators to prevent excessive hardship on the child. State law varies slightly as to what agency investigates cases of abuse and neglect outside of the child's home — protective services, the juvenile court, or law enforcement officials. Depending on the situation, the school system may be named as the alleged perpetrator.

When the parent comes to the school to report the instance, the principal should listen carefully and take notes concerning what is said. The principal should maintain an open attitude and listen without becoming defensive, accusing staff, or denying accusations. During the discussion, the principal should make it known to the parent that a report to the state child abuse and neglect hotline is the next appropriate action. The school must keep a record of the entire discussion. In most instances, the individual named in the allegation should not be told of the allegation until interviewed by the investigative worker. The school administrator should then meet with the staff member to hear his or her version of what happened. Next the administrator should meet with any collaterals named by the child or the alleged perpetrator to gather related information.

Children with special needs are at high risk for abuse from all child caregivers, including parents and teachers. Selection of teachers to work with these children is especially important. The in-service training of individuals who work with special needs children should include the particular areas they must deal with, for example, restraint, personal hygiene care, or isolation. The teacher working with a team of professionals must regularly re-evaluate the developmental appropriateness of all classroom procedures and practices. The Individualized Education Plan (IEP) should be carefully monitored to ensure that all procedures, policies, and activities are consistent with the goals stated in it.

DISCIPLINE IN SCHOOLS

Although corporal punishment is legal in many states, school districts should institute policies that prohibit corporal punishment of children. *Research shows that corporal punishment:*

— Has a negative influence on learning
— Increases aggressive behavior in children
— Increases fearfulness and anxiety in children
— Does not develop self-discipline in children

Teachers should be taught alternative methods of discipline and positive guidance techniques. Thus schools can serve as role models for nonviolent conflict resolution for this and future generations of parents.

All schools should have written policies outlining appropriate discipline techniques that have been approved by parents, teachers, and other school personnel. This policy is provided to all parents when their children enroll in school. Some schools require that parents read the statement and sign it, indicating that they have read and understand the policy. Other districts allow parents to exercise other options if they disagree with the stated policy. For example, some districts state that corporal punishment will be used unless parents present a signed statement that they do not want it used. Others allow corporal punishment only for children whose parents have given specific written consent. *Written discipline policies should include at least the following information:*

A statement of the program's philosophy regarding guiding children's behavior:

1. The goal of discipline is to help children learn self-control.
2. Discipline techniques reflect realistic expectations for children's behavior based on an understanding of child development.

215

3. Positive guidance techniques are individualized, based on the situation and the child's age and stage of development.

4. Corporal punishment and isolation of children are prohibited.

5. Children will not be subjected to verbal outbursts or remarks that are belittling or intimidating.

6. Discipline approaches will help children to develop problem-solving skills and learn the logical consequences of behavior.

   — Examples of positive guidance techniques appropriate for children of different ages.
   — Who will discipline children and under what conditions.
   — At what point parents will be asked to participate in planning strategies to help children overcome troublesome behaviors.
   — How staff will assess the effectiveness of the discipline techniques being used.

Schools should establish clear rules and expectations of students with projected nonviolent consequences for failure to comply with these rules. *Schools can institute policies that reduce the need for punishment, such as the following:*

   — Provide students with choices and options for decision-making
   — Make sure students know the school's expectations and the consequences for noncompliance
   — Provide predictable routine in attractive, orderly, and effective classrooms
   — Increase positive interactions with adults inside and outside the classroom
   — Ensure developmentally appropriate curriculum
   — Provide opportunities to assist others in meaningful ways
   — Ensure that there are opportunities for students to feel pride in themselves in a cultural context
   — Encourage all school personnel to be alert and observant of individual students as well as the total environment to ensure appropriateness of these policies

More positive reinforcement for students also emphasizes what is right and prevents the assaults on the child's self-esteem commonly seen in the use of physical punishment.

FALSE ALLEGATIONS

Abuse of children outside the home is much less common than in the home, but it does occur. After an allegation has been made and an investigation carried out, the charge may be found to be false, not factual. False allegations may come from various sources and reflect many different motivations. Children who falsely accuse usually do so for a specific reason. They may be disturbed, seeking attention, coached by someone else, or seeking revenge; alternatively they may simply be misinterpreted. Determining the reason can often help both the child and the alleged perpetrator.

DEFENSE AGAINST ABUSE IN SCHOOL

The best defenses against both abuse and false allegations are education, supervision, and openness. Education of school personnel about what is a developmentally appropriate environment for children and what is not and is, therefore, child maltreatment is needed on a regular basis. Additionally, educating children about good touch and bad touch helps them understand the appropriate adult-child relationship and their rights in such situations.

Supervision of school personnel can be an important prevention technique. Are all personnel appropriately qualified for their position? Do they have adequate in-service training and supervision? Do they have opportunities to discuss situations with a supportive individual before the situation becomes a crisis? Do personnel have opportunities to provide and receive support from peers? Are all personnel treated with respect, given opportunities to make appropriate professional decisions, and valued as contributing members of the educational team? Staff need opportunities to collaborate with peers. The collaborative effort will allow sharing of expertise and building on strengths to improve professional practice. Staff members who support each other will be better able to support and respect the strengths of the children and families they work with.

Openness means that parents are encouraged to participate in the school and that there are few, if any, places where staff can be alone with children in the school. Window shades or curtains should be removed from windows or should be readily movable, except when needed for specific purposes. Openness also means that children are only alone in a room or office with an adult where there is a specific reason, such as individual testing or counseling. Appropriate supervision of the rest rooms in elementary schools should ensure that no adults are routinely alone with one or two children. The openness of a school facilitates improved communication and support between staff and with parents.

Alternatively, access to the school should be controlled. Individuals who are not staff should routinely sign in and out of the office so that the school administration is aware of who is in the building. Additionally, the requirement to sign in may deter some individuals who have no appropriate reason for being in the school. The routine sign-in policy should not deter parents from entry, but should provide them with a feeling of safety for their children.

♦ SELECTION OF PERSONNEL

Prevention of child maltreatment in school is heavily based on the selection of appropriate school personnel. The process involves writing clear, detailed job descriptions and qualifications, conducting in-depth interviews, performing reference checks and background checks, observing candidates with children (if appropriate to the position), and doing an evaluation after a probationary period.

BACKGROUND RECORD CHECKS

All personnel who work with children must be carefully screened before employment. This screening should be complete and comprehensive. Some state statutes require both a criminal records background check and a child abuse and neglect hotline check of individuals who have the care, custody, and control of a child outside of the child's home. This requires asking the individual for permission to check with federal and state law enforcement officials, as well as the state child protective services agency. Requiring applicants to sign a form giving permission will itself screen or eliminate some who have a history of mistreating children.

The purpose of the background check is to determine if the applicant has a history of conviction or a conviction pending involving any of a variety of crimes, including child abduction, child pornography, child sexual assault, assault, murder, rape, kidnapping, and/or other violent crimes. The same screening process may be extended to include volunteers when the volunteer is not under the constant, direct supervision of a professional staff person.

Although it may seem unnecessary, school personnel should always verify the college degree and teaching credentials of each applicant with official documents — not copies or a resume.

INTERVIEWING

The interview should involve more than one interviewer. Each applicant should be interviewed in at least two situations and should be asked the same series of questions to determine appropriateness to work with children. A list of sample questions is given in **Table 13-1**. For recordkeeping purposes, when many individuals are applying and being interviewed, applicants may be asked to respond to some questions in writing. For example, the applicant may be presented with two or three typical classroom situations and asked how he or she would handle each one. Because of the intensity of the position, working with children is naturally stressful. A sense of humor may help individuals deal with the routine job stress. Therefore evidence of a sense of humor may indicate that the individual could handle various stressful situations and not mistreat children.

Table 13-1. Sample Interview Questions
Why did you choose to work with children?
What children's behaviors make you angry and how do you cope with that anger?
What would you do if a child threw a rolled up paper at another child across the room? What would you do if a child hit another child?
Give a couple of situations in which you were successful in disciplining a child.
How do you handle the routine stress of working with children?
What have you done to increase parent involvement in your classroom?
Describe a normal classroom appropriate to the grade level you are applying for. What type of routine would you follow? What would it look like? What would the children be doing? What would you be doing?

The screening process can involve interview questions relating to how the individual would handle a series of common discipline situations. These questions help determine the applicant's knowledge of child growth and development as well as methods of positive discipline. They can be especially helpful in screening for individuals who may be at risk to verbally or emotionally abuse children. Questions relating to normal expectations and classroom routine should provide insight into how age-appropriate the applicant's expectations are and how the applicant sees the adult-child relationship. Questions cannot relate to how the applicant was disciplined as a child nor to how the applicant disciplines his or her own children. It is not job related and appropriate to ask how the individual deals with stress, handles crises, or manages time and resources. It is not job related and not appropriate to ask whether the applicant has a history of maltreatment, mental illness, or substance abuse.

REFERENCE CHECKS

Checking references from previous employers is also an important part of the screening process. Reference checks should be extended beyond written letters. Phone calls to persons given as references who have worked directly with and supervised the individual are important sources of information. Specifically, all previous employers should be asked if they would re-employ the individual. Questions should also be asked about what discipline techniques the individual used, and then the answers should be compared to those given by the applicant. Other questions for professional references could include the following:

— When and where was the candidate observed working with children?
— Did the applicant routinely ask for support from supervisors or colleagues when needed?
— Did the applicant appropriately use solicited information?
— How does the applicant handle criticism and frustration on the job?
— What skills does the individual demonstrate in working with children?
— How does the applicant communicate with students? with parents? with co-workers? with supervisors?
— How does the applicant demonstrate knowledge of child growth and development?
— How does the individual build self-esteem in children?

If an applicant is employed at the time of the interview, permission should be sought regarding whether the current employer may be contacted. It is important to listen carefully to what each reference says about the applicant; the interviewer should add a written summary of each interview to the information in the applicant's file.

◆OTHER POLICY CONSIDERATIONS

IN-SERVICE TRAINING OF STAFF AND VOLUNTEERS

Routine in-service education for teachers, counselors, social workers, nurses, librarians, and administrators should include such topics as indicators of child maltreatment — neglect or physical, emotional, and sexual abuse — the reporting process, and working with victims in the classroom. Other topics to be included should relate to special areas within these more global topics. Such specific topics might include the psychosocial needs of homeless children and the impact of media and community violence on children. Building self-esteem, reinforcing assertive behaviors, praising children, and teaching interpersonal communication skills are also important topics for teachers to explore in their own career development.

SCREENING VOLUNTEERS

A specific screening process should be developed for each school district by a committee of administrators, teachers, and parents. For the safety of the children, nonparents with an open protective services case, a case under investigation, or a conviction or pending criminal prosecution should not be allowed to volunteer in the school or at school-sponsored activities. Parents with open protective services cases should *not* be automatically screened out of volunteering in the child's school. These parents need to be a part of the school district's parent involvement program to improve their parenting skills, reduce social isolation, and learn more about the resources available to them and their children. Within the parent-friendly school there should be many opportunities to learn positive parenting skills as well as improve the parents' self-esteem. The important issue is placement of all volunteers where they are appropriately supervised and never left alone with children.

SUPERVISION OF VOLUNTEERS

Volunteers add to the effectiveness of the schools. They assist the school in many valuable roles. Each volunteer needs to be specifically placed in the most appropriate role, then given a short but detailed job description and someone to periodically supervise him or her. Supervision in its most basic definition is observing the individual, anticipating any potential problems, then redirecting the individual before any problems occur. The supervision process also provides periodic feedback to the individual concerning his or her effectiveness, a very important component for volunteers. A smile and thank you helps them feel that they are needed and their time and effort are appreciated.

The supervision of a volunteer involves a quick visual check of what he or she is doing. It should not be a time-consuming process. Replacing door panels with glass or plexiglass is an easy way to increase visual contact with volunteers. The more open and visible everything is in a school, the safer both children and adults are.

◆BEYOND THE LEGAL MINIMUMS

Because of their special relationship with children and families, schools must work with the total community to support families. An African proverb states, "It takes a village to educate a child." Schools should send representatives to serve on community-based child protection teams, participate in local community councils on child abuse prevention, and initiate formation of such groups if they are not present in the community. Schools should be community leaders in developing a wide range of prevention programs. **Table 13-2** identifies some of the ways schools can support families. All parents should have access to parenting information and support services.

In their role as change agents schools are morally bound to offer prevention programs to facilitate the parenting process in this and future generations. **Table 13-3** identifies some specific long-range prevention programs that schools should consider in the planning process. In the total curriculum there should be instruction on nonviolent conflict resolution, interpersonal communication, child development, resource management, and stress management. Schools must respond to the cultural, economic, and social changes within each community to assist the children and families in coping with these changes. School personnel are morally and ethically bound to assist in the prevention and intervention of child maltreatment.

Table 13-2. Some Ways In Which Schools Can Support Families

1. Provide accessible and affordable before-school, after-school, and "school's out" child care for working parents.

2. Provide parent education and/or support groups for parents with special concerns, for example, those who are divorcing, single, noncustodial, grandparents-as-primary-caregivers, foster parents, or parents of children with special needs.

3. Provide parent education classes to help parents learn age-appropriate expectations for their children.

4. Provide evening, day, and/or Saturday parent-teacher conferences for custodial and/or noncustodial working parents.

5. Implement family play nights to allow parents free or inexpensive opportunities to enjoy parenting more and relieve routine life stresses. Open playgrounds on evenings and weekends to families.

6. Institute homework help lines to allow students and/or parents obtain assistance with homework.

7. Incorporate more parents into the school volunteer program. This builds the self-esteem of both children and parents.

Table 13-3. Long-Range Prevention Programs

1. Teach nonviolent conflict resolution skills beginning in early childhood classrooms and use peer playground monitors.

2. Involve parents and children in policy development.

3. Involve parents in lunchroom, library, and playground supervision.

4. Include a wellness curriculum that addresses both physical and emotional wellness for each grade—K-12.

5. Provide support groups to students experiencing similar life stresses, such as divorce, death of family member or friend, family or community violence, substance abuse in the family, relocation, or peer problems.

6. Initiate volunteer programs that encourage each student to use his or her skills to help others in the community.

7. Provide experiences—work and play—for each child with individuals who are different from them.

8. Allow all children opportunities to achieve their dreams!

◆ SUMMARY

By statute in all fifty states, U.S. territories, and the District of Columbia, school personnel are mandated to report to the protective services child abuse and neglect hotline when they have reason to believe that children are being abused or neglected. The requirement is not that they prove abuse or neglect occurred but that they report. School districts should, therefore, adopt policies for preventing, reporting, and working with students in the classroom. In addition, they should provide all personnel and parents of children in the district with copies of the policies relating to child abuse and neglect reporting and discipline. Beyond their legal requirements, schools have ethical requirements to support families in fostering the optimal development of each child. It does indeed "take a village to raise a child."

◆SUGGESTED READINGS

Caulfield, BA: *Child Abuse and the Law*, National Committee for the Prevention of Child Abuse, Chicago, 1979.

Caulfield, BA: *Child Abuse and the Law: A Legal Primer for Social Workers*, National Committee for the Prevention of Child Abuse, Chicago, 1981.

Koraleck, D: *Caregiving of Young Children: Preventing and Responding to Child Maltreatment*, The Circle, Inc, McLean, VA, 1992.

NCPCA policy statement on corporal punishment in schools and custodial settings, Working Paper No. 17, National Committee for the Prevention of Child Abuse, Chicago, 1987.

Tite, R: How teachers define and respond to child abuse: The distinction between theoretical and reportable cases, *Child Abuse Negl* 17:591-603, 1993.

Tower, CC: *The Role of Educators in the Protection and Treatment of Child Abuse and Neglect*, DHHS Publication No. (ACF) 92-30172, U. S. Department of Health and Human Services, Washington, DC, 1992.

Appendix I–
List of State Protective Services

Alabama
Bureau of Family and Children's Services
64 N. Union Street
Montgomery, AL 36130
Phone: (205) 261-3409

Alaska
Division of Family and Youth Services
Department of Health and Social Services
Alaska Office Building, Rm. 204
Pouch H-01
Juneau, AK 99811
Phone: (907) 465-3170

Arizona
Administration for Children, Youth and Families
1717 W. Jefferson Street
P.O. Box 6123
Phoenix, AZ 85005
Phone: (602) 255-3981

Arkansas
Department of Human Services
Division of Social Services
Donaghey Building, Suite 317
7th and Main Streets, P.O. Box 1437
Little Rock, AR 72203
Phone: (501) 371-2521
Statewide Child Abuse Hotline: (800) 482-5946

California
Office of Child Abuse Prevention
Adult and Family Services Division
Department of Social Services
744 P Street
Sacramento, CA 95814
Phone: (916) 323-2888
Central Registry of Child Abuse: (916) 445-7586

Colorado
Division of Family and Children's Services
Department of Social Services
1575 Sherman Street
Denver, CO 80203
Phone: (303) 866-2551
Statewide Hotline (other than metro Denver) (800) 842-2288

Connecticut
Division of Children's and Protective Services
Department of Children and Youth Services
170 Sigourney Street
Hartford, CT 06105
Phone: (203) 566-5506
Statewide Child Abuse Reporting Hotline: (800) 842-2228

Delaware
Division of Child Protective Services
Department of Services for Children, Youth
and Their Families
824 Market Street, 7th Floor
Wilmington, DE 19801
Phone: (302) 571-6140
Statewide Child Abuse Reporting Hotline:
(800) 292-9582

District of Columbia
Family Services Administration
Commission on Social Services
Randall Building
1st and Eye Streets, S.W.
Washington, DC 20024
Phone: (202) 727-5947
Child Abuse and Neglect Reporting: (202) 727-0995

Florida
Children, Youth and
Family Services Programs Office
Department of Health and Rehabilitation Services
1317 Winewood Blvd.
Building 8, Room 317
Tallahassee, FL 33609
Phone: (904) 488-8762
Statewide Child Abuse Reporting Hotline: (800) 342-9152

Georgia
Office of Child Protective Services
Division of Family and Children Services
Department of Human Resources
47 Trinity Avenue, S.W.
Atlanta, GA 30334
Phone: (404) 894-2287

Hawaii
Family and Children's Services
Public Welfare Division
Department of Social Services and Housing
P.O. Box 339
Honolulu, HI 96809
Phone: (808) 548-5846

Idaho
Division of Welfare, Child Protection
Department of Health and Welfare
Statehouse
Boise, ID 83720
Phone: (208) 384-3340

Illinois
Division of Child Protection
Department of Children and
Family Services
1 N. Old State Capitol Plaza
Springfield, IL 62706
Phone: (217) 785-2513
Statewide Child Abuse Reporting Hotline: (800) 252-2873

INDIANA

Division of Child Welfare-Social Services
Field Services (Child Abuse)
141 South Meridian Street
Indianapolis, IN 46225
Phone: (317) 232-4431
Statewide Child Abuse Reporting Hotline: (800) 562-2407

IOWA

Protection Services
Division of Social Services
Department of Human Services
Hoover State Office Building
Des Moines, IA
Phone: (515) 281-5583
Statewide Child Abuse Reporting Hotline: (800) 362-2178

KANSAS

Family Services Section
Youth Services
Department of Social and
Rehabilitation Services
2700 W. 6th
Smith-Wilson Building
Topeka, KS 66606
Phone: (913) 296-4657

KENTUCKY

Department of Social Services
Cabinet of Human Resources
275 E. Main Street
Frankfort, KY 40204
Phone: (502) 564-4650

LOUISIANA

Protective Services
Office of Human Development
Department of Health and Human Resources
P.O. Box 44367
Baton Rouge, LA 70804
Phone: (504) 342-4049

MAINE

Protective Services for Children
Office of Social and Rehabilitation Services
State House
Augusta, ME 04333
Phone: (207) 289-2971
Statewide Child Abuse Reporting Hotline: (800) 452-1999

MARYLAND

Protective Services
Office of Child Welfare Services
300 W. Preston Street
Baltimore, MD 21202
Phone: (301) 576-5242
H.E.L.P./Resource Project
Office of Child Welfare Services
300 W. Preston Street
Baltimore, MD 21202
Phone: (301) 576-5245

MASSACHUSETTS

Department of Social Services
24 Farnsworth Street
Boston, MA 02210
Phone: (617) 727-0900
Statewide Child Abuse Reporting Hotline: (800) 792-5200

MICHIGAN

Children's Protective Services
Office of Children and Youth Services
Department of Social Services
300 S. Capitol Avenue, P.O. Box 30037
Lansing, MI 48909
Phone: (517) 373-7580

MINNESOTA

Child Abuse and Neglect
Social Services Division
Department of Human Services
Centennial Office Building, 4th Floor
St. Paul, MN 55155
Phone: (612) 296-8337

MISSISSIPPI

Adult and Child Protective Services
Division of Social Services
Department of Public Welfare
P.O. Box 352
Jackson, MS 39205
Phone: (601) 354-0341
Statewide Child Abuse Reporting Hotline: (800) 222-8000

MISSOURI

Division of Family Services
Department of Social Services
Broadway State Office Building
P.O. Box 1527
Jefferson City, MO 65102
Phone: (314) 751-4247
Statewide Child Abuse Reporting Hotline: (800) 392-3738

MONTANA

Community Services Division
Department of Social and
Rehabilitation Services
P.O. Box 4210
Helena, MT 59604
Phone: (406) 444-5622

NEBRASKA

Child Protective Services
Human Services
Department of Social Services
301 Centennial Mall South
5th Floor, P.O. Box 95026
Lincoln, NE 68509-5026
Phone: (402) 471-3121

NEVADA

Welfare Division, Protective Services
Department of Human Resources
Capitol Complex, 251 Jeanell Drive
Carson City, NV 89710
Phone: (702) 885-4730
Youth Services Division
Department of Human Resources
505 E. King Street, Room 603
Carson City, NV 89710
Phone: (702) 885-5982

NEW HAMPSHIRE

Protective Services
Bureau of Child and Family Services
Department of Health and Welfare
Hazen Drive
Concord, NH 03301
Phone: (603) 271-4405
Child Abuse Reporting, Info-Line: (800) 852-3311

NEW JERSEY

Division of Youth and Family Services
Department of Human Services
CN 717, P.O. Box 510
Trenton, NJ 08625
Phone: (609) 292-6920
Office of Child Abuse Control/Hotline
1230 Whitehouse-Mercerville Road
Trenton, NJ 08625
Phone: (800) 792-8610

NEW MEXICO

Family Protective Services
Social Services Division
Human Services Department
P.O. Box 2348
Santa Fe, NM 87503-2348
Phone: (505) 827-4372
Statewide Child Abuse Reporting Hotline: (800) 432-6217

NEW YORK

Division of Children and Family Services
Department of Social Services
40 N. Pearl Street
Albany, NY 12243
Phone: (518) 474-9428
State Operations/Child Protective Services Hotline:
(518) 474-9607
Statewide Child Abuse Reporting Hotline: (800) 342-3720

NORTH CAROLINA

Protective Services Unit
Family Services Section
Department of Human Resources
325 N. Salisbury Street
Raleigh, NC 27611
Phone: (919) 733-2580

NORTH DAKOTA

Children and Family Services
Department of Human Services
State Capitol
Bismarck, ND 58505
Phone: (701) 224-2316

OHIO

Bureau of Children's Protective Services
Division of Family and Children's Services
Department of Human Services
30 E. Broad Street
Columbus, OH 43215
Phone: (614) 466-2146

OKLAHOMA

Child Welfare Services
Department of Human Services
P.O. Box 25352
Oklahoma City, OK 73125
Phone: (405) 521-3778
Statewide Child Abuse Reporting Hotline: (800) 522-3511

OREGON

Children's Services Division
Department of Human Resources
318 Public Service Building
Salem, OR 97310
Phone: (503) 378-4374
(503) 378-3016

PENNSYLVANIA

Office of Children, Youth and Families
Department of Public Welfare
P.O. Box 2675
Harrisburg, PA 17120
Phone: (717) 787-4756
Statewide Child Abuse Reporting Hotline: (800) 932-0313

RHODE ISLAND

Child Protective Services
Department of Children and Their Families
610 Mount Pleasant Avenue
Providence, RI 02908
Phone: (401) 861-6000 Ext 2332
Statewide Child Abuse Reporting Hotline: (800) RI-CHILD

SOUTH CAROLINA

Child Protective and
Preventative Services Division
Department of Social Services
P.O. Box 1520
Columbia, SC 29202-1520
Phone: (803) 758-8593

SOUTH DAKOTA

Child Protection Services
Department of Social Services
Richard F. Kneip Building
700 N. Illinois Street
Pierre, SD 57501
Phone: (605) 773-3227

TENNESSEE

Child Protective Services
Office of Social Services
Department of Human Services
111-7th Avenue, N.
Nashville, TN 37203
Phone: (615) 741-5929

TEXAS

Office of Services to
Families and Children
Department of Human Services
P.O. Box 2960
Austin, TX 78769
Phone: (512) 450-3448
Statewide Child Abuse Reporting Hotline: (800) 252-5400

UTAH

Protective Services
Child Abuse Registry
Division of Family Services
Department of Social Services
150 W. North Temple Street
Salt Lake City, UT 84110
Phone: (801) 533-7128

VERMONT

Protective Services
Department of Social and
Rehabilitation Services
Agency of Human Services
103 S. Main Street
Waterbury, VT 05676
Phone: (802) 241-2142

VIRGINIA

Child Protective Services
Bureau of Child Welfare Services
Department of Social Services
8007 Discovery Drive
Richmond, VA 23288
Phone: (804) 281-9081
Statewide Child Abuse Reporting Hotline: (800) 552-7096

WASHINGTON

Child Protection Services
Division of Community Program Development
Department of Social and Health Services
State Office Building 2
Olympia, WA 98504
Phone: (206) 753-0206

WEST VIRGINIA

Children's Protective Services
Division of Social Services
Department of Human Services
1900 Washington Street, E.
Charleston, WV 25305
Phone: (304) 348-7980
Statewide Child Abuse Reporting Hotline: (800) 352-6313

WISCONSIN

Protective Services
Office for Children, Youth and Families
Department of Health and Social Services
State Office Building
1 W. Wilson Street, P.O. Box 7850
Madison, WI 53707
Phone: (608) 267-2245

WYOMING

Child Protective Services
Division of Public Assistance and Social Services
Department of Health and Social Services
Hathaway Building
Cheyenne, WY 82002
Phone: (307) 777-7892

APPENDIX II–
OUTLINE OF A MODEL CHILD ABUSE AND NEGLECT POLICY FOR SCHOOLS

Sample
Child Abuse and Neglect Policy

Policy Component	Narrative
Purpose	*Family Law Article, Title 5, Subtitle 7* To inform all employees and volunteers in the local school systems of the statutory requirement to report suspected child physical abuse, sexual abuse, or neglect, and to inform employees and volunteers of their immunity from civil liability or criminal penalty for reporting. To establish procedures to be used by all employees and volunteers of the local school system in making oral and written reports to the local department of social services/law enforcement agency for suspected cases of child physical abuse, sexual abuse, or neglect.
Who Must Report	*Family Law Article 5-704, 5-705* Maryland law requires that every health practitioner, educator, human services worker, or law enforcement officer who has reason to believe that a child has been subjected to physical abuse or sexual abuse shall immediately report to the local department of social services or appropriate law enforcement agency. The report, in both oral and written form, shall be made as soon as reasonably possible, but in any case the written report must be made within 48 hours of the suspicion of possible abuse to the local department of social services and the local State's attorney. Maryland law also requires that every health practitioner, educator, human services worker, or law enforcement officer who has reason to believe that a child has been *a victim of* neglect shall immediately report to the local department of social services. The report, in both oral and written form, shall be made as soon as reasonably possible, but in any case the written report must be made within 48 hours of the suspicion of possible neglect to the local department of social services. Further, any person other than a health practitioner, educator, *human service* worker, or law enforcement officer, including any other employee of the local school system and volunteers in the local school system who has reason to believe that a child has been subjected to physical abuse, sexual abuse or neglect, shall immediately report to the local department of social services or the appropriate law enforcement agency as prescribed in the above paragraph. **Where school personnel or volunteers are unsure whether abuse or neglect has taken place, the situation should be discussed with the local department of social services.**

Sanctions for Failure to Report *Education Article 6-202, Education COMAR 13A.07.01.10*
On the recommendation of the county superintendent a county board may suspend or dismiss a teacher, principal, supervisor, assistant superintendent, or other professional assistant for misconduct in office, including knowingly failing to report suspected child abuse in violation of Family Law Article, Title 5, Subtitle 7 (Child Abuse/Neglect), Annotated Code of Maryland.

Upon the recommendation of a local board of education or the Assistant State Superintendent in Certification and Accreditation when the individual is not employed by a local board of education in Maryland, any certificate issued under the State Board of Education's regulations may be suspended or revoked by the State Superintendent if the certificate holder is convicted of a crime involving child abuse or neglect or is dismissed by a local board for knowingly failing to report suspected child abuse in violation of the Family Law Article.

Definitions *Family Law Article 5-701 to 5-715, Education Article 6-107*
A. Educator or Human Service Worker: Any professional employee of any correctional, public, parochial or private educational, health, juvenile service, social or social service agency, institution, or licensed facility. Educator or Human Service Worker includes: any teacher, counselor, social worker, caseworker, and any probation or parole officer. However, a child may not be considered to be abused solely because he is receiving nonmedical religious remedial care and treatment recognized by State law.

Family Law Article *14-101 et seq.*
B. Child: Any person under the age of eighteen (18) years. Persons eighteen (18) years of age or older who are believed to lack the capacity to care for their daily needs ("vulnerable adults") are protected by the Adult Protective Services Program. A health practitioner, police officer, or human service worker who suspects that a vulnerable adult has been subject to abuse, neglect, self-neglect or exploitation is required to report such a situation orally and in writing to the adult protective services division of the local department of social services. Any other person may make a report. Any person who makes a report under these provisions is entitled to confidentiality and immunity from civil liability.

C. Abuse: (1) The physical injury of a child by any parent or other person who has permanent or temporary care or custody or responsibility for supervision of a child or by any household or family member under circumstances that indicate that the child's health or welfare is significantly harmed or at risk of being significantly harmed or (2) sexual abuse of a child, whether physical injuries are sustained or not.

D. Sexual Abuse: Any act or acts involving sexual molestation or exploitation, including but not limited to incest, rape, or sexual offense in any degree, sodomy, or unnatural or perverted sexual practices, on a child by any family or household member or by any other person who has the permanent or temporary care or custody or responsibility for supervision of a minor child. Sexual molestation or exploitation includes, but is not limited to contact or conduct with a child for the purpose of sexual gratification, and may range from sexual advances, kissing, or fondling to sexual crime in any degree, rape, sodomy, prostitution, or allowing, permitting, encouraging, or engaging in the obscene or pornographic display, photographing, filming or depiction of a child as prohibited by law.

E. Neglect: Child neglect means the leaving of a child unattended or other failure to give proper care and attention to a child by the child's parents, guardian, or custodian under circumstances that indicate that the child's health or welfare is significantly harmed or placed at risk of significant harm. However, a child may not be considered to be neglected solely because the child is receiving nonmedical religious remedial care and treatment recognized by State law.

Examples of Child Neglect

DHR-SSA Child Protective Services Policy Manual .01.04.04

A neglected child is one who is:

- left unattended or inadequately supervised for long periods of time.
- showing signs of failure to thrive, or psycho-social dwarfism that has not been explained by a medical condition. There may be other evidence that the child is receiving insufficient food.
- receiving inadequate medical or dental treatment.
- significantly harmed or at risk of harm as a result of being denied an adequate education due to parental action or inaction.
- wearing inadequate or weather-inappropriate clothing.
- significantly harmed due to a lack of minimal health care and/or fire safety.
- ignored or badgered by the caretaker.
- forced to engage in criminal behavior at the direction of the caretaker.

Immunity

Family Law Article
Any person who makes or participates in the making of a good-faith report of abuse or neglect or participates in the investigation or in a judicial proceeding resulting therefrom shall in so doing be immune from any civil liability or criminal penalty that might otherwise be incurred or imposed as a result thereof.

Possible Abuser

Family Law Article 5-701
Any parent, guardian, adoptive parent or other person who has the permanent or temporary care or custody, or who has the permanent or temporary care or custody or responsibility for the supervision of a child or any household or family member, may be considered an abuser under the statute. Educators and other school employees having temporary care or custody or responsibility for the supervision of a child during the school day may also be deemed abusers under the statute and, when

suspected of child physical or sexual abuse or neglect, must be reported immediately to the local social services agency or the appropriate law enforcement agency, orally and in writing as prescribed by law, by the person who has reason to believe that abuse or neglect has occurred.

Reporting Procedures

(Oral Report) Family Law Article 5-704, 5-705
Any employee of the local school system or volunteer in the local school system who suspects a case of child physical or sexual abuse has occurred shall make an oral report to the local department of social services or to the appropriate law enforcement agency. In a case of suspected neglect, the oral report should only be made to the local department of social services. The responsibility of an employee or volunteer of the local school system to report suspected cases of child abuse or neglect is mandatory. The oral report must be made as soon as possible, notwithstanding any provision of law, including any law on privileged communications. In addition to making an oral report, the school employee or volunteer shall also inform the local school principal that a case of suspected child abuse and/or neglect has been reported to the department of social services or law enforcement agency. It is the obligation of the principal to insure that cases of suspected child abuse or neglect brought to his/her attention by any school employee or volunteer are fully reported by the employee or volunteer if this has not already been done.

(Written Report) Family Law Article 5-704, 5-705
The person making the oral report to the department of social services or appropriate law enforcement agency is also responsible for submitting a written report.
The written report must follow the oral report and be made within forty-eight (48) hours of the contact which disclosed the existence of possible abuse and/or neglect.

Contents of Written Report

Family Law Article 5-704, 5-705
An oral or written report shall contain as much of the following information as the person making the report is able to furnish in suspected cases of child abuse and/or neglect:

Abuse/Neglect Report Contents:

1. The name, age, and home address of the child;

2. The name and home address of the child's parent or other person who is responsible for the child's care;

3. The whereabouts of the child;

4. The nature and extent of the abuse/neglect of the child, including any evidence or information available to the reporter concerning previous injury possibly resulting from abuse or neglect; and

5. Any other information that would help to determine the cause of the suspected abuse or neglect; and the identity of any individual responsible for the abuse.

Report Distribution

Family Law Article 5-704

Copies of the written report for abuse or neglect shall be sent to the local department of social services. Copies of the written report for abuse also shall be sent to the local State's attorney office. Additional distribution shall be determined by the local school system but shall be limited to persons who have a true need-to-know and shall not violate the confidentiality requirements discussed below. The local school system shall not maintain copies of written child abuse or neglect reports.

Confidentiality

Family Law Article 5-707, Article 88A Section 6(b)
DHR COMAR 07.02.07.05E

Department of Human Resources (DHR) regulations require that the identity of the person reporting a case of suspected child abuse and/or neglect shall not be revealed. Protective services staff must protect the identity of the reporter unless required by court order to reveal the source. Educators are encouraged to share information about the reported family, but protective services staff may not identify any reporting source to a reported family unless the educator has given written permission to protective services to reveal his/her identity.

Family Educational Rights and Privacy Act of 1974 (FERPA)

All records and reports concerning protective services investigations of child abuse and/or neglect and their outcomes are protected by the confidentiality statute Article 88A, Section 6(b). Unauthorized disclosure of such records is a criminal offense subject to a fine of up to $500.00 or imprisonment for up to 90 days, or both. *Under this statute, information contained in reports or records concerning child abuse and/or neglect may be disclosed only:*

1. Under a court order;

2. To personnel of local or State departments of social services, law enforcement personnel, and members of multidisciplinary case consultation teams who are investigating a report of known or suspected child abuse or neglect or who are providing services to a child or family that is the subject of the report;

3. To local or State officials responsible for the administration of the child protective service as necessary to carry out their official functions;

4. To a person who is the alleged child abuser, or to the person who is suspected of child neglect if that person is responsible for the child's welfare and provisions are made for the protection of the identity of the reporter or any other person whose life or safety is likely to be endangered by disclosing the information;

5. To a licensed practitioner who, or any agency, institution, or program which is providing treatment or care to a child who is the subject of a report of child abuse or neglect; or

6. To a parent or other person who has permanent or temporary care and custody of a child, if provisions are made for the protection of the identity of the reporter or any other person whose life or safety is likely to be endangered by disclosing the information.

Investigative Procedure	Validation of suspected child abuse is the responsibility of the department of social services, assisted by the police. School personnel shall not attempt to conduct any internal investigation or an independent review of the facts.
School Procedure	A school employee may briefly question a child to determine if there is reason to believe that the child's injuries resulted from physical or sexual abuse, or by the child's caretaker and/or household member (e.g., What happened to you? How did this happen?). However, in no case should the child be subjected to undue pressure in order to validate the suspicion of abuse and/or neglect. Any doubt about reporting a suspected situation is to be resolved in favor of protecting the child and the report made immediately.
Third Party Presence During Investigative Questioning	*Education COMAR 13A.08.01.08* In the event that a child is questioned by the protective services worker and/or police during the school day on school premises in an investigation of either child abuse and/or child neglect, whether the child is the alleged victim or a nonvictim witness, "the superintendent or the superintendent's designated representative shall determine after consultation with the individual from the local department of social services or the police officer whether a school official shall be present during the questioning of a pupil." The school official should be selected on a case basis for the purpose of providing support and comfort to the student who will be questioned. The regulations express a preference for having a third party present during questioning except in circumstances where the superintendent or the superintendent's designee, in consultation with the protective service worker determines that a third party should not be present during the interview. This may occur, for example, where the presence of a third party may inhibit the child's responses.
	Article 88A Section 6(b) DHR COMAR 07.02.07.05D *DHR COMAR 07.02.07.17* The local department of social services shall notify school reporting sources of the receipt of the report. School personnel may request the local department of social services to call a multidisciplinary team meeting to share information and concerns to the extent permitted by the confidentiality statute and to coordinate planning for services to the child. Appropriate school personnel are expected to participate in the team meetings in accordance with the procedure established between the local department of social services and local school system.
Parental Notification	*Education COMAR 13A.08.01.08* Although the regulations express a preference for parental notification, the school principal or the principal's designee is not required to notify parents or guardians of investigations on school premises involving suspected child abuse or neglect. The principal, in consultation with the protective service caseworker, may decide

whether the parents should be informed of the investigative questioning. It may be determined, for example, that disclosure to the parents would create a threat to the well-being of the child (COMAR 13A.08.01.04B).

Emergency Medical Treatment; Access to Medical Records
Family Law Article 5-709, 5-711, 5-712
In the event that a child is in need of emergency medical treatment as a result of suspected abuse or neglect, the school principal, in collaboration with the school nurse or other health professional when available, shall arrange for the child to be taken immediately to the nearest hospital. The protective services worker or law enforcement officer should be consulted before taking the child to the hospital when feasible; in cases where the emergency conditions prevent such consultation, the protective services worker should be notified as soon thereafter as possible. In all other instances, it is the role of the protective services worker and/or law enforcement officer to seek medical treatment for the child.

Information contained in school health records needed during the existence of a health and safety emergency may be disclosed without parental consent and without violating the provisions of Federal Educational Rights and Privacy Act (FERPA) of 1974.

Educators are required to provide copies of a child's medical/health records information, upon request to the local department of social services as needed as part of child abuse/neglect investigation or to provide appropriate services in the best interest of a child who is the subject of a report of child abuse or neglect.

Removal of Child from School Premises

Family Law Article 5-709, 5-710, 5-712 DHR-SSA Child Protective Services Policy Manual .01.03.04, and Education COMAR 13A.08.01.08E
The child may be removed from the school premises by a protective services worker or police officer only if:

1. Local social services has guardianship of the child;

2. Local social services has a shelter order or a court order to remove the child. (Verification of shelter care order by school personnel can be made by calling the local juvenile services agency intake officer.) A joint decision by the principal and the protective services worker should be made regarding who will notify the parents of the action to remove the child from school. Usually this notification will occur as part of the social worker's initial family visit, or as part of the contact made to arrange the initial family interview. However, in the absence of a joint decision the superintendent or the superintendent's designated representative shall insure that prompt notification of removal from school is made to the pupil's parent or guardian.

Parental Awareness

Parents should be advised of the legal responsibility of school staff to report suspected cases of abuse and/or neglect. In order to facilitate positive interactions between the school and home/community, it is often helpful to inform parents of this before a problem arises. A letter should be sent to all parents at the beginning of the school year.

Information Dissemination

Information on child abuse and neglect should be disseminated as follows:

1. Provide annual training sessions to all school employees on child abuse/neglect policies and procedures, symptoms, programs and services, and prevention curriculum.

2. Implement, as a part of the curriculum, an awareness and prevention education program for all students.

3. Initiate a public awareness program for students, parents, and the community at large. Information may be disseminated in school newsletters or with report cards. Presentations may be conducted at PTA meetings and at meetings of other community organizations.

WORKING WITH CHILD ABUSE VICTIMS IN THE CLASSROOM

PEGGY S. PEARL, ED.D.

For every seven children in our schools, one child has experienced child abuse. With approximately 41 million children in America's elementary and secondary school classrooms, nearly 6 million are victims of child abuse and/or neglect. As staggering as these statistics are, they are merely cold impersonal numbers and don't tell the story of a child whose trust in human beings has been stripped or whose emotional stability is being destroyed by frequent verbal and physical assaults. How do we measure the damage to a child's potential by the actions of adults, often the child's caregivers? A tear is shed, a life scarred before really living, or contributions short-circuited before being made. These numbers must be thought of as human beings.

Since a maltreated child has predictable classroom behaviors, developmental abilities, and academic needs, the teacher can play a meaningful and pivotal role in providing a positive environment within which the child's maturational process can be enhanced. This chapter briefly describes the student with a history of maltreatment and then discusses some teaching techniques that may optimize the learning environment for abused and maltreated children.

◆ CHARACTERISTICS OF CHILDREN WITH A HISTORY OF MALTREATMENT

The various types of abuse result in both type-specific characteristics and shared characteristics. **Tables 14-1 and 14-2** list the characteristics of victims and the percentage of the victims demonstrating the characteristic by gender and type of maltreatment. The age of the child at the time of abuse, the length of time the abuse lasts, and the relationship of the abuser to the child determine the consequences of the abuse and characteristics evident in the victim. More problematic behaviors develop as the child matures.

In learning to survive in their environment, child abuse victims have adapted in one of two ways: (1) with externalized and undercontrolled behaviors, or (2) with internalized and overcontrolled behaviors. Most adults stereotypically see the child abuse victim as an aggressive, negative child who is incapable of playing or working acceptably with other children or adults. This is, in fact, an accurate description of only about one-fourth of the

Table 14-1. Behavioral Indicators of Maltreatment							
Indicator	Overall (N=216)		Males (N=85)		Females (N=131)		Probability
	N	%	N	%	N	%	
Poor self esteem	123	57.2	50	58.8	73	56.2	
Depression	122	56.5	45	52.9	77	58.8	
Adamance about not going home	83	38.4	24	28.2	59	45.0	p < .01
School/academic dysfunction	68	31.5	28	32.9	40	30.5	
Frequent control issues	53	24.5	17	20.0	36	27.5	
Overall runaway pattern	53	24.5	17	20.0	36	27.5	
Truancy	48	22.2	19	22.4	29	22.1	
Change in affect relating to certain adult	47	21.8	18	21.2	29	22.1	p < .05
Suicide attempt/ideation	38	18.1	10	11.8	29	22.1	p < .05
Drug/alcohol abuse	36	16.7	20	23.5	16	12.2	p < .03
Preoccupation	36	16.7	15	17.7	21	16.0	
Very secretive	32	14.8	10	11.8	22	16.8	
Assaultive/aggressive behavior	30	13.9	14	16.5	16	12.2	
Problems with hygiene	27	12.5	17	20.0	10	7.6	p < .01
Abnormal sleep patterns	26	12.0	9	10.6	17	13.0	
Sudden or chronic withdrawal	22	10.2	10	11.8	12	9.2	
Health complaints	22	10.2	6	7.1	16	12.2	
Gravitates toward abused and neglected youth	21	9.7	8	79.4	13	9.9	
Petty stealing	20	9.3	15	17.7	5	3.8	p < .001
Excessive sexual acting out	16	7.4	4	4.7	12	9.2	
Sudden change in behavior	13	6.0	3	3.5	10	7.6	
Self mutilation	12	5.6	4	4.7	8	6.1	
Abusive romantic partners	11	5.1	0	0.0	11	8.4	p < .01
Extreme modesty	11	5.1	4	4.7	7	5.3	
Criminal behavior	11	5.1	9	10.6	2	1.5	p < .01
Eating disorders	11	5.1	4	4.7	7	5.3	

(From Powers, JL, Jakllitsch, B, and Eckenrode, J: Behavioral characteristics of maltreatment among runaway and homeless youth. In JT Pardeck, ed: Child Abuse and Neglect: Theory, Research and Practice, Gordon & Breach, New York, 1989, p. 130.)

victims in any group. Since aggressive and hyperactive children demand attention, they are the children that adults must deal with. Both their language and behavior are assaultive, and these children do not listen to directions or instructions. They are impervious to disapproval and attack other children physically and verbally. The inability to delay gratification, impulsivity, and distractibility of abused children prevent any relief from their demands on teacher attention. They see themselves as bad, unlovable, and stupid. They expect punishment and will call attention to their own

Indicator	Sexual Abuse (N=47)	Physical Abuse Only (N=37)	Neglect (N=59)	PA & Neg (N=69)	Probability
Poor self esteem	74.5	35.1	54.4	61.8	p < .01
Depression	70.2	43.2	40.4	66.7	p < .01
Adamance about not going home	40.4	37.8	35.1	42.0	
School/academic dysfunction	27.7	21.6	36.8	34.8	
Frequent control issues	17.0	21.6	29.8	26.1	
Overall runaway pattern	36.2	5.4	26.3	24.6	p < .01
Truancy	27.7	5.4	28.1	21.7	p < .05
Change in affect relating to certain adult	21.3	18.9	15.8	29.0	
Suicide attempt/ideation	38.3	2.7	14.0	14.5	p < .001
Drug/alcohol abuse	25.5	13.5	19.3	11.6	
Preoccupation	10.6	8.1	21.1	21.7	
Very secretive	21.3	10.8	12.3	15.9	
Assaultive/aggressive behavior	12.8	10.8	17.5	14.5	
Problems with hygiene	12.7	5.4	10.5	17.4	
Abnormal sleep patterns	21.3	8.1	3.5	13.0	p < .07
Sudden or chronic withdrawal	12.8	2.7	12.3	10.1	
Health complaints	17.0	0.0	7.0	13.0	p < .05
Gravitates toward abused and neglected youth	12.8	5.4	8.8	10.1	
Petty stealing	10.6	5.4	7.0	13.0	
Excessive sexual acting out	19.5	0.0	7.0	4.4	p < .01
Sudden change in behavior	10.6	0.0	3.5	8.7	
Self mutilation	10.6	0.0	5.3	5.8	
Abusive romantic partners	12.8	0.0	3.5	4.3	
Extreme modesty	4.3	2.7	7.0	5.8	
Criminal behavior	10.6	0.0	0.0	8.7	p < .05
Eating disorders	4.3	2.7	0.0	11.6	

(From Powers, JL, Jakllitsch, B, and Eckenrode, J: Behavioral characteristics of maltreatment among runaway and homeless youth. In JT Pardeck, ed: Child Abuse and Neglect: Theory, Research and Practice, Gordon & Breach, New York, 1989, p. 131.)

misbehavior, appearing to gain little or no pleasure from either activities or people. Without treatment, they grow more aggressive; however, they respond best to a very calm, highly structured environment.

The remaining three-fourths of all victims are overly compliant and accept whatever happens to them. They are passive and obedient, stoic and unresponsive, withdrawn and shy, and easy to overlook. These behaviors reflect survival techniques. Abused children feel guilty for misbehaving and responsible for upsetting parents or getting them in trouble. They are very sensitive to criticism by adults and need only mild suggestions to redirect their behavior. They need an environment that is accepting, full of hugs, and encouraging. These children require a calm, predictable place in which to learn social skills and release their feelings. Often compulsively neat and overly desirous of meeting adult goals, they feel little joy or pleasure and have low self-esteem but may show indiscriminate affection for adults.

In their attempts to understand their world and avoid unpleasant experiences, abused children "stare continually," never making eye contact with anyone. It is as if they think that by not looking someone in the eye, they make themselves invisible and therefore safe from attack. The child is attempting to not be seen and, therefore, not hurt. To teachers and observers, this child may appear dull or unresponsive or may be suspected to have hearing or sight deficits. This child is often reprimanded for day-dreaming and not attending to classroom activities. In fact, the child is learning to "read" adult behavior. He or she is trying to avoid danger by carefully scanning the environment and making very detailed, accurate mental pictures of it. As these children become secure enough to talk (or later as adults), they often reveal an exceptional memory of their environment and the behaviors of those around them. Observers of child victims must be aware of this characteristic scanning behavior and not misread the behaviors or too quickly attempt to evaluate this child.

EFFECTS ON DEVELOPMENT

Frequently, child victims have not developed a basic sense of trust, and subsequent psychosocial development is delayed. The child not only distrusts self and others but also lacks positive self-esteem, all of which are needed to try new experiences. As a result, the child fails to learn the age-appropriate behaviors of the family, peer culture, or classroom. The child's need to be safe and loved causes him to become excessively responsible for himself and the adults in his world. The child's own home environment is usually the only measure the child uses to determine the typical interaction of families in homes. Following the role models present in the home gives the child abuse victim few opportunities to learn positive coping, decision making, or interpersonal communication skills and provides few opportunities for enjoyment of life. **Table 14-3** summarizes some of the characteristics exhibited by child abuse victims.

Table 14-3. Characteristics of Students with a History of Maltreatment

Lack sense of trust

Have low self-esteem

Guess at what is normal

Poor interpersonal communication skills

Overly responsible

Lack positive coping skills

Don't enjoy life

Aggressive, hyperactive, or withdrawn, passive, overly compliant

Apathetic, unresponsive

Developmentally delayed

Lack decision-making skills

Self-defeating, self-mutilating behaviors

Substance abusing

Excessively manipulative

Undercontrolled, feel powerless

SEXUAL ABUSE

Sexual abuse victims share many of the characteristics just described but exhibit some additional behaviors. You may find in them an extreme external locus of control evident by attributing responsibility for their actions to others. They have experienced an exaggerated imbalance of power or control and may exploit other children. The child's sexual behaviors may be connected to feelings of anger, rage, frustration, humiliation, poor self-image, powerlessness, and/or lack of control and may be supported by irrational thinking. These children often have unresolved losses and exhibit boundary problems. They become sexually active at an early age and engage in more masturbation than age-mates. Victims of sexual abuse are often deficient when compared to other children, including other victimized children. They are also unable to identify and/or label feelings, so they lack the ability to express feelings. Since they may not have had their own feelings consistently validated, they may have difficulty in distinguishing their own feelings as being separate and different from the feelings expressed by others. Nondirected, compulsive, and aggressive behaviors are often exhibited as a reaction to the child's sense of helplessness and lack of control.

Acting-out adolescents are often victims of maltreatment. Because of their lack of maturity and mobility, they are often chronic runaways engaged in disruptive and criminal behavior, including prostitution and involvement in the drug trade to survive. These young homeless victims are at high risk for AIDS, drug overdose, suicide, and murder. Sexually acting-out adolescents are frequently victims of sexual abuse. Early pregnancy and prostitution are two common evidences of attempts to survive sexual abuse, but unfortunately victims tend to become victimizers, with approximately 20% of sexual abuse by adolescents. As many as 70% to 80% of adult sexual abusers were abused as children.

Summary

Child abuse negatively impacts normal development. Without intervention, the impact grows increasingly serious. The longer a child experiences abuse, the more serious the impact on each area of development. Recognizing behaviors manifested by victimized children is the first step the teacher must take in playing a meaningful role by providing the necessary learning environment for maltreated children. Although all abused children exhibit common patterns of behaviors and developmental delays, children who are abused and controlled through the maltreatment of a close family member demonstrate more problematic behaviors than children abused by acquaintances or strangers.

◆ CHARACTERISTICS OF THE TEACHER

Teachers' perceptions of themselves and their abilities to work with children are strongly related to their enthusiasm for their own childhood and sense of self-esteem about their early lives. Teachers rated as effective by students identify their own families as close, supportive, loving, and secure. Effective teachers commonly feel good about their own family's care and support of them. Research consistently identifies the effective teacher as a person with high self-esteem and the ability to nurture children.

This should not imply that teachers who do not have this family background cannot be effective. However, it does imply that before any teacher can be effective in working with victimized children in the classroom, he or she must come to terms with emotions relating to child maltreatment. Likewise, a teacher who was a victim will need to work through his or her own problems before being able to be effective with students. The best solution is not to repress these feelings but to attempt to understand them. Local community mental health/support services may be valuable resources for the teacher. Self-help support groups, often patterned after the Alcoholics Anonymous (AA) model, have a history of effectiveness with individuals who feel isolated by their problems. Adults Molested as Children was designed for past victims of incest. Writers' groups have also evolved for individuals with abusive histories. Support groups provide the victim with peer support that can lead to understanding and recovery. Additionally, there are numerous self-help books for people who have survived abusive childhoods. A teacher who has lived in or who is living in a chemically abusive family must also recognize the dangers of this situation and seek aid. As with any helping professional, a teacher must have good mental health to effectively work with or teach those who do not. Individuals who have been maltreated or lived in dysfunctional homes often fail to recognize indicators of abuse in children because of their own lack of understanding of what is normal.

Teaching is nurturing. To be effective at nurturing, the individual must have had a wide range of positive experiences and a strong basic sense of trust. Assuming the teacher is prepared to objectively and professionally work with maltreated children, the question arises, "What do I do when I suspect that a child has been maltreated?" All states have mandatory reporting laws. It is, therefore, incumbent upon the teacher to report the suspected child abuse or neglect.

♦ ONCE A REPORT IS MADE

Once a report to the state child abuse and neglect hotline has been made, school staff should continue to be supportive of the child. Telling about child abuse, especially sexual abuse, by its very nature becomes a crisis for the child and family. *The following can be supportive responses to the child:*

— Treat the child as you did before the report. Many times a child is treated as if he or she has been "broken" or "damaged" or is pitied.

— Treat the child with respect and understanding; be sensitive to the child's needs.

— Be sensitive to times when the child may need to be alone or to talk.

— Be aware of mood changes. Children often feel depressed or anxious after a report. Frequently, especially with sexual abuse, this rethinking and depression or anxiety lead the child to recant the story. When a child recants the story of abuse, the professional should not assume that the abuse did not occur.

— Redirect the inappropriate touches of others by the sexual abuse victim. Then define appropriate behaviors.

— Listen when the child appears to want to talk, but do not quiz. Observe and respond to nonverbal communication.

— Praise the child for her courage in reporting and assure the child that it was not her fault. However, don't promise the child that the abuse will never happen again.

— Provide the child opportunities to feel in control of self and the environment.

Maltreated children have been manipulated into silence. A powerful, often trusted, and assumed knowledgeable individual may convince the child by statements such as the following:

— "It is OK not to tell this secret. No one else will understand."

— "Your mother knows and approves."

— "If you tell, it will break up your family."

— "If you tell, I will kill your mother."

— "If you tell, I will go to jail."

These are powerful statements! Children need permission and authority to tell their secret. After they share the secret, they need support. Whatever the secret, children fear what will happen next, that no one will believe them, or that they will be punished. Children need a nonpunitive, nonconfrontational environment in which they are valued and given control over their lives following the report.

♦ TEACHING TECHNIQUES

Teachers need to make each classroom developmentally appropriate with a curriculum guided both by their understanding of the developmental abilities of children within the age range being taught and by a responsiveness to individual differences in growth, individual personality traits, learning style, and family background. The following teaching techniques are most effective with victims of maltreatment while being appropriate for all children. The topics and techniques are divided into separate sections for ease of discussion only; in the developmentally appropriate classroom, they are integrated.

BUILD A SENSE OF TRUST

Children learn to trust themselves, and therefore others, when they predictably have their needs met by caring adults. When children have been maltreated in their own homes, where this basic trust normally develops, they frequently fail to develop trust. Trust can be learned later in life, however, when adults act in consistent, caring ways. The structure and routine of the classroom also provide predictability and facilitate the development of a sense of trust. Teachers help children develop a sense of trust when they keep their promises. By observing teachers plan, implement, and evaluate routine activities, children gain confidence that adults can meet their needs. Maltreated children are often unable to delay gratification because they have not been able to trust that the adults around them can or will carry out promises. Teachers should call each child by name, listen to what each child says both verbally and nonverbally, anticipate each child's needs, and then respond to these needs. Children who know that someone is listening begin to feel safe. To maintain the trust of children, teachers must maintain confidentiality and be someone "you can always count on."

The adolescent is developmentally asking all adults, "Can I trust you to do what you say you will?" "Do your actions agree with my ideal concept of what should be?" "What do I believe, as compared to what you believe and what I think I should believe?" For the adolescent who was abused at an early age and lacks a basic sense of trust, this is an especially difficult task. Because the victim comes from a family where roles are nondistinct, the child is uncertain about what is "normal." The child needs to learn what is appropriate and positive. Because the basic sense of trust is lacking, the adolescent cannot rely on adults and therefore cannot sort out what he or she believes and values. To improve their sense of trust in themselves and others, children need adults who are consistent and dependable. The teacher also needs to respect privacy, protect confidentiality, and routinely "practice what he preaches."

Expect Success

As simple as it sounds, one of the most effective ways to build success is to expect success. Children who feel that others care about them doing well are more apt to achieve. To build success in children, teachers must say they care about each child and act like they care about each child. Many abused and especially neglected children have never known what it is to have others support their efforts and direct them toward achievement. Abused children commonly suffer from intellectual delays due both to the maltreatment and to the general home environment. Even when the home provides materials and opportunities for intellectual development, stress and anxiety impede the normal acquisition and use of knowledge. However, the environment usually has lacked age-appropriate learning opportunities, guidance, and reinforcement of learning. The classroom must provide an environment in which intellectual skills can be learned when the child is emotionally ready.

Abused children initially lack the intrinsic motivation for learning and the joy from learning experienced by normal children. In an environment in which they are accepted as they are, allowed to succeed, and encouraged to meet their own needs rather than the needs of adults, these children eventually experience the joy of learning and develop curiosity.

Students should be placed in learning situations in which they are not valued or assessed according to their performance but rather as individuals — "just for being." Academic performance or product of effort is evaluated as a separate issue by comparing performance to a predetermined standard of performance. The teacher should evaluate the product, not the producer. "Not all of the math problems are worked correctly" is an objective statement about the math problems. However, the statement "You failed to work all of your math problems correctly" devalues the student rather than evaluating the product.

When teachers require students to evaluate their own work against a predetermined evaluation scale, they are providing an environment that enhances the child's internal locus of control and allows the student to feel successful and self-determining. Programmed instruction also places the student in control of progress and minimizes teacher evaluation. Students need a learning environment structured to build successes rather than directed toward correcting failures.

Teachers should provide a wide variety of opportunities for children to construct their own ideas. Children, regardless of background, need multiple opportunities to improve their knowledge base. Different learning styles as well as different emotional states influence the acquisition of knowledge.

Teach Social Skills

Social skills allow maltreated children to reduce their isolation and to build a web of relationships. Children need to feel connected to others in a mutually supportive system. Most abusive families are isolated, untrusting, and fearful of the outside world. The children of such families have no role models except those they see at school. The feelings of connectedness help build bonds of trust and reduce fear—another example of the interrelatedness of human development.

Teachers should encourage abused children to stand up for themselves and should support them when they do. Initially an aggressor may listen only because the teacher is literally standing behind the victim, but the notion that people have rights and can assert them appropriately and effectively is important. These are children whose personal rights have been violated. They need a place where this does not happen and a role model to show them how to prevent it in a nonviolent manner. Efforts must be made toward helping the child develop assertiveness and resistance. Opportunities should be provided for the child to interact with a small group of age-mates. The adult working with this small group must defend and support each individual's rights while directly teaching skills that will assist each group member in successful group interaction. Mainstreaming the victimized child into a group of normal children allows the victimized child to see models of appropriate behavior. Due to the interrelatedness of development, the child's ability to learn social skills is directly related to emotional development.

TEACH LIFE SKILLS

Teachers should set realistic standards, not ideals, because students who have lived in dysfunctional homes already have difficulty with "what is" and "what should be." The curricular content of all classrooms should allow students to learn life skills without racial, ethnic, or gender bias. Self-esteem develops in the context of mastering changing life tasks and challenges.

The curriculum should include basic life skills such as health and physical education, money management, stress management, nonviolent conflict resolution, nutritional competence, food preparation, and interpersonal communication. Students need to learn that all families have money management problems and that planning to prevent the problem is a better course of action than merely blaming other family members. Older students in math, business, and home economics classes can have classroom exercises based on case studies of individuals and families solving money management issues to offer opportunities to practice resource management, communication, and negotiation skills. By practicing problem solving and decision making in the classroom, the student experiences an alternative family lifestyle. Simple group projects in any discipline allow the student to construct knowledge relating to the subject matter content as well as learn interpersonal communication and negotiation skills. Students should be allowed to make age-appropriate decisions and live with the consequences, for example, "Would you like to work with Erin or Sandy?" or "Which of these three books would you like to read for Monday?" All of the choices must be real and require students to accept the consequences of their decisions. All classroom activities must reflect various socioeconomic levels as well as cultural and ethnic backgrounds.

TEACH COMMUNICATION SKILLS

In most abusive homes, interpersonal communication is poor. The curriculum should include units on interpersonal communication, conflict resolution, and family/personal resource management. All of these units are especially important to young people who have no role model for appropriate interpersonal communication. In abusive families the person in whom ultimate power is vested usually communicates in vague terms and expects no two-way communication. The child may have been routinely punished for replying to adults even conversationally; therefore, the curriculum must begin with the basics. Additionally, the classroom must be structured to give all students opportunities for communication with peers as well as with the teacher.

In giving instructions, adults should make sure the directions are clear and simple. Since children feel that which is nearer is more important, adults should be physically near the child when giving directions. Teachers should use a clear, quiet voice, while looking directly at the child. Children who have lived with many commands and general uneasiness will not respond well to general directions given from across the room. As with all children, teachers should give some latitude when giving instructions, to allow the child to make simple decisions. It is important that the adult's words and body language convey the same message. Child abuse victims are not easily fooled by people who say one thing and do another. Calm body language will placate and relax the child more than words. Voice tone is more important than what is said. The teacher should be careful to make sure that the voice says what is intended. "Time to begin writing now?" spoken with a questioning voice leads the child to disobey the spoken words. "It is time to begin writing now" spoken in a clear, calm manner will tell the child specifically what to do.

The adult should tell the child what behavior or actions are appropriate and expected, rather than what not to do. "Clean up your desk and get ready for lunch" is too vague. "Place the writing papers in your folder, place the folder in your desk and return all books to the shelf in alphabetical order, wash and dry your hands, and then go to the lunch table" provides the child with directions for appropriate action. The more concise and specific the directions, the better they define appropriate actions. After each appropriate action, teachers need to provide lots of praise, smiles, and hugs to the child. All staff should model calm behavior. Additionally, the staff should exhibit an appropriate sense of humor.

Puppetry can be used to facilitate language development and communication skills. Puppets provide nonthreatening opportunities to gain new experiences for students at various developmental levels. Young students may use them for storytelling, acting out stories, or free play. Secondary school students may be involved in the preparation of puppet shows or simple presentations to younger students. Puppets may also allow an avenue for victims to release feelings and gain relief from disclosure. Puppets are a versatile educational tool that facilitates development in many areas.

ALLOW STUDENTS TO BE STUDENTS

Because they have been reared in an environment in which they parented their parents as well as younger siblings, victimized children may be overly helpful to teachers and classmates. This may be the student that you "love to have in class," the "assistant you so desperately need." However, don't succumb to the temptation to accept the help this student seems to need to give and seems to enjoy giving. The student is demonstrating the only survival technique that has previously brought acceptance and praise. Because the child was praised and accepted for doing responsible helpful tasks, especially cleaning, he or she learned that the same helpful behavior will earn predictable and needed praise in school. As important as it is for children to learn helpfulness, they also need to develop skills in relating to peers as equals and adults as caregivers. When academic and social skills are lacking, this student tries to succeed by cleaning and helping. While this behavior gains approval and perhaps passing grades from the teacher because it is easy to reinforce, the cyclic pattern of repetition fails to teach appropriate communication or social skills and often allows the student to become further victimized by peers.

The teacher must be alert to the student who is "excessively" responsible and redirect that student to more appropriate behaviors. This often involves observing the group activity and assisting and encouraging the victimized student to say, "I have done my assigned tasks. I'll help you complete yours but I won't do them for you." This says to the victimized child, "You have rights and responsibilities just as each member of the group does." Since other students frequently recognize the vulnerability of the victimized child, comments such as "Sandy didn't do her part . . . " may be a common response when the victimized child asserts herself. The teacher must verify what the assigned tasks were and what tasks were left uncompleted. You must not automatically come to the aid of any child because you "feel sorry" for him or her. Defending the rights of the victimized child shows that you value the child and her or his rights, teaches assertive behavior, and allows the child to see appropriate means of resolving peer conflict that will be needed when the victim encounters sibling conflict as a parent.

In working with this extremely helpful student, you must remember that this student needs positive interactions with adults; the teacher, librarian, coach, or principal are all appropriate for this role. However, special attention must be paid to the part the role model plays. You must be careful not to become another adult that the child "cares for" or fall into the easy pattern of allowing the student to take care of you and pick up after you to the extent that you come to treat the student like an adult, creating yet another situation of role reversal. Rather, you should tell the student that you can use a "student assistant" during a specific hour of the day or before school, etc. The student is then responsible for specific routine tasks, rather than for remembering what you need to do next or what you have forgotten to do. It is useful to carefully outline in writing and post in a specific place the appropriate tasks for the student assistant. Following each task, you should identify the expected level of proficiency on which the "assistant" will be evaluated and periodically evaluate the level of proficiency exhibited in completing the tasks. Praising the student for specifically completing tasks is better than making general comments such as "You're working hard, that's good" or "You're super to have around and you do so much hard work." Specific praise allows the student to feel good about herself or himself, learn skills for the world of work, and gain additional insight into the "normal world." This type of "businesslike arrangement" is mutually beneficial to the student and the teacher.

TEACH POSITIVE COPING SKILLS

Behaviors such as empathy, understanding the points of view of others, good verbal skills, good attentional processes, reflectiveness, problem solving, inner locus of control, frustration tolerance, and appropriate responses to success appear possible to teach. Some other behaviors seem to be more complex and global and do not easily lend themselves to an instructional and training approach. Among these latter are having the ability to detach from the dysfunctional behaviors of others, being personable and well liked, being a creative thinker, practicing autonomous thinking, being optimistic, having a sense of humor, being aware of personal power, having a future orientation, and having a well-developed value system.

Students need instruction in good management and coping skills, including various opportunities to practice those skills. Students with a history of maltreatment have routinely developed dysfunctional coping skills that lead to additional victimization, self-defeating behaviors, and maltreatment. Such children and adolescents frequently follow poor role models. The resulting behavior is either inappropriately acting out or depression. Because of the number of hours teachers spend with children each day, they are the ideal role model for positive coping skills. Appropriate coping skills can be taught by modeling, role playing from scripts, or allowing students to view videotapes that set up a situation and then require the students to discuss the alternative solutions.

Resource management should be integrated into the curriculum. The individual can be taught how to avoid many stressful situations with good management techniques. Many resource management and stress management programs are available in a variety of formats. Some interactive computer programs may be especially helpful for students who lack the language skills necessary for verbal role playing.

When alcoholism is present in the family, confrontation skills are essential to each victim's ability to learn positive coping strategies. However, this requires more involvement than the classroom teacher can provide and these situations are best handled by referral to community resources, including mental health professionals or support groups such as Alateen. The classroom teacher can educate students about the resources available to individuals and families with chemical addiction problems but cannot cure or treat the student (*see list of state protective services in Chapter 13, Abuse, Schools, and the Law*).

The teacher should provide a role model of positive responses to stress and ensure that the classroom environment does not cause additional stress for the child. Good coping skills are perceiving yourself in control of your life and having good self-esteem.

Provide Pleasurable Experiences

There is educational merit to making learning fun or at least pleasant and enjoyable. Victimized children have had few, if any, experiences of pleasurable activities, and then often when they do have fun they are not allowed to appropriately enjoy the pleasure. The school is an especially important place for the student to develop new interests, hobbies, and skills that provide pleasurable experiences. All students, but especially maltreated students, need to hear the role model (teacher) speak about the pleasant odors, flavors, and touches in the world around them. The pleasant smells— paints, crayons, flowers, colognes/aftershaves, lemon oil, chlorine cleaners, etc.—have frequently been missing or not appreciated in the maltreated child's home. Common positive sensual experiences are frequently lacking for maltreated individuals. The child or adolescent needs opportunities to have these experiences and see an adult enjoying or appreciating them. The physical education, art, music, science, and home economics classrooms routinely provide a wide variety of these experiences. Firsthand exploration of the world through the senses is required by the adolescent who has "missed childhood" if that individual is going to be able to nurture the next generation. The teacher must continually offer extra attention to ways of adding pleasant sensory experiences to the curriculum.

The child with a history of maltreatment has for so long been made to feel guilty for enjoying even the simplest of activities that he or she may no longer be able to feel or express joy. When a teacher observes that a student enjoys an activity, it should be acknowledged along with a brief discussion of similar experiences that the student might enjoy. The teacher must give the student permission to feel good about the things he enjoys. By providing a wide variety of learning experiences, the teacher gives students more opportunities for success as well as more opportunities for having pleasurable experiences. It should be recognized that what one student enjoys may not be at all pleasant to other students. Many students find pleasure in tasks that most students see as "very distasteful," for example, dissecting a frog, doing math, performing messy art activities, doing research in the library, or writing poetry. The teacher should acknowledge student enjoyment, praise successes, and encourage students to feel pride and pleasure even when it involves doing what is "different." (As an encouragement, every classroom should have, as standard equipment, multiple colorful posters stating "it's OK to be different.") An environment in which students are encouraged to enjoy learning will always be an environment in which more learning takes place.

All students need the role model of an adult who enjoys the everyday world. Children who have grown up in a dysfunctional family urgently need to see adults who can laugh when things are funny and who "live" to care for special plants, play the guitar or piano, go fishing, golfing, or running, make Christmas cookies, sew with the latest fabric, listen to the rain on the roof, or enjoy the songs of the birds. They need role models who take pride and pleasure in the things they do well, who willingly try new activities, who read and enjoy learning, and who demonstrate pleasure in their interactions with people of all ages, sexes, races, and ethnic backgrounds. Teachers can provide that role model for their students.

BUILD SELF-ESTEEM

Self-esteem is a complex, multifaceted phenomenon integrally related to the development of values, moral character, and personality. It includes feelings about the social, cognitive, moral, and physical/motor aspects of the individual. The four major aspects of self-evaluation are acceptance, power/control, competence, and moral virtue.

All teachers should be aware of the importance of student self-esteem and include in the curriculum ways for children to improve their self-images. To children who have been victimized and who have experienced extreme external control and manipulation, these activities are especially important. The activities included should encourage students to focus on their positive abilities and actions, to learn positive behaviors, and to seek methods for self-improvement. In *"He Hit Me Back First!" Creative Visualization Activities for*

Parenting and Teaching, Fugitt provides a variety of activities for inclusion in lesson plans to build student self-esteem and help students progress from victim to survivor. Improving their knowledge of the world around them also provides students with information on community resources and how to access those resources for personal growth in areas such as athletics, dance, physical education, art, and music. For all students, knowledge brings with it the feelings of power and being in control, which are essential to building positive self-esteem.

As children gain mastery over their bodies, their feelings about themselves as unique individuals improve. Physical education, recreation, drama, and movement/dance provide valuable opportunities to gain greater body awareness, define personal boundaries, and improve self-concept. Additionally, physical activities allow the individual to stimulate the senses, release feelings and anxiety, engage in communication, experience physical and emotional joy, and know feelings of both control and freedom. When these activities are done with others, there are additional opportunities for developing decision-making, problem-solving, coping, and communication skills as well as a sense of trust. Programs such as Outward Bound that involve survival training are especially helpful to participants in developing trust, cooperation, impulse control, self-confidence, and self-sufficiency. If properly structured, physical activities may also allow individuals to feel the joy of success.

To build their sense of worth, all children need opportunities to be responsible, caring members of society. Children of all ages need opportunities to feel that they are capable of helping others, for example, by listening to younger students read, acting as a student librarian, volunteering at the recycling center, or working as a stage hand for the school or community theater. Teachers need to empower children to understand that they can choose to make a difference by "public service." Choosing to care is different from perpetuating the role reversal and overly responsible behavior learned as a survival technique in the child's home. If it is done out of choice, service to others allows the individual to feel personal value.

Improve Academic Skills

Because of prior experiences, victimized children often lack dispositions for learning, such as curiosity, resourcefulness, independence, initiative, responsibility, and goal-directed behaviors. One third of all abused and neglected children repeat at least one grade in elementary school. Ideally, the school experience allows children to slowly develop these abilities. Early maltreatment interrupts the normal growth of trust, autonomy, independence, and initiative; child abuse robs children of their childhood. The child must go back and work through each of these psychosocial stages and construct the knowledge necessary for academic competency. Teachers must structure the environment to allow for children with varied backgrounds and dispositions for learning and mastery to acquire knowledge.

As already noted, abused children need a learning environment that is calm, structured, and predictable. An individual study area may assist some children in focusing on the academic tasks before them. The environment may overly stimulate children who have spent much of their life in chaos. Other children may have or may develop learning disorders and need to be evaluated for special services. Teachers must structure the environment for success.

Instructions may need to be written and clearly divided into simpler tasks to allow the child to complete parts of the total assignment and then move to the next one rather than be overwhelmed by complex tasks. Clearly, children who have not lived in calm, ordered environments need special attention.

PROVIDE AVENUES TO GAIN INSIGHT

Bibliotherapy is one way to help children who are the victims of abuse gain personal insight; bibliotherapy literally means to treat through the reading of books. The goals of bibliotherapy are to teach students to think constructively and positively, to encourage them to talk freely about their problems, to help them analyze their attitudes and modes of behavior, to point out that there is more than one solution to a problem, to stimulate an eagerness to find an adjustment to problems that will lessen conflict with society, and to assist them in comparing their problems with those of others. Although the teacher is not a therapist or a counselor, he can request that books about children who have dealt positively in adverse circumstances be available in school libraries and can include some readings as part of required and optional assignments (**Table 14-4**). High school students can gain insight into their own lives by reading or acting out with puppets such books with younger children in child development laboratories, as teacher assistants, or by working in the school or community library. In addition to providing therapeutic value to students who have been maltreated, these books teach all students what is appropriate treatment of children and become part of a child abuse prevention program.

◆ RESILIENCY OF CHILDREN

Despite their prior life experience, some children overcome the odds. *Researchers have called these children invulnerable, stress resistant, or vulnerable, but invincible. These children share the following four characteristics:*

1. An active, evocative approach to solving life's problems, enabling them to negotiate successfully an abundance of emotionally hazardous experiences

2. A tendency to perceive their experiences constructively, even if the experiences caused them pain or suffering

3. The ability to gain other people's positive attention

4. A strong ability to use faith in order to maintain a positive vision of a meaningful life

Teachers can assist these resilient children in turning their vulnerability into resiliency by actions such as the following:

1. Encouraging children to reach out to friends, teachers, and others

2. Accepting the children and assisting them in building on their strengths, rather than expecting failure and allowing them to become overwhelmed with their problems

3. Conveying to the children a sense of responsibility and caring and rewarding them for helpfulness and cooperation

4. Encouraging the children to develop a special interest, hobby, or activity that can serve as a source of gratification and self-esteem

5. Modeling coping skills

6. Providing dependability

"Beating the odds" occurs when someone cares enough to reach out to the child, providing an alternative to giving up.

Table 14-4. Examples of Books for Bibliotherapy

Benedict, H. (1985). *Recovery: How to survive sexual assault for women, men, teenagers, their friends and family.* New York: Doubleday. Ages 11-18; Gr. 5.

Cole, B. S. (1987). *Don't tell a soul.* New York: Marian.

Crutcher, C. (1986) *Stotan.* London: Greenwood.

Declements, B. (1987). *No place for me.* New York: Viking.

Hayden, T. L. (1987). *One child.* New York: Putman.

Jocoby, A. (1987). *My mother's boyfriend and me.* New York: Dial Books.

Klein, V. (1986). *Bad-mad boy, honey bear and the magic waterfall.* Somerville, NJ: Hage Publications.

Klein, V. (1986). *I-am, pa-pah and ma-me.* Somerville, NJ: Hage Publications.

Kropp, P. (1987). *Take off.* St. Paul, MN: EMC Publications.

MacLean, J. (1987). *Mac.* Boston: Houghton.

Madison, A. (1979). *Runaway teens.* New York: Elsevier/Nelson Books.

Miklowitz, G. D. (1987). *Secrets not meant to be kept.* New York: Delacorte Press.

Miller-Lachman, L. (1987). *Hiding places.* Madison, WI: Square One Publishers.

Page, C. G. (1987). *Hallie's secret.* Chicago, IL: Moody Press.

Posner, R. (1987). *Sweet pain.* New York: M. Evans.

Quinn, P. E. (1986). *Renegade saint: A story of hope, a child abuse survivor.* Nashville: Abingdon Press.

Rosa, G. (1978). *Edith Jackson.* London: Viking.

Seixas, J. S., & Youcha, G. (1985). *Children of alcoholism; A survivor's manual.* New York: Harper & Row. Ages 11-14; RL Gr 6.

Swan, H. & Mackey, G., (1983). *Dear Elizabeth: Diary of a survivor of sexual abuse.* Leawood, KS: Children's Institute of Kansas. Ages 11-18; RL Gr 6.

Woolverton, L. (1987). *Running before the wind.* Boston: Houghton.

◆TRAINING AND SUPPORT FOR ALL EDUCATIONAL STAFF MEMBERS

Teachers working with child abuse victims require additional specific training in the special needs of abuse victims. Teachers also need support and encouragement as they attempt to meet the needs of child abuse victims. Teachers not specifically trained to work with these special needs children can quickly become frustrated because the traditional methods of working with children do not produce the desired changes. The progress is slow and the behaviors of these children are extreme. To prevent becoming overly frustrated, teachers must be aware that although abused children respond negatively to friendly overtures, teachers need to continue to be warm, encouraging, and accepting, with lots of hugs and smiles. An adult model of sharing, helping, and comforting is important in assisting children to develop trust and empathy.

All staff members require training specifically for interactions with child victims. When special needs children are mainstreamed into the classroom, the teacher-child ratios must be lowered to allow staff to individualize instruction and to prevent their being overwhelmed by the demands placed on them. Volunteers and aides are vital to making the classroom more effective.

Teachers need the support of principals, school nurses, and counselors to provide evaluation of techniques being used and to allow all input into each child's developmental record and/or individualized educational plans. Further, this process allows the teacher an appropriate release for feelings of anxiety and frustration. The ability to verbalize frustrations and laugh with accepting co-workers helps relieve stress.

Maintenance of short, daily logs on each child provides the needed data for preparing progress reports as well as serves to document for the teacher the progress that each child is making. To be effective, teachers should be provided with a work environment in which everyone can feel good about themselves and valued for their contributions to the program, an environment in which they have the opportunity for meaningful input, and an environment in which there is evidence of progress toward definable goals.

◆CONCLUSION

With general knowledge of the characteristics and classroom needs of the child abuse and neglect victim, the teacher can effectively select and utilize teaching techniques that will enhance the learning environment for this special student. The victimized student commonly lacks a sense of trust, good self-esteem, and an understanding of age-appropriate behaviors, especially communication skills. Fortunately, children spend many hours in school, time that can be used to promote individual growth and progress toward survival. Knowledgeable teachers can select content and teaching strategies and techniques that will benefit all students, including those who have identified themselves as victims and those who have behaviors consistent with a history of victimization. Although classroom teachers are not therapists, they can guide the victimized student to facilitate personal growth and insight through specific classroom assignments and make referrals to other sources of assistance in the school system. Most importantly, teachers can provide an all-important role model of predictability, trustworthiness, and joy in living for the maltreated child.

♦SUGGESTED READINGS

American Association for Protecting Children (AACP): *Highlights of Official Child Neglect and Abuse Reporting 1984*, The American Humane Association, Denver, CO, 1986.

Anthony, EJ: The syndrome of the psychologically invulnerable child. In EJ Anthony and C. Koupernick, eds: *The Child in His Family: Children at Psychiatric Risk*, Wiley, New York, 1974.

Cicchetti, D, and Carlson, V, eds: *Child Maltreatment: Theory and Research on the Causes and Consequences of Child Abuse and Neglect,* Cambridge University Press, New York, 1989.

Fugitt, ED: *"He Hit Me Back First": Creative Visualization Activities for Parenting and Teaching*, Jalmar Press, Rolling Hills Estates, CA, 1983.

Helfer, RE: *Childhood Comes First: A Crash Course in Childhood for Adults*, ed 3, Ray E. Helfer, East Lansing, MI, 1991.

Kempe, RS, and Kempe, CH: *Child Abuse*, Harvard University Press, Cambridge, MA, 1978.

Lawrence, D: *Enhancing Self-Esteem in the Classroom*, Paul Chapman Publishing, Ltd, London, 1987.

Lynch, MA, and Roberts, J: *Consequences of Child Abuse*, Academic Press, New York, 1982.

Powers, JL, Jakllitsch, B, and Eckenrode, J: Behavioral characteristics of maltreatment among runaway and homeless youth. In JT Pardeck, ed: *Child Abuse and Neglect*, US Department of Health and Human Services, Washington, DC, 1989.

Chapter 15

PREVENTION

PEGGY S. PEARL, ED.D.

Child abuse prevention depends on neither a program nor a system of services, but must be founded on a society valuing its children. Within such a context the society will be willing to fund preventive services, programs, and policies rather than merely "attempting" to solve the crises caused by the lack of interest in children's welfare. Table 15-1 lists some of the indicators that are apparent when a nation makes its children a high priority.

◆PROGRAMS INVOLVING GOVERNMENT, THE JUDICIAL SYSTEM, AND THE PRIVATE SECTOR

The prevention of child abuse involves providing all parents with the necessary resources for successful parenting. The basic national commitment to children and the prevention of their maltreatment begins when the nation's leaders take the initiative to support families. However, society cannot assume that child abuse prevention is a function of government alone. The leaders must represent both the public and the private sectors. The private sector must support families through interventions and prevention programs offered in the workplace as well as encourage and fund community-wide efforts on behalf of children. Workplace policies supportive of families include job sharing; flextime; mental health, medical, and dental insurance; parental leave; employee assistance programs; and dependent care assistance programs. Recognizing the correlation between unemployment and child abuse and neglect, job training and full employment are important segments of a societal commitment to children.

Comprehensive child abuse prevention includes action taken within the judicial system. The legal system—criminal, civil, and juvenile courts—must support laws and procedures both to ensure the protection of children and to support families. Judicial procedures should be sensitive to the needs of children and families. Additionally, there must be adequate numbers of well-trained judges, lawyers, and court support staff, as well as manageable caseloads, to address the complex and demanding nature of child abuse and neglect litigation. The legal system must be sensitive to the needs of abuse victims to prevent additional maltreatment of these vulnerable individuals within the system as well as to protect children from continuing in abusive, dysfunctional families. To continually monitor the effectiveness of the legal and protective service systems, each community should have active citizen advocacy groups. These groups continually work to ensure that the policies of the private and public sectors offer the most appropriate support for families and children.

Table 15-1. Indicators of a Nation with Children as a High Priority

Outraged citizens are motivated to action when they hear that children are being maltreated.

Adequate and affordable housing is available for all families.

Recreation and esteem-building activities are available to all children and families.

Mental health, medical, and dental care are accessible to all families.

Social service delivery systems are accessed by families in need of assistance before maltreatment occurs rather than systems that treat after abuse occurs or punish for maltreating.

Universal instruction in the care and guidance of children is found in the curriculum of all public and private schools (kindergarten to grade 12 as well as adult continuing education).

Instruction in interpersonal communications, nonviolent conflict resolution, and resource management is provided all students (kindergarten to grade 12 as well as adult continuing education).

Job training and education programs provide all workers with access to jobs as an avenue out of poverty.

Workplace policies support families, i.e., parental leave; job sharing; flextime; employee assistance programs; dependent care assistance programs; mental health, medical, and dental insurance; career ladders; and employee wellness programs.

Nonviolent societal role models are highly visible.

All parents have access to self-help and support groups.

Adequate funding exists for research to build the data base regarding environments that facilitate optimal development of individuals throughout the life span.

Legal systems, both criminal and civil, are properly funded, staffed, and trained to promptly and fairly resolve maltreatment cases.

Culturally and ethnically sensitive home-based parent education programs are available to all new parents.

Adequate salaries are provided for professionals who work in all child-related professions to attract and retain the best and the brightest in jobs caring for the nation's priority—children and their families.

Each individual is equally valued without regard for sex, race, ethnic background, ability, disability, or economic status.

♦ PROGRAMS AND SERVICES NEEDED BY FAMILIES

To prevent child maltreatment, a wide range of training, services, resources, and policies must be available to parents. *These preventive strategies are commonly classified as primary, secondary, or tertiary:*

> *Primary prevention:* provides training, resources, and policies to all parents to enhance their parenting and keep abuse from occurring. Examples

include health care, adequate child care, supportive workplace policies, and life skills training for children.

Secondary prevention: provides training, resources, and policies to targeted high-risk populations to enhance their parenting skills, including training and services to victims to keep abuse from occurring in the next generation. Secondary prevention includes self-help groups for parents who consider themselves at risk for maltreating their children, home visitor programs for new parents, and parent education programs for adolescent parents.

Tertiary prevention: provides training, resources, and policies to enhance parenting to keep abuse from recurring once it has been identified. Among the programs included are respite day care for parents, treatment for abused and neglected children, crisis intervention services, and stress management training.

Within our society basic prevention programs should be available to all parents before any maltreatment begins. All parents require access to parenting information, especially when they have their first children. Perinatal coaching, home visitor, and parent aide programs have proven effective for parents with young children. Additionally, all parents must have access to health care both for themselves and for their children. All schoolchildren require life skills education, and all parents need stress management training and access to positive support services to help them cope with the stress of parenting. In our highly mobile society, many families lack the positive support of family and friends and, consequently, this support must be supplied by other sources, for example, the church, social organizations, or mental health agencies. Accessible and affordable child care must be available to all working parents, but especially to single parents and the "working poor." Treatment programs should be added within the penal systems for individuals of all ages—especially adolescent offender—to prevent the abuse of children and women after incarceration. Additionally, all programs must be respectful of cultural issues in order to be effective.

In both private and public schools, children need instruction regarding positive ways to interact with others as much as they need instruction in math, English, and science. Life skills education should be integrated into the curriculum beginning with kindergarten and continuing into adult education. Life skills education includes nonviolent conflict resolution, stress management skills, resource management, effective decision-making, and effective interpersonal communication, as well as information regarding child development and guidance. Additionally, the basics of substance abuse prevention education currently advocated must be a component of education for parenting or life skills. Schools should provide the role model of positive discipline and not use corporal punishment.

Every community must make the accessibility of parent education classes part of a comprehensive adult education program. Topics suggested for these parent education classes include principles of child development, positive child guidance, and basics of child care, such as child nutrition and safety. One vital area that should be addressed with parents of children at any age is techniques to improve the parent-child interaction. Learning to play with and enjoy their children enhances both this interaction and the parents' pleasure in their parental role.

Corporal punishment can easily become abuse when administered by parents who are angry and under stress. Therefore, instruction in the positive methods of child guidance is required. Additionally, parents need to know constructive methods of coping with stress. Self-help groups such as Parents Anonymous (PA) give parents alternatives to abusing their children, emotionally or physically, and provide positive support networks when stress occurs. PA uses the Alcoholics Anonymous (AA) model of self-help, which has proven successful. Both primary and tertiary support groups should be developed to prevent and combat abuse.

To enhance parenting skills and competence as well as prevent child abuse, new parents benefit from various instruction and support services. *The specific content and structure of these programs will vary, as well as the sponsoring agency or institution; however, the goals for new parent programs include:*

1. Increasing the parent's knowledge of child development and the demands involved in parenting

2. Enhancing the parent's skill in coping with the stresses of infant and child care

3. Enhancing parent-child bonding, emotional ties, and communication skills

4. Increasing the parent's skill in coping with the stress of caring for children with special needs

5. Increasing the parent's knowledge about home and child management

6. Reducing the burden of child care

7. Increasing access to social and health services for all family members

Parent education offered as tertiary prevention for various types of maltreatment differs in informational need from primary or secondary programs and responds to separate service delivery systems. All programs should be culturally sensitive and targeted to the appropriate developmental level of the parents. Group parent education that emphasizes impulse control and alternative methods of discipline is particularly successful with physically abusive parents, whereas one-on-one, home-based services founded on individual counseling and problem solving techniques are more effective with neglectful parents. Neglectful parents need instruction in practical child care tasks, for example, diapering and feeding an infant or distracting and communicating with a two-year-old. Programs successful in preventing emotional abuse include group-based services that define nonphysical methods of discipline; emphasize the need for consistency in determining and implementing rules; and offer parents ways of demonstrating affection toward their children.

♦ ROLE OF THE MEDIA

The media must play a key role in the prevention of child abuse. As a major force in shaping public opinion, the media can offer responsible programming and reporting to de-emphasize the current societal acceptance of violence. Additionally, through judicial programming, the media can reverse the current trend toward a desensitization of individuals to the horrors of violence. As the acceptance and glamorization of violence are removed, a new message can be sent—that violence in all forms is inappropriate. The media can depict nonviolent methods of conflict resolution. The media has been involved in and should continue to play a role in educating the public as to the magnitude of the consequences of violence in the lives of families and possible alternatives. The media may also advocate policies beneficial to children and families. One important step involves portraying parenting as the important and valued job in our society it is and thereby increasing parental esteem and helping prevent child abuse.

◆PROGRAMS TO PREVENT NEGLECT AND SEXUAL ABUSE

Although different in form, child maltreatment practices share common causes and therefore the societal approaches to prevention impact most types of maltreatment. However, specific mention should be made about prevention programs for neglect and sexual abuse, since the causes of these types of maltreatment differ slightly from those of physical and emotional abuse.

PREVENTION OF NEGLECT

To prevent child neglect, parents require the basic resources to provide proper care for their children. At some income levels parents cannot provide the necessary food, shelter, clothing, or mental health, medical, and dental care for their children. At this poverty level of existence, parents are also experiencing stress and are usually without adequate support systems. Currently in our society many individuals are employed full-time at jobs that do not pay enough to provide the basic needs for the family. Many more parents lack the job skills necessary for entry-level jobs; even if they had these skills, many entry-level jobs fail to provide medical and dental insurance. At the same time, national and state governments provide fewer mental health, medical, and dental services for citizens. The consequences of these two trends is that growing numbers of children are without adequate health care services.

When society makes adequate child care a national priority, it ensures, through various public and private sector means, that all parents have access to the basic resources to care for their families. To care for our nation's children, all parents must have access to decent and affordable housing; adequate mental health, medical, and dental care; nutritious food; and developmentally appropriate child care services. The cycle of poverty that results in the disintegration of families and an atmosphere of chronic violence must be interrupted with culturally sensitive programs that work, addressing housing, jobs, substance abuse treatment, family support, etc.

To prevent neglect, parents must also function at optimal levels so that they can focus on their children's needs. Many parents are impaired in their ability to parent because of substance abuse or psychopathologic disorders. To prevent child maltreatment, these adults and adolescents must have access to culturally sensitive, developmentally appropriate substance abuse prevention and treatment programs and mental health services. These services must be available to all parents either free, at fees based on ability to pay, along sliding scales, or under provisions of employee insurance or employee assistance programs.

PREVENTION OF SEXUAL ABUSE

In the last decade many programs to prevent sexual abuse have been developed and widely implemented. Generally these sexual abuse prevention programs teach children how to protect themselves from abuse. Researchers and clinicians caution that the major responsibility for prevention of sexual abuse cannot be placed on the victims or potential victims because they are children. Sexual abuse prevention programs must focus on the perpetrator. The National Committee for the Prevention of Child Abuse has developed a comprehensive strategy for preventing adults from becoming child sexual abusers.

This prevention strategy includes the following:

1. Education for adolescents and young children that provides all adolescents with quality sex education, including healthy sexuality, during the preteen and teenage years to enhance their knowledge of what is normal and abnormal.

2. Training for professionals and volunteers who work with children that teaches these individuals how to identify and help children who are being abused, how to teach children to protect themselves from abuse, and how to detect those who may be potential molesters.

3. Education for parents that provides all new parents with quality education and support to enhance early attachment and bonding when their first babies are born. This should include information about appropriate and inappropriate touch and what to do about it. Parents need to know how to detect and handle in their own children symptoms that may indicate that sexual abuse has occurred.

4. Institutional changes that ensure that all child-serving institutions and programs, e.g., schools, boys clubs, Girl Scouts, day care, etc., train children in self-awareness and self-protection. Guidelines and regulations must be in place to screen, train, and monitor all volunteers and staff.

5. Media messages that create an environment in which the prevention programs and concepts just outlined will be effective by communicating two messages.

   First, for adolescents and adults, messages that say:
   Child sexual abuse is a crime.
   Help is available.
   Abuse is a chronic problem unless you get help.
   Children get hurt when you sexually abuse them.
   Children cannot consent to this kind of behavior.

   Second, messages to children, including:
   It's okay to say no.
   It's not your fault.
   Reach out for help if this begins to happen to you.
   Help is available for you.

The comprehensive child sexual abuse prevention strategy just outlined, like all prevention programs, strengthens individuals and families by enhancing parenting skills.

Since many sexual abuse perpetrators are former victims who commit their first offense during adolescence, it is essential that all victims receive treatment. In addition, all offenders must have treatment before being released to offend again. In the current era of increased criminalization of sexual maltreatment, all segments of the penal system must have mandatory treatment programs for individuals eligible for parole. Perpetrators who refuse to participate in a meaningful way in prison treatment programs should be denied their right to return to full community participation.

◆ SUMMARY

All parents should have available to them the resources, education, and services needed to parent effectively. A comprehensive multidisciplinary approach to prevention is needed. No specific program or plan is most effective with all parents. A mix of family support programs is needed in both the private and public sectors to enhance parenting. Once abuse has occurred, various resources, educational programs, and services are needed to prevent additional abuse. Each family needs a culturally sensitive and developmentally appropriate individualized approach, with some requiring intense and ongoing services to prevent maltreatment. Research has shown specific gains in the following areas after parental participation in secondary and tertiary prevention programs: improved mother-infant bonding and maternal capacity to respond to the child's emotional needs; demonstrated ability to care for the child's physical and developmental needs; fewer subsequent pregnancies; more consistent use of health care services and job training opportunities; and decreased reliance on the public welfare system, higher school completion rates, and higher employment rates.

Prevention requires society's commitment to the welfare of children. This commitment begins with individual attitudes that equally value all individuals. Additionally, the commitment must be backed by both the public and the private sectors and must extend beyond mere rhetoric to include allocating resources as well as changing existing policies that do not conform to this commitment. Society must recognize the importance of parenting and then commit resources to assist all parents in performing this challenging and rewarding job.

◆ SUGGESTED READINGS

Cicchetti, D, and Carlson, V, eds: *Child Maltreatment: Theory and Research on the Causes and Consequences of Child Abuse and Neglect*, Cambridge University Press, Cambridge, England, 1989.

Cohn, AH: Our national priorities for prevention. In RE Helfer and RS Kempe, eds: *The Battered Child*, University of Chicago Press, Chicago, 1987.

Daro, D: *Confronting Child Abuse: Research for Effective Program Design*, Free Press, New York, 1988.

Kempe, CH, and Kempe, RS: *Child Abuse*, Harvard Press, Cambridge, MA, 1978.

INDEX

A

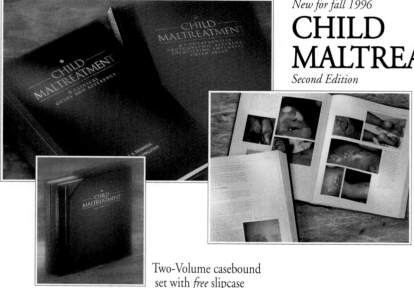

Child Maltreatment Order Form

✄ *Photocopy or detach this order form and mail or fax today.*

❑ **YES!** send me _____set(s) of *Child Maltreatment* at $189.00* per set, **saving $30 by buying both books.**

Please check payment option:

Bill my credit card: ❑ MasterCard   ❑ VISA

Acct. No. _____

Signature _____

Exp. Date_____

❑ Bill me.   ❑ Purchase order _____

detach and mail to: **G.W. Medical Publishing, Inc.**
2601 Metro Boulevard • St. Louis, MO 63043 • 314 298-0330
Order Toll-Free 1-800-600-0330 or FAX orders 1-800-339-2385

Shipping Information

Name _____

Title _____

Institution _____

Address _____

City _____

State _____ Zip_____

Daytime phone (____) _____

* All orders are billed for postage, handling, and states sales tax where appropriate. All prices subject to change without notice. If using a purchase order, please attach to this card.

Money-back Guarantee: Your satisfaction means everything. If you are not 100% pleased, simply return the book(s). Your money will be promptly refunded without question or comment.

✄ *Photocopy or detach this order form and mail or fax today.*

❑ **YES!** send me _____set(s) of *Child Maltreatment* at $189.00* per set, **saving $30 by buying both books.**

Please check payment option:

Bill my credit card: o MasterCard   o VISA

Acct. No. _____

Signature _____

Exp. Date_____

❑ Bill me.   ❑ Purchase order _____

detach and mail to: **G.W. Medical Publishing, Inc.**
2601 Metro Boulevard • St. Louis, MO 63043 • 314 298-0330
Order Toll-Free 1-800-600-0330 or FAX orders 1-800-339-2385

Shipping Information

Name _____

Title _____

Institution _____

Address _____

City _____

State _____ Zip_____

Daytime phone (____) _____

* All orders are billed for postage, handling, and states sales tax where appropriate. All prices subject to change without notice. If using a purchase order, please attach to this card.

Money-back Guarantee: Your satisfaction means everything. If you are not 100% pleased, simply return the book(s). Your money will be promptly refunded without question or comment.

✄ *Photocopy or detach this order form and mail or fax today.*

❑ **YES!** send me _____set(s) of *Child Maltreatment* at $189.00* per set, **saving $30 by buying both books.**

Please check payment option:

Bill my credit card: ❑ MasterCard   ❑ VISA

Acct. No. _____

Signature _____

Exp. Date_____

❑ Bill me.   ❑ Purchase order _____

detach and mail to: **G.W. Medical Publishing, Inc.**
2601 Metro Boulevard • St. Louis, MO 63043 • 314 298-0330
Order Toll-Free 1-800-600-0330 or FAX orders 1-800-339-2385

Shipping Information

Name _____

Title _____

Institution _____

Address _____

City _____

State _____ Zip_____

Daytime phone (____) _____

* All orders are billed for postage, handling, and states sales tax where appropriate. All prices subject to change without notice. If using a purchase order, please attach to this card.

Money-back Guarantee: Your satisfaction means everything. If you are not 100% pleased, simply return the book(s). Your money will be promptly refunded without question or comment.